'In *Shamanic Dimensions of Psychotherapy*, Robin van Löben Sels artfully weaves together personal narrative and clinical experience, along with threads from art, poetry, literature, analytical psychology, and psychoanalytic theory, to articulate the shamanic elements underpinning the psychotherapy experience. However, this volume is not a dry, academic treatise on shamanism. Throughout the volume, van Löben Sels reveals how the "shamanic complex" functions to facilitate healing in the space created between therapist and patient. In addition to having significant implications for the practicing psychotherapist, her careful and astute articulation of "shamanic attributes" might well serve as a template for the practice of conscious living. Rather than simply explaining shamanism, van Löben Sels utilizes the patterns found in shamanism as a means of amplifying important elements of life and the depth of the therapeutic encounter. *Shamanic Dimensions* is an important and satisfying contribution to our understanding of shamanistic experience, depth psychology, and the unfolding of life.'

– Mark Winborn, PhD, NCPsyA, Jungian psychoanalyst, psychologist, and author of *Interpretation in Jungian Analysis: Art and Technique*

'Robin van Löben Sels has the rare gift of being able to capture with words our primary, felt experiences that often have an ineffable quality and, as such, elude verbal description. In this poetic and evocative book, van Löben Sels provides us with anthropological, clinical, and personal descriptions that illustrate, as well as evoke, aspects of the shaman archetype and its operation in the therapeutic situation – especially in the form of the seven shamanic attributes she explores. To pay attention to these attributes is to work mostly at the level of what is non-conscious yet experienced and manifested bodily; it is to be present to the language of sensations and is foundational to moving towards ego consciousness and a growing capacity to name one's experience – what the author calls a yoga of consciousness.

As I read her book, I was repeatedly aware of links between her shamanic attributes and the work of current neuroscientists such as Schore, Damasio, and Porges; as well as infant researchers such as Stern, Trevarthan, and Reddy. Her emphasis on the physical/somatic attributes of the shaman also link with somatic therapies such as authentic movement, dance therapy, art therapy, and the somatic psychotherapies of Somatic Experiencing, Hakomi, and Somatic Transformation. More specifically, van Löben Sels's seven attributes have a natural deep link to the seven archetypal affective systems that neuroscientist Jaak Panksepp suggests are the "ancient ancestral wisdom" of humans, and indeed all mammals. Both the shamanic attributes and the affective systems are core, essential components of our moment-to-moment experience through our nonverbal, implicit system. The depths of primary and secondary shamanic experience are multi-dimensional, and if you want to explore the full noetic reality of shamanic experience, this magically lyrical and well-grounded book is a must read.'

– Julie Kilpatrick, MD, Jungian psychoanalyst and educator of attachment theory and affective neuroscience

Shamanic Dimensions of Psychotherapy

In *Shamanic Dimensions of Psychotherapy: Healing through the Symbolic Process*, Robin van Löben Sels uniquely and honestly recounts her personal journey toward a shamanic understanding of psychotherapy. Exploring the disruptive breakthrough of visions and dreams that occurred during her analysis, personal life, and psychoanalytic training, van Löben Sels illustrates how the phenomenology of ancient shamanism is still alive and how it is a paradigm for the emergence and maturation of the psyche in people today.

This original book delves into van Löben Sels's personal experience of the shaman, identifying such eruptions as a contemporary version of the archaic shaman's initiatory call to vocation. The book is split into two parts. It begins by outlining the shamanic personality in history, recognizing this as an individual that has been called out of a collectively sanctioned identity into a creative life, and the unconscious shaman complex they consequently face, especially in psychotherapeutic relationships. Practical as well as theoretical, the second part outlines the shamanic attributes that underline psychotherapeutic relationships – silence, sound, mask, rhythm, gesture, movement, and respiration – and usefully describes how to use them as *asanas* for consciousness, or vehicles toward psychological awareness. With clinical examples and personal stories throughout, this book's unique Jungian perspective addresses contemporary expressions of the shaman complex in our current world.

Shamanic Dimensions of Psychotherapy: Healing through the Symbolic Process will be essential reading for Jungian analysts and psychotherapists in practice and in training, as well as for academics and students of Jungian and post-Jungian studies. It will be especially helpful and illuminating to those who have experienced an involuntary plunge into the depths and who seek ways to articulate their experience.

Robin van Löben Sels, PhD, is a Jungian analyst teaching and consulting in New Mexico, USA. She is the author of *A Dream in the World: Poetics of Soul in Two Women, Modern and Medieval* (Routledge, 2003) and has written several other books and poetry.

Shamanic Dimensions of Psychotherapy

Healing through the Symbolic Process

Robin van Löben Sels

Routledge
Taylor & Francis Group
LONDON AND NEW YORK

First published 2020
by Routledge
2 Park Square, Milton Park, Abingdon, Oxon OX14 4RN

and by Routledge
52 Vanderbilt Avenue, New York, NY 10017

Routledge is an imprint of the Taylor & Francis Group, an informa business

British Library Cataloguing-in-Publication Data
A catalogue record for this book is available from the British Library

Library of Congress Cataloging-in-Publication Data
A catalog record for this book has been requested

ISBN: 978-1-138-09571-7 (hbk)
ISBN: 978-1-138-09572-4 (pbk)
ISBN: 978-1-315-10558-1 (ebk)

Typeset in Times New Roman
by Apex CoVantage LLC

'Never was anything in this world loved too much but many things have been loved in a false way: and all in too short a measure.'

– Thomas Traherne

For Don

Contents

Illustrations

Acknowledgments

Publishing this book gives me a chance to thank three stalwart New York colleagues – Phillip Zabriskie, Walter Odajnyk, and Jonathan Goldberg – who read my early efforts to formulate my experience of the shaman complex as my thesis for the C. G. Jung Institute of New York, then titled *Shaman: A Differentiation of Image from Instinct*. It also gives me a chance to thank Ann Belford Ulanov, without whose encouragement I would not have discovered the joy of completing a doctoral program in psychiatry and religion at Union Theological Seminary in New York. Thanks to my long-ago voice coach, Joseph Ruff; I can't imagine what my analytic training experience would have been had I not worked with Joseph at the same time, and by some miracle he was in Manhattan when I needed him. Thanks also go to the C. G. Jung Institute of New York itself, first for making it possible for me to spend a winter auditing classes at the Jung Institute in Zurich, Switzerland, and then – when I began formal training in New York – for many years of training and fellowship with other candidates that followed.

Special thanks to Mark Winborn, from The Interregional Society of Jungian Analysts, and Julie Kilpatrick, from the Santa Fe Society of Jungian Analysts, for reviewing this version of the shaman, and to Monika Wikman, who dubbed the heavy manuscript I hauled out of a back closet my 'dinosaur egg' and encouraged me to start working on it again. Thanks also to my friend Mark Richardson, whose painterly response to my poem *Shaman Song* became the cover art.

I also owe a special note of thanks to my patients, who journeyed with me over these many years. None of this would have been possible without their courage and companionship. Nor could I have done without the tutoring of my husband Don, who persistently helped me translate my characteristic, 'circular' (poetic?) style of writing into more 'linear,' readable, psychological prose, over many mornings and many cups of coffee. Without Don's help, this book would not have been possible.

Introduction

Personal background

When I was in my early thirties, a constellation of disastrous circumstances in my life led me through a kind of breakdown in my sense of identity through a process that completely deconstructed my personality (as I then knew it) to eventually reconstruct it on a truer, more embodied foundation. Over time, I've come to understand this experience as my small, personal version of Dante's midlife descent into hell and reemergence 'on the other side of the world,' as Dante imagined it, or C. G. Jung's creative illness (Ellenberger) that followed his break with Freud, initiating a prolonged series of visionary experiences that Jung later recorded in his *Red Book.*

Overall, my creative illness followed a cascade of cataclysmic events that plunged me, on the one hand, into three years of oblivion, and, on the other, into 'another world,' a world of spirits, ancestors, dreams, and visions – in short, into the precincts of the ancient shaman. Precipitating events included the dangerously complicated and almost fatal (to me) caesarian birth of my son, followed by twelve days of anesthetic stupor because of a botched spinal block, and, on the day I came home from the hospital, the revelation of a shocking betrayal by a close friend that first rendered me briefly unconscious on the floor, and eventually led to a painful separation from my children. A day or two later, as I drove home from grocery shopping, I had a definitive, almost visionary experience of being sliced in two: the felt image was of myself as a kind of taproot, like a carrot, and I felt myself cut, sliced through horizontally, right below my ribcage. Throughout this 'vision,' I held tight to the steering wheel with both hands and simply kept driving, for I had to get home to nurse my infant son. But after that experience I entered a period of numbness, psychological homelessness, and loss of soul, for which – for a long time – I would have no words.

In my self-sufficient tradition of muscling my way through, I first tried to manage all this by myself. For the better part of three years I staggered through life, job after job after job, desperately trying to support myself and stay in touch with my children, who now lived in another part of the country. I remember no dreams during this time. I ended up in Manhattan, and some evenings I frequented the

Kristine Mann Library, a major repository of Jung's work, which was located in a suite of rooms in the Peter Cooper Hotel. One evening, alone in the library just before closing time, I remember that I leaned into a full-length closet door mirror, one hand on either side, and said aloud, 'Robin, you *must* contain yourself.' But clearly self-containment was something I couldn't continue much longer, for I also found myself unconsciously walking into traffic, I had become dangerously thin, and I knew that I desperately needed to talk to someone who – I hoped – would not find me completely crazy.

When I finally found my way to a kind and generous female Jungian analyst, my inner floodgates opened and what felt to me like a huge gap in my very being began to flood with powerful imagery and numinous experiences that eventually began to herald the possibility of a new life. For example, early on in my work with Dr. P. I dreamed

> *I am alone in a dark cellar or basement, where I see a huge garbage can, the lid of which lifts up and down, up and down, while out of the can flashes a red light – 'danger, danger, danger.' At the same time, enormous wheels of light are moving across the dark walls, white and golden lights, wheeling one after another, higher than I can reach, yet they do not light up the interior.*

Even then I knew that this dream pointed to a large volume of repressed and dissociated 'shadow material' that I was somehow required to process, but the great whirling wheels of light also intimated a kind of potential wholeness, perhaps even healing, that somehow lay ahead. Inwardly, my shamanic journey had begun.

I worked with Dr. P. for a year or so, and that work was followed by regular and difficult work with several others, including one other wise person (with a lot of personal analytic experience) whom I have come to think of as a shamanic personality. Joseph Ruff was actually a voice coach, with whom I also worked for almost ten years. During this entire tumultuous time, I also became involved in a community of likeminded seekers who were involved in various stages of analytic training within the C. G. Jung Institutes of Zurich and New York. Needless to say, the combination of all of this was highly psychoactive, and my already fragmenting self was dissolved in a kind of communal bath with others: a bath consisting of shared experiences, symbolic images, personal narratives, theoretical understandings, and hours upon hours of personal analysis, all of which served as lifebuoys in the stormy sea in which I found myself struggling to survive. After attending one class, for example, I dreamed that while I sat in a seminar, everyone (including me) left up to flee an enormous tidal wave approaching from the distance – a huge tsunami. I escaped with others to higher ground, but I also realized that I would have to return to this place alone, because from higher ground I saw my familiar handbag, now under water, entangled in the bottom of a large, rope-woven net that had been anchored into the sandy seafloor. The net stretched vertically, up, up, up, through the heaving water to a surface I couldn't make out.

Discussing this dream with my analyst, I could only conclude that the dream forecast *something* that lay ahead. Even though I felt lost, *some* sense of self (my handbag, a sense of personal identity?) was safely snagged in a net that somehow spanned the depths, now stretched taut within the raging waters. I alone could fish my bag (myself? my identity?) out again, but I could not imagine how I would be affected by submersion in such a storm. Still later, I came to understand the woven-rope net (psyche itself?) in terms I will present herein – as the shaman complex, for example – a particular archetypal constellation from which I've been disentangling a personal story of my own ever since.

By the time this 'midlife' crisis occurred, I had made a reasonably successful adaptation to the outer world, or so I thought: I had an educated mind that was well furnished with ideas *about* the psyche, I had a dance-honed, though underappreciated and undervalued body, and I had a heart that was chock-full of sadness that I couldn't bear to feel and couldn't imagine how to talk about. But never mind. In retrospect, I was yet to experience the reality of the psyche as I now understand it. Apparently, back then, the seed of a truer self was nested in a state of *participation mystique* with the world around me (the outer collective) as well as with the objective psyche within me (an inner collective), and I experienced both of these collectives as one and the same. One could say that I was unconsciously identified with unconsciously held images of myself in the eyes of others – the eyes of parents, lovers, teachers, and public figures – and/or, that I was unconsciously identified with the inner world of the objective psyche, a world of collective ideas, collective images, and religiously sanctioned beliefs. One could also say that, unknowingly, I had been leading a life that was more generic than it was personal – that I had been immersed in what the sociological psychologist John Haidt calls society's 'consensual hallucination,' by which Haidt means an unconscious participation in the symbols and rituals of the society around me, without realizing that I was doing so (Haidt, 2012).

I came to think of this entire tumultuous time as a shamanic initiation, and only now can I be somewhat more articulate about it all. I now see that what was so blatantly missing in an ego seed that hid in my apparently normal outer personality was *personally embodied feeling*. A full flowering of personally embodied feeling could happen only in real-world relationships later on, but back then, the stage was set for its emergence, and I entered a course of analytic training that was interlaced with powerful shamanic experiences activated both with my analysts and with Joseph, my voice coach with whom over a period of years I weekly sang myself into embodiment.

For the most part, all these experiences were mediated through the agency of what I've come to think of as various shamanic attributes – silence, sound, movement, mask, respiration, gesture-posture, and rhythm. Because these attributes were major vehicles of activating my own shaman complex, I spend the latter part of this book reflecting on them in the seven meditative chapters that make up Part II.

My personal experience of the shaman complex happened over years, and I was able to track it through many dreams. My experience of the activated complex was also marked by visceral, sensate body experiences that I interpreted only through the vocabularies of the 'spiritual' disciplines I knew: Kundalini energies spiraled up and down my spine, and spiritual emergencies of various kinds made themselves felt, along with repeated eruptions of enormous (archetypal) feelings that apparently had been locked away in a body that I suddenly had to learn much more about, inhabit more deeply, and experience more fully.

Eventually I emerged out of this maelstrom with a profoundly different feeling of identity, a deepened sense of personhood, a more differentiated psyche, and an experience of physical embodiment that *felt* different, almost as if my flesh and bones had been remade. Additionally, the physical world into which I emerged was extraordinarily vivid: and it was a world that I experienced with more gratitude than I had ever imagined possible. Allusions to death and dying were everywhere. Early on I walked into Dr. P's office and declared, 'Do you know what I want engraved on my headstone? "She loved *this* world!" (as opposed to another world?)' What I really meant by this statement would clarify only over time. In the moment I said it, however, the fact that I actually said out loud what I was feeling to another person felt miraculous.

I don't want to overstate this revolution of consciousness. Of course I am the same person that I was before I had these experiences, but over the time of their happening, it didn't feel that way. In some profound manner that I then understood metaphorically, life as I had known it before became dismembered and I 'died.' Later I would come to feel reborn, reconfigured, and reconnected to myself in ways that hopefully anyone who has undergone a deep analysis will understand. And out of all of this commotion, gradually I came to imagine the psyche itself as kind of fifth element, as a kind of alchemically connective tissue that allowed me to undergo experiences that felt shot through with being *fully* human, for the first time ever, as if were psyche's very reality that wove my healing, whole-making experience of mind, body, spirit, and soul – an experience utterly unimaginable before it actually occurred.

Some Jungian analysts might describe this 'death and rebirth' process as a realignment of a misaligned, or poorly aligned, ego-self axis. Edward Edinger (*Ego and Archetype*) suggests that such a realignment is engineered by what Jung called the Self in a process that is carried in projection by an analyst. The gradual evolution of the analytic relationship allows this externally constellated process to be internalized, to take up residence within, thereby to become a source of inner sustainment. Other depth psychologists (including Jung) might refer to the 'death' I underwent as a loss of soul, the new sense of myself to be later reconfigured as a recovery that became the soul's return, as if a return of soul connected my formerly collectively functioning ego with a newly reachable core of embodied affect and aliveness that either I had lost or had never developed in the first place.

Object relations theorists like D. W. Winnicott, Michael Balint, and others might understand my experience as a profound regression out of a false self-identification and into the new beginnings of a more deeply grounded personality, or into a true self. Self-psychologist Bernard Brandschaft might see the same progression as movement from a defensive position of 'pathological accommodation' into an inner differentiation of personal boundaries and a more vital sense of personhood. All of these formulations are useful. But in the following pages, I will try to give an account of my experience from the inside out, which means what the experience was like for me subjectively. And from *within* my experience, the thing that most surprised me was my encounter with the *reality of the psyche per se* in a full-bodied experience of an everyday world that I had always known, yet with another world folded into it. Poet Paul Eluard's phrase 'There is another world, and it is in this one' comes pretty close. As revelation after revelation of the psyche's reality hit me like proverbial tons of bricks, I wandered into one early analytic hour muttering to my first analyst, 'Oh my God! Just because something is invisible doesn't mean that it isn't real, right?' She just grinned.

Through a shamanic lens

Five or six years later, trying to digest all that I had experienced and understand it in terms that made room for the language of soul and spirit, I was naturally led to Mircea Eliade's *Shamanism: Archaic Techniques of Ecstasy*. I owe Eliade's book thanks for grounding my early attempts to articulate the connections I was able to intuit between my personal experience and the phenomenology of shamanism, both ancient and contemporary. From Eliade, I learned that for centuries, and all over the world, shamanism has existed as a phenomenon of outward behavior and inner experience that shares a language of soul loss and recovery, thereby acknowledging the soul's transitory life between the 'two worlds' of spirit and matter. Eliade's work underlay the writing of my 1980 thesis for the New York Jung Institute, and that thesis in turn served as a ground plan for formulating this book forty years later.

In many ancient cultures the shaman was someone whose call to vocation came in the form of illness that involved loss of soul. Black Elk, for example, fell seriously ill as a young boy, thrashing about with a high fever and delirium for the better part of a week, completely unconscious. Although he was given up for dead (or insane), eventually Black Elk recovered from his illness, and he reported later that for the entire time he had been gone from this world he traveled in an alternative reality filled with spirit beings. Black Elk met ancestors and gods, and strange, daimonic animals and apparitions similar to the spirit beings that Jung met in active imaginations that were to become the contents of his *Red Book*. Black Elk also described how his soul was lost in this visionary 'other' world, how he found his soul again, and how he brought it back through a series of sacred stories and songs that instructed him about the origins of his people, the great dangers they were facing, and how to heal the sick by recovering the soul.

Black Elk also understood that the other world into which he disappeared was unquestionably sacred, full of spiritual power both light and dark. Hence the spirit world was to be both feared and revered. One could get lost there, or the soul could get stuck, in which case an initiate might disappear into what today we would call a psychosis. But with help from his community, and because he was flexible and resilient, Black Elk learned *to relate* to this mythopoetic realm – how to enter it and return, first with his own soul and then with the souls of others – rather than to be completely overtaken by it. This learning is what made Black Elk into the shaman he became, and as an initiate, he could then initiate others.

So as my search for a language with which to understand my experience unfolded in the training community of the New York Jung Institute, I glimpsed strong parallels between the metapsychology of shamanism and the metapsychology of psychoanalysis, especially Jungian analysis. It was from shamanism and a shamanic worldview, I realized, that psychoanalysis borrowed its understanding that alongside or beneath our familiar rational world lies another world, a world that can temporarily take over the familiar world, causing symptoms or acute illnesses that shamans described as loss of soul. *Freud and Jung simply relocated this world of 'non-ordinary reality' within the psyche and called it the unconscious.* They also discovered how dreams can bridge these two worlds, and they discovered that when dreams are shared and experienced within the container of what came to be known as a psychotherapeutic relationship, 'bridging two worlds' facilitates the healing of an injured, misaligned, or divided soul. The history of psychoanalysis itself began as a world of cultural and scientific endeavor that is fewer than 150 years old (Ellenberger, 1970).

Ultimately, a wide range of what I came to think of as shamanic experience condensed into the outlines of what I offer here as the shaman complex – a psychological complex that is deeply activated in any truly transformative relationship – which informs the title of this book: *Shamanic Dimensions of Psychotherapy*. On a level of personal experience, it seemed to me that the symbolic image of the archaic shaman stirred within the depths of psyche until it literally erupted into my inner world, usurping any sense of personal, individual life. I was mostly inarticulate about this entire experience for a long time. But perhaps three years into it all, I remember saying one day to Joseph, who was at the piano, 'It's like the big shaman is healing the little shaman!' to which Joseph replied exactly nothing. We simply kept on singing.

The shaman in psychotherapy

For me, the image and dynamics of the archetypal figure of the shaman have everything to do with what happens in a therapeutic relationship, and I will try to explain this in the following pages. First let me say that by psychotherapy I simply mean a process through which one person is companioned through stages of growth and psychological development by way of shared consciousness in a creative dialogue with another person, a therapist. This definition assumes that the therapist (or analyst) has studied and knows about working within the unconscious, transference/countertransference field that emerges in any relationship, as well as working with intrapsychic products of the unconscious that emerge in such a context: dreams, visions, voices, and wild imaginings. Of course personal relatedness and personal history are taken into account, but so too are collective contents, meaning archaic and typical (archetypal) complexes and cultural works like fairytales, myths, and religious texts. Whether we are aware of it or not, contact and connection with unconscious psychic reality (inner and outer) is critical for all of us, and a skillful therapist not only knows about the unconscious psyche but is sensitive to fact that psychotherapy participates in the *ongoing formation* of psychic reality, and this holds true for both parties in any psychoanalytic adventure.

In other words, as therapists, we don't just fix something in the past; the process of building and rebuilding psychic reality goes on every moment. This means that the privileges and responsibilities of therapists are great and can be troubling. Whereas other people turn to a beloved form of art or other engrossing activities like gardening, traveling, or fishing – indeed, any symbolic medium through which sustenance and revitalization draws from the depths into consciousness – therapists are faced with a peculiar circumstance, for therapists call on their own personality as a primary instrument in professional work. Thus therapists may use professional analytic work itself as a major form of symbolic expression, participation, and creative exploration of the unconscious not only for others, but for themselves as well. Day by day, all of us are unconsciously tempted to exploit life for the sake of connection to the psyche, but the therapeutic situation is particularly tempting, and a therapist's unawareness of these potent psychological dynamics can be dangerous. Just as in daily life, the less personalized a therapist's form of connection to the psyche is, the greater is the possibility that they tend to displace their unconscious needs onto others, seeking fulfillment through their patients. When a therapist falls prey to this temptation, it is at the patient's expense, since unconscious processes of the analyst's personality will be projected within the symbolic field. The patient, burdened by issues that properly belong to the personality of the therapist, then struggles with unasked-for material to the detriment and possible neglect of their own personality development. Children saddled with unconscious shadow issues do the same, unconsciously living out the 'unlived life' of a parent or other ancestor from even generations before their time.

The danger of such a constellation exists not so much in the archetypal dynamics of a therapeutic relationship that unfold willy-nilly, but rather in an individual therapist's *lack of awareness* of how and why an activated shaman complex has been constellated. In the following pages, then, I will suggest that familiarity with the symbol of the shaman and the various attributes through which the shaman complex makes its presence known in therapeutic situations is not only practical knowledge, guarding against every therapist's inherent unconsciousness, but functioning as an aid, even a teaching tool, for the person sitting in the other chair. This is because the symbolic image of the shaman that can constellate between two people in dialogue functions as both mirror and guide.

Here let me clarify that my essential subject in these pages is therefore not shamanism per se, nor even the historical shaman, no matter how persistently those images occur. The essential subject of this work is the contemporary shamanic or shamanistic person, the person who carries a personality through which the 'instinct' to shaman consistently seems to manifest. All therapists who enter this field as a vocation or 'calling' fall into this category, myself included. But so do artists, performers and creative people in general, for creative persons also experience their profession as a 'calling' and a vocation. Thus I propose that the image and 'instinct' to shaman express a paramount personality configuration about which it is necessary to become aware *so that it can be held in consciousness*, particularly for those who work in any of the helping professions.

Broken pots and mending gold

When I first wrote about the archaic shaman and their experience, I prefaced my diploma thesis with the following story: in ancient China, working with earth, air, water, and fire in great kilns, artisans produced porcelain vases of extraordinary delicacy. These vases, despite their beauty as they emerged from the kilns, were considered incomplete, and they were to be used in ordinary cooking, or as water jars. No matter how extraordinary (or ordinary, for that matter) any vase might look, it was considered primitive and raw until, in its own time, and in the random banging-about of everyday living, it broke. The owner of the broken vase then gathered all the pieces and returned them to the artisan, who painstakingly pieced the shards together again with ribbons of molten gold. Broken and mended, each vase then became beautiful, for the ribboning gold allowed the pot to shine with manifest justification for its own existence. Not until then was any vase to be considered whole.

I relate this story now, because although I wasn't prepared to talk about it back then, as I ended my experience of analytic training, I felt as if I understood – or even were – one of those water jars, broken and mended again, and finally – maybe – able to be seen as something of worth. While I could blame no one but myself for my 'broken life,' I also felt that perhaps I had found a way to make my experience worthwhile to other people. My entire process had been held in therapeutic relationships and a training community, and I thank God that in those early years, my Jungian analysts (including Joseph) knew how to make space for an inner healing process without unnecessary interference. Although generally speaking, in my early analytic hours we fussed around endlessly at the ego level with all my struggles in life and relationships, that was not really what seemed to mend the broken places: by the way my therapists held the space between us, honoring the autonomy of an emerging psyche and its symbolic processes, they let me know that it was not *they* who did the healing, but rather, that we were in the unfolding presence of a meaningful mystery. It was as if with the help of analytically trained people I slowly found a way to gather together the pieces of my broken pot, my broken self, and then 'handing them back' to a mysterious artisan in the psyche, who painstakingly fitted the fragments together again, resulting in molten gold.

Over time, I thought of the molten gold in many ways. Early on, perhaps because I was so relieved to rejoin human community, I thought of it as the community itself. Then I began to think of it as my *feeling* for my analysts and analytic colleagues, my finding value in training and psychotherapeutic work. An alchemical transformation of *prima materia* into gold was an analogy close at hand, and I was deeply glad of the energies I experienced as rising up from within myself. I poured these energies into therapy, into dreaming, into painting my dreams and writing (poetry again!) and into working any and all kinds of spare jobs to financially support myself and my studies. All this energy was *life,* an experience of aliveness and an all-out, no-holds-barred acceptance of life again that was mediated by an activated shaman complex. In addition to feeling profound relief that not only my dreams but my whole life finally made sense in a way I hadn't seen before, as well as feeling healed, reborn, and gifted with a second chance, I discovered the companioning presence of the shaman – an historical, albeit ancient human being as the symbolic process itself, flowering into my personal experience of inner and outer psychological development.

So, running through these pages like Ariadne's thread, and manifest in various excursions in the following chapters, is what I have come to think of as the evolution and differentiation of *a shaman instinct as central in the formation of the creative human personality*. This formulation is theoretical and speculative, to be sure, but it has become the way I make sense of the evolving experience of personhood that emerged in my own process through an activated shaman complex. In short, I propose that as it constellates within the field of psychotherapy or any other form of healing partnership, the figure of the shaman evolves into a symbol of the symbolic process itself, knitting together and making meaning out of fragmentation. If, as is often the case in our field, we understand psychopathology as an injury to the capacity to feel as well as an injury to the psyche's symbolic function (breaking the pots), then *when the activated shamanic complex is held in an appropriately honoring fashion, it restores the capacity to feel on which the psyche's symbolic function depends*. Restoration happens with the psychic equivalent of molten gold, a substance that adds value and meaning to a 'suffering into wholeness' that is part and parcel of what it means to feel fully a human religious imagination. Poets like Yeats may remind us that 'nothing can be whole that has not been rent,' but such wisdom as Yeats describes emerges only while, in theologian Barbara Brown Taylor's lovely phrase, 'lying flat on the dirt floor basement of one's heart' (Taylor 2010).

To summarize, the ancient shaman was historically the first to discover, and later comes to represent (as an archetypal image), the fact that in touching (and exposing) the deep roots of human nature, we see that an essential part of what it means to be human may be to be broken – and not just broken, but broken open, or broken into – an experience of having one's original sense of self and identity fractured as one is catapulted toward the possibility of a different kind of wholeness. The history of the shaman gives us an image of the first historical human figure that we know of who was initially part of a tribal culture, then alienated through a destabilizing eruption of visionary material ('broken'), and finally reassembled through what appears to be a unique process of evolving ego capacity and a growing possibility of witnessing consciousness that made them whole again; not 'whole' as the shaman was before, but whole in a way that includes the molten gold of conscious suffering and the ensouled wisdom that suffering can bring. In today's language, while unconscious suffering indeed leads to feeling 'broken,' conscious suffering can render us feeling 'whole.'

Perhaps – to avoid intimations of perfection – a better word than 'wholeness' is 'completeness.' Wholeness is never 'oneness,' a characteristic that is often applied to the original, unmarred condition of infancy and/or a naïve, unthinking identification with collective and heroic values like 'fitting in' that I had clearly been caught up in before my own breakdown into a shamanic initiatory process. Historically, the ancient shaman was the first to discover that such a breakdown was also a breakthrough into another world. This discovery made the shaman a religious figure for others and a healer and restorer of souls. We might say that in the archaic shaman's story, human religious imagination is born.

The shamanic personality and the experience of nonbeing

Consider the origins of the contemporary shamanic personality: at some time or other – time that stretches from conception in the womb to old age – and consciously or unconsciously, a shamanic personality is one that undergoes an indescribable experience. When and if memories of this experience emerge into ego awareness, the person who struggles to describe this essentially indescribable, subjective, experience tends (as did the earlier historical shaman) to name it death, saying in essence, 'I died.' Sometimes they say, 'I died and was reborn.' Saying 'I died and was reborn' after such an experience has to be saluted as a gallant acknowledgment that the person who 'died' speaks at all, but it also contains an important human truth: we can have a subjective experience of dying and being reborn, and apparently there are no other words for it. Often the person will add, 'I am a different person now,' or, 'I've never been the same.' William James called such people twice born (James, 1936).

We can say that at some time or other, a shamanic personality has experienced consciously or unconsciously, once or several times, a 'cessation in Being,' or an extraordinary, subjectively undergone experience of 'before, and after.' This gap in Being (a gap between before and after) may have been caused by any number of things – uterine or birth trauma, childhood trauma, accidents, illnesses, or any or all of the unexpected and uncontrollable circumstances human beings undergo. Hamlet's 'slings and arrows of outrageous fortune' are not choosy and target us all.

We must keep in mind, however, that a shamanic personality responds to their general share of human trauma with a particularly sensitive and resilient constitution. A shamanic personality seems to come equipped with a genetically receptive, neurologically wired *readiness*, a kind of inborn ability to stamp a collective reaction with a uniquely individual response. In turn, this highly individual response forms a kernel, or a core, or a secret seed of something that later flowers into a shamanic personality configuration. Perhaps this seed generates the shaman instinct, or perhaps the shaman instinct itself generates the kernel of the shamanic personality's remarkable grasp of 'relevance to something yet unknown' – a faculty that probably underlies what Jung called intuition. Here I want to emphasize that an individual's subjective response to whatever objectively happens to them seems to be an essential ingredient in their apprehension of reality. In fact, I even suggest that the possibility of subjective experience was probably born with the shamanic personality.

If the aforementioned gap in Being happens while the person is an infant, or very young (before what we call normal ego development), all this psychological experience is unconscious and may remain so for years *or even forever*. For patients who have suffered the kind of death-in-life that we call dissociation, this fact carries important implications for the psychotherapy process. Asking our patients to step into an essential gap in identity, where they experience and suffer a symbolic 'death,' is equivalent to expecting someone to step into a place of nonbeing. This huge expectation ought not be taken lightly. A therapist may speak glibly about a patient's 'resistances,' but glibness can dishonor the essential courage it takes to step voluntarily into nonbeing of any kind. Those who suffer through a shamanic initiation know this and remembering how important the tribe as a containing 'other' was to the archaic shaman who undertook a similar journey to an 'other world' should help us understand today how important training communities can be. Trainees often 'fall apart' and reassemble their 'broken pieces' in the containing relationships and rituals that are aspects of any psychoanalytic training process, and without the security and guarantee of such a sustaining community, an eruption of shamanic material can feel disastrous. No wonder the gratitude I held toward my training community felt like molten gold, helping me mend my broken pot!

Even more important for those who must step off a cliff into nonbeing is the analytic container. Because shamanically informed practitioners have 'been there' before, they know that when we step into nonbeing, we do not step into a total void; just as a shaman's tribe did for an archaic shaman, we analysts have to imply (in effect, 'say') to such a patient, 'I will remember you while you are gone, and I will remember you until you return.' Perhaps we are able to assume (with David Bohm) that an 'implicate order' underlies the Void, and this gives us confidence that if a patient retains courage and curiosity as they enter these gaps, most likely they will be met by *images of energies and spirit forms* that can terrify and enlighten, and probably will do both. As a patient, however, we can't know.

Much suffering from early trauma is necessarily mute, unimagined, unstoried, and untold, especially if it happened early – before eighteen months, for example, when the left (verbal) hemisphere comes online and a more integrated, coherent ego begins to form (Schore, 2019). Suffering like this is likely to be first experienced in and as a body simply weeping, or convulsed with terror, and nothing but endurance is expected. Witnessing raw, archetypal affect by both partners in the therapeutic situation seems to be a necessary and crucial ingredient by which a mute body begins to gain images that somehow contain embodied but inarticulate agony or chaos.

In my work with Joseph, there were three months in which I seldom spoke. We exchanged few words at all. I didn't even want to sing aloud the words of songs: all those silly love songs and clichéd phrases in the music Joseph chose for me were too painful to utter. I could only hum. So, hum we did. The sound and rhythm of the piano kept me going, and even though I couldn't speak, words unspoken and their collective meanings rushed through my mind and heart and body, and I agonized. Sometimes Joseph and I moved about the studio, enacting a kind of sign language or body language (see mask, posture, gesture, movement, etc.), but always we hummed, and all around me, the sound of Joseph's voice and the sound of the piano merged with sound coming from inside me, carrying me into and through feelings – preverbal, deep, inarticulate feelings that didn't *need* to be put into words but *did* need to be felt and uttered . . . as if I were an infant, crying.

Later came dreams and visions. Poet Theodore Roethke tells us that, 'in a dark time, the eye begins to see.' What the mind's eye of the historical shaman began to see were outlines of a spirit world intimating psyche's reality. The shaman is our earliest historical example of this discovery, and shamans emerged all over the world thousands of years ago, as if to mark a major evolutionary step in the history of consciousness itself, as hitherto mute agonies of human existence began to be given meaning in image, story, and song, for mute suffering becomes meaningful suffering only as it is felt into, and given form.

In depth psychotherapy today, we try to keep in mind that the panoply of archetypal imagery from the spirit world that floods imaginal space opening in analysis happens as the psyche attempts *to bring unconscious pain into awareness*. Our minds need to see images – that's the way we're constructed – and any heart's mute agony eventually needs images to pour itself into. But it is dangerously easy for our minds to become enchanted with archetypal images, and when that happens, we may overlook plumbing Roethke's 'dark time' in ways that only the heart and a feeling sensitivity explore, forgetting that human suffering cannot be encompassed by the human mind alone. The moments of true *coniunctio* are moments when minds and hearts come together, moments of alchemical gold that mend the broken places.

The archaic shaman's images emerged from the gap of nonbeing that archaic shamans bravely entered, thousands of years ago. An archetypal world flowed in to bridge gaps in Being itself, as if death, as inexpressible as it may be, ignites the depths of our human capacity to imagine. Perhaps the symbolic process awakens first as psyche, bridging before and after, and if any of this reaches consciousness, we too tell stories of 'what it was like.' The shaman's heights and depths of 'another world,' (the collective unconscious) exists, says Jung, in both somatic and celestial form (cf. Jung's *Nietzsche Seminars* on the living body); in Jung's understanding, extremes are unified by images of wholeness that unify body and mind, heart and soul, and spirit and matter into a transcendent 'third.' Jung called such unifying images of wholeness evidence of the self, and he called the process through which they emerged the psyche's transcendent function. In other words, when today Jungians say that the shamanic archetype is constellated in a person, the self is constellated too, and in alchemical language, the personality itself is *prima materia* transforming through various alchemical operations. A shamanic personality emerges from a death/rebirth process through alchemically incorruptible substance. In simpler psychotherapeutic language, however, the shamanic personality forms in, by, and throughout an honest suffering of Jung's process of individuation.

From body to psyche

Because it offers us an historical analogy to a process through which mute suffering begins to speak in moments of modern psychotherapy, albeit in images instead of language, the image of the ancient shaman is relevant to our preverbal, pre-imaged, wordless suffering. In an archaic shaman, we witness someone who was seized by the symbolic process without a developed ego capacity or psychological resources to either contain or become conscious of what was happening to them, very like a patient who is being flooded by terrifying imagery, awake or asleep, who doesn't understand that – or how – such images relate to them and their individual history. Such persons are apt to think that whatever is happening is coming from the outside, or from other people. To an aware analyst, however, emotional flooding in another can indicate that a patient's innate capacity for a sense of psychic reality is stirring in 'archaic mind,' just as it did in the disturbing visions of an archaic shaman.

In the maturing ego typical of later childhood, erupting images can be contained and – as language provides words – may be interpretable as related 'having to do with me,' e.g., to the patient's personal history. Up to this point, however, such a patient doesn't really have a *personal* history, they have a *generic* history. In my own case, for example, I underwent significant early trauma even *in utero*. Five months into my mother's first pregnancy she miscarried my twin and was sent to bed for the rest of her term. Her pregnancy and miscarriage occurred while her young husband (my father) was being shipped from state to state for military training. After the partial miscarriage my pregnant mother went to live with her mother, and when I was born, I was covered with a thick caul. Perhaps not surprisingly my mother's breast milk never 'came in,' so she was unable to nurse me. Apparently (I'm told) I survived on a combination of goat's milk and mild tea, given to me every few hours on a strict feeding schedule (long before Dr. Spock).

Until I was four years old, I had severe eczema all over my body, perhaps from food allergies: Who knows? Throughout toddlerhood, so that I wouldn't scratch myself bloody, I wore braces on my arms, and to ease the agony of itching skin (again, I'm told), I rolled around on carpets. Years later, I saw a picture of my small self at a family wedding: perhaps I was two years old, and I wore a sign around my neck that read, 'Please Don't Feed Me!' And I don't look happy. I'm also told that when I was two and a half, without prior notice even to my mother, my father was sent into active duty in South Pacific (World War II), and when I discovered him gone I cried myself into a fever. I didn't see my father again until I was seven, when he was shipped home with a Bronze Star and a Purple Heart for having been wounded in Leyte, in the Philippines.

I have few memories of my early years and was unaware of much history except as it came to me through occasional stories from my parents or grandparents. As I began analysis, somatic images erupted that – at least in retrospect – seemed to point back to difficult, unremembered times: I dreamed that I saw a naked woman walking on a beach. It looked as if fire burned and rippled under her skin on one side of her body – one hip and shoulder. On waking, possible body memories of the loss of my intra-uterine twin came into my mind. Did those inflamed areas indicate where we had nestled together in the womb? In light of recent prenatal and perinatal studies, it does not seem farfetched to imagine that I must have experienced prenatal loss – not only the physical, bodily loss of my twin, but the loss of my mother's birth-giving, mothering attention. She was young, grief-stricken, alone, and frightened herself. Decades later, other signs of early trauma appeared, including dream images of areas of my own body spontaneously coming back to life. Patches of childhood eczema erupted at different times, and kundalini energies coursed up and down my spine, making my body glow with what felt like blue light. Eventually I've came to understand such happenings as constituting the emergence of psyche itself, 'filling in gaps' with its own being. For a long time, all my dream images seemed symbolic of early trauma and deprivation – images precipitating themselves out of pre-symbolic experience.

I grew around such wounds, of course. Most of us do. Over time, my ego became relatively strong and resilient. But if we are lucky (at least in terms of psychological maturation), unlived life has a way of catching up with us. In my early twenties, I saw in a newspaper a picture of a starving infant in Africa, a girlchild sitting in the dust with outstretched, twiggy little legs, her belly distended from starvation and her face a mask of rage, grief and hunger. As I looked at the picture I thought 'that's me,' and I was shocked to experiencing recognition: where had *that* come from? That wasn't at all how I *thought* I felt – or even how I imagined 'seeing' myself. But someone, somewhere deep in my own body, clearly felt, or knew, or recognized, what the starving, weeping African girlchild in that newspaper picture must have felt: emotionally deprived, undernourished, enraged, and alone. I cut the picture out of the paper, folded it up, and kept it with me for a long time. That image of an anonymous starving child drew my awareness toward feelings I had no idea existed within my realm of experience.

Before the time we become aware of psychic reality, perhaps there is only a body, the mind a process of becoming intelligent. Perhaps – before psychic reality makes itself known – everything that is to *become* symbolic lies encoded in the flesh. Modern psychology refers to this encoded reality and encoding process as the *somatic* unconscious. In the somatic unconscious, it is said, all life occurs simultaneously, and all experiences exist together in the flesh. 'For what are we, if not a body taking a mind for a walk, just to see what's there,' says Cory Taylor in a moving account of her own dying: 'And, in the end, where do we get to, if not back to a beginning that we've never really left behind?' (Taylor, 2017, 124).

In modern depth psychotherapeutic work, the therapeutic relationship is considered to be symbolic from the get-go. We simply assume that the relational field will constellate renewed attachment longings between analyst and patient, provoking recapitulations of early experience not yet imagined, storied, or felt. This crucial aspect of a therapeutic relationship can be captured in two small words: '*as if*.' It is 'as if,' when winged psyche enters the therapeutic picture. It is as if, while encoded bodily experience is slowly released, hour by hour, images arrive in dreams, or while waking, or both, pointing both parties in an analytic endeavor toward gaps of unremembered and unformulated life. In that a body holds the truest record of all we see and feel and do, perhaps we can say that at bottom, a 'body' is a journey that all of us take. Everything that we experience goes somewhere, even if to become a rune in the flesh or the memory of a cell: 'this place' is the place my body *is*, has been, and will be – the site of all my apprehensions, all my misapprehensions, all my blinding insights and my wounds of bright surprise.

The shaman and the Anthropos

In describing the death and rebirth process of my own shamanic breakdown and breakthrough, I used the imagery of misalignment and realignment, and I referred to Erich Neumann's important image of the ego-self axis to support my reflections. Neumann suggested that the ego is an 'affiliate' of the self (just as Christ is an 'affiliate' on earth of his Heavenly Father) and that the ego-self axis constitutes a binary field evolving over time toward the realization of a sense of life's meaning and fulfillment – a sense referred to as wholeness, or self-realization, or (for Jung), individuation.

An image for this wholeness frequently referenced by Jung is the ancient idea of the Original Man or Anthropos, variously translated as the *inner spiritual man* of the Gnostics, (CW14:490), the *true man* of Chinese alchemy, the *incorruptible substance* of Western alchemy, the *man of light* imprisoned in Adam in Sufism (CW13:168), the *primordial (or astral) man* of Paracelsus, and so on. The basic idea behind these various conceptions is that there is an ideal, pre-existent form of each individual that is more or less faithfully incarnated in the empirical personality and that the empirical personality must struggle to actualize that ideal by suffering and sacrifice. The idea of the Anthropos was similar to Jung's idea of the self, but Jung emphasized the Anthropos as 'natural man,' as if an experience of wholeness might embrace an experienced return to one's 'original' nature as well.

Jung also held that the unfolding of a true or spiritual self was a sacred mystery at the center of the individuation process, or as he put it (CW 6:755), *individuality has an a priori unconscious existence*. In another reference, Jung says, 'The Self, like the unconscious, is an *a priori* existent out of which the ego evolves. It is, so to speak, an unconscious prefiguration of the ego' (CW 11:139). These references are abstract versions of the Gnostic idea that each person has their own heavenly star, a kind of celestial counterpart that represents their cosmic dimension and destiny (see Edinger's *Ego and Archetype*). One's name, in other words, is 'written in Heaven!' The star over the Christ Child in Bethlehem is an example familiar to many. Lines in Wordsworth's great 'Ode' capture the same idea:

> The soul that rises with us, our life's star,
> Hath had elsewhere its setting,
> And cometh from afar . . .

Such considerations lead us to understand that wholeness is much more than a unification or integration of our dismembered parts and that *alignment* of these parts with a spiritual principle from another world or dimension of being may be required. Hence, we do not think of the Anthropos, or 'whole human being,' as a symbol of the self *per se* but rather as a symbol of the ego-self axis, or the ego-self *field*.

It's not hard to translate the understanding of the shaman as a person who has been 'broken,' or threatened with a 'gap' or cessation of being, into our experience of someone who has suffered a broken or misaligned ego-self axis. Similarly, the image of a shaman journeying to the top of the World Tree in search of a star that represents their soul easily translates into the present-day experience of searching for a celestial point of orientation and a center in oneself, a center that feels aligned with one's destiny. Jung even titled one of his books *Modern Man in Search of a Soul* (1933). However, to me, this center is more than celestial or spiritual, just as I have to understand the Anthropos as more than a Platonic ideal. In language that I hope will become more intelligible as we proceed, what I mean by an experience of 'the Anthropos' is a *visceral experience of a symbolic premonition*, a prefiguration of an experience of wholeness that happens when psychic reality becomes embodied or discovered 'in person': in other words, when the 'star' that the shaman sought 'out there' enters a human heart. Here's my experience of this event:

> Stepping out of the shower one morning, I saw an image on the shower wall. I literally lifted my eyes to discover a great Eye looking back at me from the shower wall. The experience was momentary, and when I described it to my analyst, he poked around, wondering, I suppose, whether I might be feeling persecuted or exposed, but I truly wasn't. I explained that what struck me most was the beauty of the Eye, because 'there was a star in the heart of the pupil.' Later that week, I made a painting of this vision (Illustration 1). Both my analyst and I were aware of double meanings to the words 'a star in the heart of the pupil' – for example, me as a pupil of the psyche with a star in my heart, in addition to simply pointing to a central point of light in the pupil in the center of the Eye.

Now, looking back in light of the thesis of this book, I think that this vision also recorded my dawning awareness not only of psyche's reality, but of an intuition that for me, my realization of psyche's reality would have a great deal to do with bringing heartfelt suffering into consciousness. My vision of an Inner Eye with its flowering star was to become a kind of bridge for me to suffering that I had yet to fully feel. Of course I was tempted to simply amplify the image, (e.g., the Eye is also considered an archetypal image of the Eye of God, and/or Plato and Christian mystics have called Eye the eye of the Soul or the Soul-center in the unconscious. Even Jung comments that as a mandala, the Eye represents a reflection of insight into our selves!) But this vision with its 'star in the heart of the pupil' was to give truth a new slant for me – a slant that indicated that perhaps I, too, could begin to 'see,' as well as sense, a truer, more honest center in myself, as I slowly developed a capacity to feel my way into an unremembered history that made sense out of my present life. In some deep sense, this process continues. Only as I reached for this vision to illustrate this section did I notice that the centering star emerging from the white, many-petaled flower might indicate a feeling for life that flowers as a whole – a feeling that now makes all the sense in the world: thus the title of this vision, Inner Eye, Flowering.

The outer (heroic) and the inner (shamanic) journey

As an archetypal image of the Anthropos falls into embodiment, it not only takes on patterns of universal human experience but also a pattern of individual experience that heads toward personhood in the individual that is experiencing incarnation or embodiment. The universal story of the hero and their trials may be the most familiar archetypal pattern. Depth psychology has interpreted the hero's story as paradigmatic of human ego development and more specifically, the development of ego consciousness. By bringing into focus remarkable parallels in the myth of the hero from every epoch all over the world, Joseph Campbell outlined the function of the hero myth and the hero's journey for both individual and cultural development. Campbell also made a persuasive case that the hero myth is the central image for what Jung means by individuation – becoming an individual in relation to the collective – something that the history of shamanism shows that a shaman did instinctively, by nature.

So where does the archetypal image of the shaman fit this picture? While it is possible to force the phenomenology of shamanism into the heroic paradigm, when we do so, something unique about the shaman's experience is lost. In the case of the shamanic personality, understanding what it means to be fully human according to the hero's journey alone falls short, because it leaves out the inner life – an entire province of human experience – and that won't do. Usually, the hero's story is a story of mastery and confidence – at least, the hero's story *includes* a period of victory and dominion – even if a particular story ends in death. Generally, the hero's image endows everything that points to triumph over life and triumph over the unconscious background from which consciousness springs. For all the hero's dominance, however, an heroic perspective limits and distorts our view in that it skews our engagement with 'human being' away from darkness, mystery, and any experience of life's innerness that can reconnect us to each other and to our beginnings.

So, just as the image of the hero points us toward a heroic, almost classical development of ego and ego consciousness, I suggest that the image of the shaman emerging from the Anthropos points us toward the development of a *qualitatively different ego* possibility in the human personality. As a 'chosen one,' a hero goes out in search of adventure, slays the dragon, rescues the maiden, and is usually celebrated as a leader of his group. We may *interpret* the hero's conquests (as Jungian psychology has done) as an inner journey along the path of individuation, but the story itself is about outer conquest. In contrast, a shaman's discoveries and adventures take place in an inner world, and a shaman learns to relate to the spirits, not vanquish them. If a shaman's inner journey is to succeed, they must win the spirit's help, particularly in turning the hurt of damaged instinct into a helpful ally.

Within the difficulties of every life, the hero's way of coping is to overcome, triumphing over adversity and deprivation. In contrast, a shaman usually starts out as a misfit – the child who stands out or is in some way extraordinary – as someone who is 'marked' (like Cain), not 'chosen'. Perhaps they are disabled or oddly alienated. Perhaps they plunged into an inward journey because they were ill and had no other choice. Somehow they are broken or invaded, taken over by spirit, by what theologian Walter Wink calls 'the Powers that Be' (Wink, 1984, 104–105). If a shamanic personality does not get entangled in the fear and terror that lead to feelings of helplessness and victimization (a constant danger), they will become not a heroic leader but someone who copes with bridging the gap between worlds, someone who becomes a transformational 'cope-er,' transforming others as she helps them do the same.

The shaman's story, then, is one of resilience and flexibility, and of suffering transformed. This is the person who, in turn, becomes a wounded healer, meaning that they find ways and means to use difficult, individual experience in a manner that helps others who suffer similarly. They become someone who transforms seemingly random events of life into a coherent story that somehow preserves integrity, compassion, and hope: they cope with a difficult life by transforming suffering into wisdom. These are people who become 'stronger in the broken places,' people whose wounds become blessings, though they may never heal.

In summary, the hero has an *ego story*, and the shaman has a *soul story*. The hero's story gives us a mythic paradigm for the birth of ego agency and ego consciousness, and the shaman's story gives us a mythic paradigm for the discovery, loss, return, and development of the human soul. Because the human soul both represents and embodies spirit, it is the shaman in us that reconnects us to our bodies and to all we have in common with each other. In the *Zarathustra Seminar*, Jung goes so far as to say that body and soul are one and the same, two sides of the same coin, soul being in essence the *psychological experience* of body (Jung, 1988, 355). So the shaman also reconnects us to the unconscious, especially to Jung's somatic unconscious. Symbolically speaking, as a personification of mind-body linking, shamanic energy seeks to integrate body and spirit, inner and outer, consciousness and unconsciousness, head and heart, and psyche and soul, and it does so *by way of soul,* on behalf of a 'celestial counterpart' that Jung called the self.

Those of us who find ourselves uncomfortably embedded in our fast-paced, externally oriented, temporal culture (Jung called his experience of this, 'the spirit of the times') may recognize how badly we need a shamanic sensibility to balance the sensibility of the hero. Now more than ever, and particularly in times of overwhelm, only an inner world can balance our relentless extroversion. We need to know how to turn *in* and cultivate creative imagination. From the inside out, transformative personalities know that we cannot reach a place of authentic suffering without our bodies, and in teaching us how embodied authentic suffering is, a transformative personality helps us suffer our authentic selves. Every shaman knows how authentic suffering is flensed from flesh and bone, until mind and heart meld into soul.

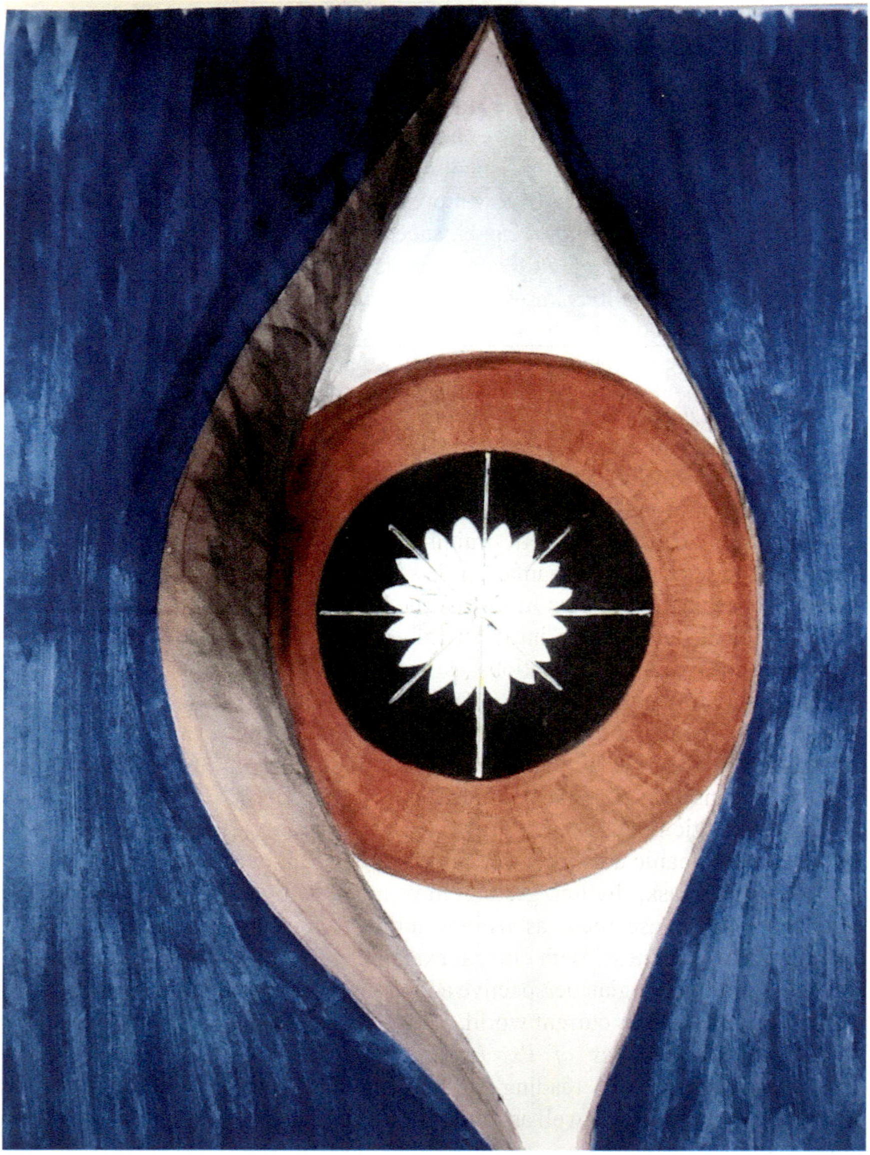

Figure 0.1 Inner Eye, Flowering Center (Robin van Löben Sels)

Figure 0.2 The Skin of the Angel (Robin van Löben Sels)

Part I

Personal, cultural, and historical aspects of the shaman

Chapter 1

The shaman in history

The shaman and cave art

One of the first things we notice about our Cro-Magnon ancestors is that they drew, and they were skilled. The walls of Northern Spain's Alta Mira Caves and the Caves of Lascaux in Southern France are covered with petrographs, painted with colors that so expertly employ already-existing stone formations in the cave walls that when I saw them I could imagine that the standing bison and the running deer still lived. Scholars suppose that the roots of shamanism reach back to the Paleolithic era, thirty to fifty thousand years ago, and they also suppose that these painted caves were the work and province of archaic shamans; apparently, in addition to the shaman's role as healer, balancer of society, maker of songs, dances and rituals, the archaic shaman gives us our earliest example of the 'artist.' Images of animals drawn by shamans conveyed a world of spirit as well as matter. Unlike the sleepers that we are today, scanning our memories as if our dreams were pictures in a book, archaic shamans painted instinctively, drawing the first figurative images we know of and presenting them to the impressionable eyes of other human beings around them – images that are now visual traces in our present, collectively evolving human memory.

Most scholars recognize that the whole primitive world must have been flooded with mystical experience. But what we interpret as a 'constellation of mystical images' was no such thing to an archaic shaman, for typical archaic societies recognized no dichotomy between the sacred and the profane. Then, as now, the holy welled forth from the unconscious rather than appearing by means of conscious intent. What an archaic shaman depicted in the secret recesses of a Paleolithic cave sanctuary signified immediate contact with the spirit world – what Giedion (1962, 279) called *contact immediate* with *realities invisibles*. Shamanic images were concerned with far more than the tribe's hunger and the hunt: there were spirits to be propitiated and souls to be found. Seen through a psychological lens, the distinction we make between 'sacred' and 'profane' occurs only with the development of an ego, but an archaic shaman did not have an ego as we understand ego and consciousness today.

The bird-masked man

In addition to the extraordinary animals found in the Caves of Lascaux, one engraved tableau depicts a small anthropomorphic figure of a naked, ithyphallic, bird-headed man, clearly lying in trance. With him are an *auroch*, wounded, its intestines spilling out, and a bird-topped pole, perhaps representing a tutelary spirit. In 1952, Horst Kirchner published a symbolic analysis of this pictograph, interpreting it from the point of view of his studies of shamanism (Eliade, 1964, 481). We can read these images concretely, as a man, a wounded beast, and a bird stick, but by taking them altogether instead of one by one, Kirchner understood them to represent the interior process of an archaic shaman, reasoning that the naked man was caught at a precise moment of ecstatic metamorphosis, his aroused body fallen into rigid trance and his soul embarking on a celestial journey. The *auroch* or bison that accompanied the shaman, then, was not hunter's prey but depicted the shaman's instinctive *animal self* sacrificed to ecstasy and the shaman's self-transcendence. Additionally, the bird-pole lying alongside the bird-headed man symbolized the shaman's simultaneous, subjective experience of transcendence and celestial ascent (*ibid*., 503). In other words, this shaman left his body behind in the form of a wounded animal self as the shaman's spirit ascended.

Historically, the bird-pole symbol is directly antecedent, and comparable to bird staffs long known to be an essential piece of shamanic paraphernalia in the Americas and elsewhere. It is also antecedent to the bird-topped World Tree found in the Americas and the myths and cosmic schemes of many peoples. We will return to the motifs of bird and flight in some detail in Chapter 3: The shaman and the vertical hierarchy of worlds. For now, what is striking is the possibility that even so long ago, instinctive human conflict and/or conflicting instinct – what psychoanalysts call 'the dynamics of a divided mind' – appear to have been imaged *by the psyche* in a tension between a spirit-possessed human being and a wounded animal. We can imagine this early drawing in Lascaux as a depiction of an entranced human being as *a living battlefield* between colliding archetypal energies, one energy represented by the wounded animal self, the other energy represented by invading spirit (the bird.) Although no observing ego is depicted, each spirit has become, in effect, an 'object' of knowledge and perception to the other, and in the ensuing collision, both the entranced shaman and the shaman's unconscious animal nature are broken *into*. The entire constellation of images – masked, entranced human being, and the gathering of wounded animal, bird, pole, soul, and spirit – may be understood as a self-portrayal of the psyche as it leans toward the possibility of slowly accruing ego consciousness developing in an individualizing human being – the 'individual' person that this particular shaman in trance was in process of becoming.

Apparently, this evolution in consciousness started with an invasion by the spirit world entering a wounded body self – impossible to say whether the invading spirit created the wound, or whether such a wound was simply a ready site for spirit's penetrating impact. But through such wounding, and the imagery that floods into such wounding, the contemporary ego also gradually accrues its own agency as an 'affiliate' of Jung's self, and through similar imagery the psyche gradually evolves and develops from such collisions. Therefore we sometimes say that a wound is 'a blessing in disguise,' as was the situation in Genesis into which Jacobfell when he wrestled with an angelic being who dislocated his hip at the River Jabbok:

> Then (the angel) said, 'Let me go, for the day has broken.' But Jacob said, 'I will not let you go unless you bless me.' And (the angel) said to him, 'what is your name?' And (Jacob) said 'Jacob.' Then (the angel) said 'Your name shall no longer be called Jacob, but Israel, for you have striven with God and with men, and have prevailed. . . . The sun rose upon (Jacob) as he passed Penuel, limping because of his hip.'
>
> (Genesis 32:22–32)

Jacob's body bore the mark of transformation into Israel.

In later Christian tradition, this often-painful conjunction between the human world and the spirit would be referred to as the Incarnation, and beyond the understandings of Christianity our contemporary psychological understanding emerges that the conscious suffering of affect *in the body* builds up ego resources, thereby uniting spirit and matter into a mysterious 'third.'

The roots of shamanism

As mentioned earlier, the roots of shamanism reach back approximately thirty to fifty thousand years. Yet ethnological and prehistoric documents go back to the Early Stone Age, so we can imagine that as a species we had not only healing practices but a vivid and variously experienced religious life during thousands of years preceding. Seventy-five thousand years earlier, Neanderthals left remains designated by paleoanthropologists as exhibiting religious sensibilities in that they buried their dead with flowers, and marked ceremonial areas have been found in and near Neanderthal dwellings, so perhaps the human shamanic sensibility goes that far back. Having found a skeletal structure identical to our own in Cro-Magnons, however – and because we assume that present-day human consciousness had to evolve from psychosomatically similar human beings, most writers place the recognizable beginnings of shamanism here too.[1]

Late Paleolithic tribes inhabiting the vast Central Asian steppes ranged in race from Caucasoid Finnish and Turkish types to pure Mongolians in the East. We also suppose that American Indian immigrations began from this geographical matrix, so perhaps that is why Indigenous tales from the Algonquins, Athapascans, Navaho and the Apaches perfectly match the structure of tales told in Siberia, and Navaho sand paintings suggest sand paintings found in the Tantric colleges of Tibet (Alexander, 1967, 56). Shamanic motifs have been traced in the religious systems of the Near East, in Islam, in North Africa, and in the religions of India, while Tibetan Buddhism is permeated with shamanistic relics (Lommel, 1967b, 10). Whether such structured expressions of human experience were carried from place to place by immigration or sprang *sui generis* in each location, scholars find ideas derived from shamanism (or first cryptically manifested) in the myths, philosophies, and religions of many later cultures, including those we think of as 'high' civilizations. With this in mind, I propose that in the history of the archaic shaman we can see an evolving image of the original human mouthpiece and enactor of what Frederick Myers would come to refer to in 1903 as 'the mythopoetic function of the unconscious psyche' (Ellenberger, 1970, 314).

The functions of shamanism

For Joseph Campbell, in early societies the archaic shaman stands out vividly against a backdrop of almost complete cultural conformity. Apart from the tribal group, Campbell says,

> individuals would neither have come to maturity nor been able to survive on their own. Nature was then very hard: society, therefore, too. Youngsters found to be intractable were simply wiped away. Conformity in the narrowest sense was an absolute necessity. And yet even then there was an allowance made for a certain type of deviant, the visionary, the shaman; the one who had died and come back to life, the one who had met and talked with spirit powers, the one whose great dreams and vivid hallucinations told effectively of forces deeper and more essential than the normally visible surface of things.
>
> (Campbell, 1970, 384–385)

These visionary gifts, Campbell notes, were put to practical use in early hunting societies – such as in healing the sick, influencing weather, causing game to appear, vanquishing enemies, and so on. But this was not the shaman's central purpose:

> it was, in fact, from the insights of just these strangely gifted ones that the myths and rites of the primitive communities were in largest part derived. *They were the first finders and exposers of those inner realities that are recognized today as (the realities) of the psyche.* Hence the myths and rites of which they were the masters . . . touched and awakened the deep strata and springs of the human imagination.
>
> (*ibid.*, italics mine)

The depth of a shaman's visionary perceptions gives them their historic importance, and for Campbell, this had nothing to do with mental instability:

> Although the temporary unbalance precipitated by such a crisis may resemble a nervous breakdown, it cannot be dismissed as such. For it is

> a phenomenon *sui generis*; not a pathological but a normal event for the gifted mind in these societies, when struck by and absorbing the force of what for lack of a better term we may call a hierophantic realization: the realization of something far more deeply interfused, inhabiting both the round earth and one's own interior which gives to the world a sacred character, an intuition of depth, absolutely inaccessible to the "tough minded" honest hunters
>
> [. . .]
>
> The crisis, consequently, cannot be analyzed as a rupture with society and the world. It is, on the contrary, an overpowering realization of their depth and the rupture is rather with the comparatively trivial attitude toward both the human spirit and the world that appears to satisfy the great majority.
>
> (ibid.)

This access to depth and the collective foundations of the mythopoetic psyche is, for Campbell, both a source of the shaman's superior vitality of spirit and physical stamina over normal members of their group and also the powerful source of their overall significance as a historical figure in the history of human culture in general:

> This crisis, consequently, has the value of a superior threshold initiation; superior, in the first place, because spontaneous, not tribally enforced, and in the second place, because the shift of reference of the psychologically potent symbols has been not from the family to the tribe, but from the family to the universe. The energies of the psyche summoned into play by such an immediately recognized manifestation of the *field of life* are of greater force than those released and directed by the group.
>
> (Campbell, op. cit. 252–254, italics mine)[2]

> In a profound sense, then the shaman stands against the group and necessarily so, since the whole realm of interests and anxieties of the group is for him secondary. And yet, because he has gone through – in some way, in some sense – to the heart of the world of which the group and its ranges of concern are but manifestations, he can help and harm his fellows in ways that amaze them.
>
> (*ibid.*)

Mircea Eliade suggested that archaic shamanism consisted of archaic 'techniques of ecstasy' that were at once mystical, magical, and religious in the broadest sense of the term (Eliade, op. cit. xix). Historically, a shamanic experience has been understood to manifest a basic primordial phenomenon that belongs to being human *as such*, not necessarily to a human being as a particular historical individual. Eliade also implies that an experience of ecstasy as a primary phenomenon that is fundamental to the human condition was known to the whole of archaic humanity: what *has* changed over time, and continues to change, modified by different cultures and different religions, are the interpretations and evaluations of this basic human experience.

Commenting on present-day differentiations between the crisis undergone by someone experiencing an initial shamanic call and modern forms of personality disturbance, San Francisco analyst John Layard muses that even though a liability to fits of unconsciousness might have been a necessary precondition of archaic shamanism – the important difference is that for a shamanic person today, this experience comes about *nolens volens*, almost as if it were an inherited disease. So to be called a shaman today is only *generally* equivalent to being afflicted with hysteria, and as in shamanism per se, acceptance of the 'call' can mean recovery: today, that includes gaining an ability to make use of such 'seizures' in the service of a craft – as artists do, as actors do, as psychotherapists do – rather than continuing to turn them against one's self. Bluntly, Layard concludes that

> The shaman is one of those persons, not absent among ourselves, who knew how to turn their affliction into an asset. Indeed, the period of preparation for office appears to consist largely in an artificial heightening of nervous tension. . . . Such psychic 'forcing' ends either in disaster or in some kind of 'revelation' [whereas] acceptance of a 'call' [leads to] a redirection of power and the ability to control it in the service of something within us which is stronger than ourselves.

This is how a shaman's wound was a blessing in disguise.

A shamanic predisposition

Generally speaking, ancient cultures recognized that a shamanic 'gift' or predisposition was inborn, but it had to be realized only by ordeal, initiation, and revelation, or by a spontaneous experience of vocation. Sometimes the profession might be designated by hereditary transmission, evidence from a big dream, or an involuntary trance or illness. Designation also occurred by 'divine election,' like being born with a symbolic deformity or being 'marked' by an accident or a strange misfortune.

In my own case there were several signs of 'shamanic inclination' early on, unrecognized as such. Had I been born into in an early tribal culture, for example, the fact that I was covered with a birth caul, or the fact that I was a surviving twin might have been considered a shamanic 'mark.' Another factor might have been the eczema that covered my body, or the extreme sensitivity and porousness that later identified me as 'too sensitive.' Or my solitary, dreamy childhood might have been noticed: by the time I was four, I had pretty much disappeared into a world of books. Back then as now, illness can be seen through several lenses. Early on, our ancestors seemed to think that illness came about from breaking taboo, or from the activity of evil spirits. But not all illness was thought to be retributive: even if inadvertently evoked, a mere touch by a spirit, evil or good, could cause illness or catastrophe. For an incipient shaman, however, such an illness might be deemed desirable. Where a shaman's neighbor might feel victimized by the circumstances of falling ill, a shaman-to-be might experience that same illness as a struggle, a kind of 'training' exercise that taught them how to appease a spirit.

Sometimes the shamanic profession was gained through personal quest or (more rarely) decreed by the will of the clan. Sometimes an experience of being called was described as a dream in which the shaman journeyed not to foreign countries or to the underworld (the world of the dead), but to the deepest interior of the earth, where the creative power of the world – imagined as an enormous snake – dwelled in a deep cave or in watery depths.

And apparently, even among the earliest hunters, the shamanic experience was distinguished by its entirely individualistic nature. Because the archaic shaman stood apart *as* an individual, alien within their society because of their odd characteristics and formidable powers, the genesis of a shaman out of early hunting communities the world over offers us a psychological testament of an ineluctable evolution of the individual from the collective, an individual who is pictured as someone who is simultaneously in a process of separation from, and active relationship to, their tribe. An authentic shaman attained this position of centrality through a series of subjective experiences that we now deem 'psychological,' by which we mean subjective events that opened new areas of inner experience (hence, powers of 'knowledge') that were not available to others. In exchange, a shaman's dances, songs, and paintings activated mythological and cosmological images for the tribe, rendering them productive in individual variation by the single person of the shaman.

Vocational power

Even in Paleolithic times, individuals who were chosen to become shamans did not differ from others of the tribe in their eagerness for power. Rather, a shaman was marked by an individual capacity for personal experience of magico-religious power in depth and by their having little choice in the matter of vocation. For someone so 'fated,' premonitory dreams could become mortal illnesses were they not rightly understood and piously obeyed. Possessed by spirits, shamans-to-be either died, or they recovered and accepted a vocational call. In whatever way the shamanic calling might be translated, it was truly obligatory, and were a shamanic vocation refused, ancestral spirits might torture the children of the tribe, making them irritable and nervous, subject to crying in their sleep. For whatever reason, historic shamans-to-be were individuals who had an involuntary experience of the 'as-is' depths of the psyche – depths that today we designate as an experience of the *numinous*.

Also, to archaic peoples, initiation conferred power, but power was bivalent, which meant that it could work for good or ill: the more evolved an individual's extraordinary faculties were, the greater the maleficent factor might be, and this held true even for the power to heal. A shaman could kill, as well as cure. And even this division wasn't always reliable, for at times, an evil shaman might perform miraculous cures, while even the most reliable healer could occasionally resort to fierce supernatural combats with competitors, cast love spells, or hire out as a spiritual assassin. Thus, in Europe as well as throughout the immense areas that comprise Central Asia and Northern Asia, wherever the individual ecstatic experience was highly valued, the magico-religious life of a tribe centered on the shaman. While priests and heads of families might coexist, the shaman became a dominating figure who was separated from the rest of the community by an intensity of felt religious experience.

San Francisco analyst William Reed (Reed, 1978, 47) comments upon how well this historically ambivalent attitude toward power can elucidate the *healer's shadow* even today. For example, in archaic societies, to the degree that a shamanic initiation remained a prerogative of the spirit, shamanism seemed to maintain its integrity. However, when and where initiatory powers were usurped by individuals or institutions, shamanism tended to become debased, leading to all manner of ethical transgressions and power abuses. Although many writers and researchers today may disagree, Eliade believed that the use of psychotropic drugs also corrupted authentic shamanic initiation (Eliade, 1964, 401), for in a psychological culture the use of psychotropic drugs can be understood as an attempt to control spirit itself, not to mention numbing one's feeling life, or the insidious way addiction scars the soul.

The shaman versus the spiritual healer or priest

Eliade's excellent study of shamanism documents the fact that apparently at all times, and all over the world, magico-religious powers have been believed to be obtainable either spontaneously, through sickness, dream, or chance encounter with a source of power, or deliberately, by quest. But these beliefs have also been accompanied by deeply ambivalent attitudes toward the sacred: a desire to contact the sacred is counteracted by a perfectly natural fear of being obliged to renounce the simple human condition in order to become a pliant instrument for whatever manifestation – god, spirit, animal or ancestor – happens to seize one's life. We've seen that while in one sense a shaman was adapted to and needed by the community, in another sense, they lived on the fringes, alien and almost in exile, feared and loved, and respected and despised, because of magico-religious power. The lack of ordinary, warm, secure relationships with fellow human beings was only one of many prices a shaman paid for the individual power that they inadvertently accrued.

By virtue of the intellectual and emotional intensity with which the inner world was experienced, the shaman differed from a spiritual healer. A shaman acted under inner compulsion, seized and oppressed by spirits despite (often) having little or no desire to become a shaman. Within the shaman's psyche, unconscious energy could erupt so strongly that she could find no way to contain it other than by escaping into what we recognize today as creative activity –singing dancing, drawing, acting – any activity that would both contain and express the invading imagery. Recognizing the historical shaman as prototypical of the artistically productive personality – a 'shamanic' personality or a person acted on by creative energies – Andreas Lommel suggests that this inner intensity or inner compulsion is the primary difference between an early shaman and an early spiritual healer or priest – a difference that counteracts usual inexact historical distinctions.

While both shaman and priest might perform similar functions and employ similar techniques, for example, there were marked differences in the form and intensity with which each person experienced the vocational call as well as in the relationship of each to techniques used to influence others (Lommel, op. cit., 54ff). Like the shaman, a spiritual healer might also occupy a central position vis-à-vis the tribe, but first and foremost, a spiritual healer was a doctor in a role more nearly approaching that of our spiritual guide, priest, or medical psychiatrist. Usually such a person was (and is) of high intelligence and possessed definite ambition. In addition to a capacity for performing tricks, suggestion and hypnosis, a spiritual healer usually had solid medical ability along with knowledge of plants, herbs, and archaic healing techniques.

Both the shaman and the spiritual healer exercised great influence on their community, and the social function of both was to supervise and maintain the psychological equilibrium of the community. Traditionally and socially defined, disease had strong social components, so traditional medicine was predominantly but not exclusively seen to be an art derived from human relationships, morals, and society. If one behaved well, nearly all forms of illness and disease, individual, and communal, catastrophes or accidents or unusual happenings that befell human beings – even death – were easily attributed to the machinations of enemies or to the malicious influence of spirits inhabiting the world around the tribe.

Unlike the spiritual healer, however, a shaman acquired influence as a result not of an ambition toward a consciously chosen profession, but of a particular kind of psychological development. Whereas a spiritual healer was apt to allay disease through an understanding of the human body, a shaman worked primarily with imaginal realms behind the scenes of the visible world. The shaman's main provenance was the supernatural, and the shaman's main concern was the loss of soul. While a shaman could also function as priest, doctor, and spiritual guide to the group, in *contrast* to the spiritual healer, therapeutic efforts were never carried out in a state of clear consciousness. Shamans acted in a state of trance, so psychic phenomena tended to predominate – mysteries, like clairvoyance and telepathic phenomena. As proof of individual power, a shaman relied on synchronous phenomena wherein coincidence could carry meaning in an affectively subjective conception of a world that went far beyond the usual effect of the spiritual healer, who used suggestion without going into trance. The shaman's trance, and the trance-like participation of their audience thus defined a plane of communication on which healing psychological effects took place, and unlike a spiritual healer, shamans had intense personal experience of such psychological phenomena.

Strengths of the shaman

Shamanism came into being when the first early humans began to carry on the struggle for existence by 'spiritual' means. An archaic shaman attached special importance to the state of one's soul as a condition for surviving, and a variety of rituals and traditional behaviors and beliefs were formulated and systematized to promote specific favorable conditions for the soul. From the soul's point of view, reality is to be found not in mastery of self or of outer things but in an acceptance of a life and acquiescence with beings and essences on a spiritual scale. *Reality is found in regions of the psyche.* Feeling relatively helpless in the face of hidden things, and relatively powerless in relationship to the environment, early tribal peoples related themselves above all to what we would call a primary reality of psychic dominants, primordial images, instinct, and archetypal patterns of behavior, and these factors became the objects of the shaman's 'science.' It could have been no mean psychological feat to keep onlookers in awe and mystery; by employing solitude, higher mental capacities, and (I propose) a burgeoning sense of ego cohesion, shamans protected themselves by allowing shamanic activities to seem otherworldly, thereby creating an atmosphere or ambiance of spiritual power and omnipotence.

From the tribe's point of view, when illness occurred because of spirit intervention – meaning when the spirit world intruded into the human world of morals and society, whether because of broken taboo or because of the intentions of the evil spirits themselves – a shaman was summoned because shamans dealt with illness that manifested itself through the interface between the known and the unknown, the world of human beings and the world of spirits. A shaman first learned how to deal with such illness through an involuntary vocation and an initiation that pushed to an extreme a shamanic person's innate, instinctive capacity to cope with such an invasion in an individual fashion. Importantly, although the purpose of the shaman's initiation experience was to enable them to function effectively for the tribe, shamans underwent initiation in solitude. In order to survive, in order to survive, shamans have to be able to survive alone.

William Reed's summary of early notions of shamanic initiation and power include ways that these notions affect contemporary shamanic personalities today:

1 The shaman's profound initiatory upheaval is neither a response to maladaptation nor to a state of life; instead, it represents a particular spirit's need for actualization through a human partner.
2 Initiation and the spontaneous occurrence of death and rebirth imagery with its attendant illness is the first act in a life-long subjective relationship with a spiritual principle or agency called the helping spirit. The figure of an initiation master (or helping spirit) appears not simply to effect transformation but to assert its identity and demands affirmation.

3 The ego's hegemony (or in the case of the archaic shaman, the shaman's mundane life as part of the tribe) is overturned by a helping spirit on the occasion of its first manifestation. Living in close quarters with death is the ineluctable demand that an ally makes of the shaman for the rest of their life.
4 Although the human subject of all this upheaval has no choice in the matter, a particular kind of power was the consolation prize. The shaman was not better, kindlier, or more accepting of others than other tribal members were, simply more psychologically powerful, although the choice to do good or evil was never fully the shaman's to make (Reed, op. cit., 47–48).

Back to Lascaux

Let us imagine Reed's list as articulating what happened to the archaic shaman pictured in the Lascaux Cave drawing, lying in trance with his bird stick and a wounded beast: to all appearances, the shaman's life has been taken over by an invading spirit (symbolized by their bird mask and the bird on their staff) that transforms subjective experience and demands the shaman's affirmation; the shaman's experience of an everyday world has been flooded with an experience of dying to one world and rebirth into another, and a capacity to *internalize the experience of interaction between these two worlds* is what will imbue the shaman with an 'aura of the sacred' (mana) that will reposition the shaman within the tribe in a memorable fashion. When this particular shaman lived, none of this would have been consciously articulated. All of this would have simply been *affectively enacted by* the most shamanic person of the tribe, the one *individual who was most porous to a collective influx and able to contain it.*

Perhaps wearing the bird mask intensified the shaman's intentional identification with spirit/instinct, for not only does wearing a mask intentionally put the shaman in touch with spirit, it enables spirit to speak to the tribespeople *through* a mask: thus, in effect, the Lascaux shaman communicates experience *by way of the unconscious,* using an image we recognize, attributes that we will explore (mask, posture, respiration, and the bird stick), and common human emotions that shamanic attributes make accessible. Not until the nineteenth century will the field of psychoanalysis develop methods of conscious investigation and study of the dynamic unconscious that includes the growing conceptual network of helpful words and cloaks of ideas that we use today.

Notes

1 Bataille, George: *Lascaux, or The Birth of Art*. Translated by Austryn Wainhouse. *SKIRA: Great Centuries of Painting*. Cleveland: The World Publishing Company. 17.
2 'Field of life' tends to describe the archetypal field' of the *Anthropos* that underlies the image of the shaman. Here, 'field of life' refers to human-being-ness *as such* rather than a more particular or localized experience.

Chapter 2

Initiation and vocation

Initiation

Eliade's vast study of shamanic initiation brings home the sheer anthropological importance of initiation as an indispensable acculturating process through which we become mature, human people. Culture has always been a world of creative play in which imaginations become social realities, but only by way of a culturally sanctioned initiatory experience does an individual become a fully spiritual person, meaning someone who understands the difference between the sacred and the profane, for example, or someone who acknowledges social customs and cultural taboos, and knows the difference between them. In our present cultural malaise these differentiations are less apparent: a look at the history of our shamanic ancestors may help us gain perspective.

Generally speaking, the initiatory experience of an archaic shaman consisted of overlapping phases of the following important elements: (1) an election or vocational call (often with vows of secrecy) involving estrangement from life as it was before; (2) purification and preparation followed by an ordeal that usually included tortuous dismemberment of the body and renewal of the blood and organs; (3) a journey or an odyssey that included a period of apprenticeship, instruction, and mastery over various powers, including learning secret languages, during which some journeys were spent in the underworld where teachings were received from animals or other spirit entities like the souls of dead ancestors or ancestral shamans;[1] and, finally, (4) a renewal, rebirth, and/or revelation that often involved an ascent to heaven to obtain consecration from a god of heaven. Daniel Merkur tells us that in Inuit culture, ascent to heaven might be accomplished by a visit to The Moon Man.[2] I attempted to express something of my personal experience of initiatory descent and ascent in a poem titled 'Shaman Song,' written long ago (see Chapter 9, Rhythm); at the end of this poem I address the 'high deity' as Lord of the Narrow Gate and Needle's Eye.

In early days, tribal life was so deeply centered on the figure of the shaman that the shaman's trance itself was considered to be a religious rite. Shamans were thought to emerge out of initiation and training with means of access to the spirit world perfected and a relationship firmly established with one or more helping animal spirits. Commencement into the shaman's new identity also signified the mastery of a profession, which meant that they acquired titles that reflected new strengths: master of ecstasy, master of fire, or lord of magical flight. The areas of collective human experience to which these titles refer are still alive and relevant to contemporary shamanic personalities (especially in a shamanic profession like psychotherapy), so I will describe them in some detail in this chapter and several others.

Election and vocational call

Election of a shaman-to-be by the spirit world was usually preceded by marked changes in a person's demeanor. Sometimes a kind of syndrome occurred, during which a young person began to attract attention by their strange behavior, seeking solitude and becoming absentminded. Roaming the woods or unfrequented places, a shaman-to-be might have visions or be found singing in their sleep. Symptoms of this incubation period might be marked by fits of fury or unconsciousness, or by a severe crisis during which they physically harmed themselves. Scourging and scarification (ritual scarring) were also common, and while a person undergoing such ritual was understood to be 'beside themselves,' it was also understood that a soul was in a process of being named or instructed. Someone so chosen could not escape the compulsion of spirit that sought to make them into a shaman, and spiritual demands might drive the person deeper and deeper into mental confusion or physical illness.

Overall, shamanic transformation involved experiencing a shattering psychological process that went to the limits of physical endurance. During the process of being cut apart and put back together again, a shaman-to-be was primarily unconscious in what we now call an altered state. Often the person went into a kind of prolonged swoon, undergoing a genuine experience of death and rebirth. As the shaman-to-be began the tormenting ordeal in which even their bones would be fit together anew, they could not possibly conceive of eventual rebirth, and the dramatic experience of 'death' was exactly what allowed the disorder provoked in the future shaman to be valued as initiatory. In other words, the agonizing news that a shaman-to-be was chosen by the spirits began – and the gift of shamaning was obtained – by a solution of the very psychic crisis that brought about early symptoms of election or call in the first place. For both the tribe and the individual, the conclusion would appear to be an enforced process of maturation that manifested itself in a profoundly mystical experience, the results of which ultimately increased personal and psychological potency.

As with every real parting from the old, and in every depth transformation, real and prolonged pain is inevitable. A shaman-to-be participated in a plane of experience revealed by sickness wherein such fundamental data of human existence as solitude and suffering, the danger and hostility of the surrounding world, and the overall precariousness of human life were aggravated and utterly intensified by the symbolism of initiatory death. Our later ego development tends to defend itself against such depths of experience. But now as then, only psychic isolation, ritual solitude, and physical pain seems too bring about the involuntary and transformative experience of death and rebirth that is profound enough to meet the criteria of *self-sacrifice* seemingly demanded by the gods.

Ordeal and trance

As I mention in Chapter 1, an essential aspect of the archaic shaman's initial calling was being overtaken by an initiatory experience of death and rebirth that involved trance and an experience of being transported out of the body: an experience of *ecstasy*. The word itself comes from *ekstasis*, meaning 'to be drawn out of oneself.' In turn, the Greek word *stasis* means 'a standing'; hence *ex-stasis* implies a displacement or a standing apart from the ego. E. R. Dodds[3] suggested that this definition be expanded to include *any* abrupt change of mind or mood and any state of awe or stupefaction, but especially a state of possession, whether benign or diabolic, and whether by a god or by a demon. In any complete description of ecstasy today, psychologists would have to include the phenomenon of dissociative possession by various 'part-personalities,' whether malignant or benign.

The phenomenon we characterize today as arctic hysteria, marked by extravagant crying, wild singing, and passive withdrawal alternating with passionate activity, is interpreted by the Inuit as possession by spirits and regarded as an indication of a vocation to be a shaman (Merkur, 1992).[4] If the condition recurs in response to stimuli such as drumming, a shamanic vocation is confirmed: now, rather than being possessed by the spirits, the shaman demonstrates access to them (turnabout) as if the shaman possesses them, and formerly uncontrolled possession has become 'controlled possession.' The difference is important: to be known as a technician of ecstasy means that a shaman can bring about ecstasy at will, rather than simply being overtaken.

Gradually becoming familiar with the various languages and techniques of the profession, an archaic shaman learned to intentionally free soul from body. As they learned to will what originally happened involuntarily, they became, in Eliade's words, 'technicians' of ecstasy. Above all else, a shaman learned to enter trance at will, because only in trance could they perform miraculous deeds. Today we might call this entering a state of willed dissociation – or even, in Jung's language, active imagination.

The primary way a shaman could gain control over a spirit was by giving it form. A shaman might portray spirits by dancing them, or by identifying and interpreting them through enacting their lives and interactions with people. That the shaman's images were recognized as real and used as such clearly demonstrates that then, as now, much of the instinct to heal consists of the impulse to create an enabling space wherein innate order might occur, where form can arise out of confused and chaotic imagery. Whatever the content might have been – ecstatic, inspiring, or terrifying – the impact of imagery flooding into the realm of possible realization was an inner experience of such intensity that it was taken to be a real event in the outer world and described as such. A shaman's state of trance allowed inner imagery to shape itself as it would, thereby fulfilling the object of all shamanic techniques, which was to enable communication with the spirit world, foster spiritual powers and insight, foretell the future and issue oracular truths, heal disease, propitiate the spirits, and clear the way for the souls of the dead. And all of these were inner adventures – not outer, heroic ordeals.

Today it is understood that trance states and states of spirit communication activate levels of imagination that are not easily available. Shamans employed such levels of imagination first out of necessity, and then out of inherent knowledge of – and an instinct with regard to – the relevance and possibility of creative dialogue with the unconscious. We might say that an early shaman's training enabled their progression from a negative experience of ecstatic possession to an increasing capacity to hold a positive attitude toward states of possession, an attitude that is in itself helpful in mastering trance states at will.

With a capacity to identify imaginatively with invading spirit entities, a shaman enacted 'theatrical' demonstrations of extraordinary inductive power, transmitting their experience in trance and their increase of psychological potency directly to the unconscious of others by a variety of deeply affective, primarily nonverbal means. Shamanic communication took place through such emotion-arousing techniques as painting, drawing, poetry, music, singing, dancing, drumming, and the sheer spectacle and presence of an entranced or possessed person, usually including pictorial representations of symbols, vivid colors in clothing, arresting masks, and dramatized portrayals of myth.

Comparing the American spiritual healer and the Asiatic shaman, Clarence Quinan categorizes what he calls the learned auto-hypnotic techniques of shamanism according to three degrees of dissociation – slight, partial, and complete – taking into account the divination agency, the productive action, and the posture and sensorium of the shaman.[5] For example, scrying and scapulimancy are two oracular activities that involve slight dissociation: to 'scry' means to gaze fixedly into a quartz crystal or a piece of crystal until a peculiar light is seen, and scapulimancy consists of divination with the shoulder blades of animals. Often the scapula was burned and an oracle was deciphered from how the bone cracked under intense heat, cross-wise or length-wise, fully broken or not.

These two shamanic activities are not as arcane as they might seem; I place such activities in a practice of intuitive disciplines, along with psychologically informed astrology. Scapulimancy persists in the Muslim religion today,[6] and both scrying and scapulimancy are imaged in dreams and popular culture: Dumbledore, Harry Potter's beloved wizard, had an extraordinarily effective scrying setup, and in Philip Pullman's *His Dark Materials,* Lyra's wonderful gift for puzzling out messages from the alethiometer accompanied her throughout her 'other world' adventures in. To add a personal reference, a dream I had during training simply presented me with oracle-like markings that covered a large, plate-like bone in front of me, and I knew that I had to 'scry' charcoal markings that had been burned into the dry, white shoulder blade of a giraffe. Today in retrospect I see this small dream image as part of my own call into the shamanic life that I've led as a psychotherapist for the past forty years, struggling to read opaque and suggestive markings of the symbolic world in the dreams of my patients as well as my own. At the time of this dream, my only association was to an article I'd written in my early teens, titled 'How To Move Like a Glass Giraffe.' The article described how hard it felt to recover from stiff, sore muscles after acrobatics or classes in ballet and modern dance. When I had this dream I mused that perhaps my bones held some unconscious knowledge about where I had come from that I couldn't see, or some unconscious knowledge about where I was fated to arrive; had I then been more psychologically astute, the sheer anonymity and impersonality that were implied by the image of a dead giraffe's scapula (not even a human-shaped bone!) might have alerted me in to deeper shamanic implications, as it does now. But at the time, like many athletes and dancers, I was out of touch with how prone I was prone to *use* my body rather than relate to my self in a personally embodied manner, knowing something about a body that I 'had,' but far less about the body that I *was*. Choctaw and Huron lore understands that the real seat of the human soul is in the bones, so perhaps my psyche felt that a 'giraffe-bone-scapula' *did* hold the secret of my soul. The ancient Hebrew had a similar idea: the Hebrew word for bone, *etzeu*, means 'a man's self, a man's person,'[7] and the *Talmud* states that the bone of Luz, one of the bones of the spine, is indestructible. From the Luz, the entire body can be recreated at the resurrection.[8]

In archaic times, techniques for inducing partial dissociation might require the use of bells and rattles, along with accompanying activities like singing, dancing, fasting. These techniques enabled archaic shamans to dream aloud and talk to spirits. Amulets and prophetic voices in themselves, bells were believed to be curative agents as well as musical instruments. The sounds of a bell could summon the gods, and a shaman often wore bells and rattles for incantations and prophecies. Since ancient times, the sound of bells has also been believed to protect hearers against being struck by lightning, or other evils. Considered to be the voices of spirits, rattles were known as *idiophones*, meaning 'self-sounders.' And fasting has been a regular aspect of the training and initiation of seers and divines the world over. Immediately affecting the body, fasting brings a body into consciousness in a manner such that ideas themselves seem to 'take on body.' As with flagellation or other physical ordeals, experiences obtained with the aid of fasting are seldom forgotten. When fasting is combined with prolonged and strenuous dancing, it enables entry into a partial dissociation that is comparable to what can be achieved on drugs. In the time of archaic shamans, such aspects of ascetic life essentially lent witness to the experience of a non-material dimension to living, becoming a kind of shamanic, second-world entry into what was repeatedly experienced as a form of death.

Another auto-hypnotic technique that even today induces states of more complete dissociation (Quinan's third category) was drumming. Often shamans drummed, danced, and sang until they fell to the ground in trance. Whether the attempt was to induce spirits or repel them, drumming opened the possibility of direct communication with the spirit world. It might take a training period of two or more years to perfect drumming techniques and overcome the natural tendency to exhaustion. Specialists in such archaic techniques for achieving ecstasy used the ecstatic states they reached for many purposes: for purely empirical matters of survival in the material world like finding game or improving skills, or for predicting weather changes and the outcome of ritual actions, or for influencing the course of natural events and knowing things beyond the scope of the physical senses. Others were intended to heal illness and injury, and still others might relate to the specialized guidance of troubled souls, either the sick and disturbed, or the souls of people who had died.

Contra-sexual encounters

The psychological motif of androgyny or bisexuality is central to the shaman complex. Presiding over this motif is Hermes, the familiar figure of transition whose most essential characteristic is changeability. As the ithyphallic Kyllenic Hermes, Hermes is called Logos and Original Man and is a symbol of generation (CW:9i:313, 331). Black and white at once and essentially paradoxical, Hermes rules over the duality of appearance, over sexual duality, and over deviousness and duplicity (e.g., the double-faced-ness of Hermes as thief). The hermaphrodite was the double-sexed child of Hermes and Aphrodite.

While in an ecstatic trance of willed dissociation, an archaic shaman might contact a contra-sexual element, and reversal of sex is a common theme in North American Indigenous and trickster tales. Sometimes the shaman of a tribe was a transvestite. In the arctic, male shamans were thought to obtain spirit wives during training, whereas female shamans obtained spirit husbands. Because all shamans were thought to be born – and initiated – at the North Pole, spirit mates might come from the North Pole, as well. This kind of material points us toward the sexual *dual-unity* of the field of the Anthropos.

Initially, perhaps, such contra-sexual imagery evolved because of the increased intensity of sexuality, or the heightened sexual arousal that can happen under trance - remember the aroused, ithyphallic Bird Man in Lascaux. Later, in more subtle dimensions of ecstatic trance, ecstatic communion can be understood as mystical union, as illustrated by the biblical *Song of Solomon* and other mystical poetry. A second widespread archetypal theme that has come down to us through the canons of mythology and religion is the notion that sexual intercourse occurs between mortals and supernatural beings, and perhaps a shamanic experience of ecstasy is the forerunner of our earliest, most literalized belief in such a possibility. Possessed by a spirit mate, an archaic shaman might undergo a psychological change of sex, becoming either a 'soft man' or a 'hard woman.' Later on, clothing might indicate such transformation: a man put on a skirt, or a woman brandished a hunting spear. Special markings or ritual behavior could also designate such interchangeability. Forced to proceed through neuropathic training from an experience of involuntary possession and trance to become a technician of such an experience, we can imagine a shamanic progression from involuntary possession by a spirit mate to a more voluntary marriage and commitment, all performed in obedience to their calling. Then as now, however, spirit marriages were thought comparable to being unconsciously overwhelmed, and such an experience can be harsh, to say the least.

Writing about *The Woman Who Became A Spider*, an Inuit fairytale reported by Knud Rasmussen, Marie-Louise von Franz relates a story about a young girl who married a spirit mate.[9] Rejecting the usual human fate of an ordinary marriage and a continuing instinctual life within her tribe because she wanted something 'special,' this girl deliberately 'broke taboo' by marrying a talking head (an autonomous spiritual factor) instead of a human being. Indeed she experienced the unconscious and was initiated into a world beyond the Copper Moon Man, von Franz tells us; however, when the girl returned to earth she did not open her eyes quickly enough, and so she was changed into a spider.

Such a tale suggests that if consciousness is too weak – essentially, meaning that if we cannot face a return to reality – then a shamanic, initiatory experience of the unconscious can be negative instead of positive. Von Franz suggests that had the girl opened her eyes to reality, perhaps she would have become a female shaman, or a priestess who knew from her own experience about the mysteries of the beyond. Perhaps the girl would have gained the status of an 'initiated one' who, through special experience, really knew what was happening in the unconscious. Then she might have been able to tell her tribe about the 'other side, the other world.' Instead, this particular girl became a spider, weaving webs of illusion for others and self-deception for herself.

At any rate, it would appear that historical shamans had little choice in matters of spirit marriage or androgyny, and it was also said that this matter might be more difficult for a woman than for a man, because the spirit husband of a female shaman was apt to desert her during childbirth or menses, wanting nothing to do with such matters. The real point of von Franz's small tale seems to be that whenever, and however, we encounter the dark powers of dark places, we must keep in mind that such powers can be hypnotic, seductive, and entangling. Love for one's ordinary, everyday life may be the most potent force we can summon to free ourselves from trance.

Drug experience

Research during the past sixty years indicates that many drugs, including psychedelics that are common to our time, were used to alter consciousness in early cultures as well. But this did not (and does not) mean that drug experience gave then, or gives now, a shortcut to spiritual consciousness. This is because drug experience may weaken the ego rather than strengthen it – and only ego awareness can attain, and ground, and maintain authentic spiritual consciousness. Drug-induced transformation may help us get in touch with dissociated feeling, but such experiences do not necessarily carry over to normal states of consciousness, and a person who uses drugs may well fear becoming dependent on drug use in order to bring about ecstasy again. As a master of ecstasy, an archaic shaman was not dependent on drugs, even if they used the drugs for enhancement. In the third book of *Journey to Ixtlan*, for example, Carlos Castaneda recants the earlier implication of his first two books – that psychedelic experience can be equated with spiritual awareness or meditative ecstasy. His earlier beliefs that this must be the case then become part of Castaneda's naïveté and intellectual arrogance, aspects of personality that Don Juan, Castaneda's teacher, works to transform. In still later work, Castaneda claims that all the experience that was crucial to his maturation involved non-drug-related, meditatively induced, altered states of consciousness. And in a different account altogether, Lame Deer, who participated for six years in peyote sessions of the Native American Church, came to a similar conclusion. Lame Deer told his biographer,

> I found out that it was not my way. It was a dead end, a box canyon, and I had to find my way out of it . . . And if you take an herb – well, even the butcher boy at his meat counter will have a vision after eating peyote. The real vision has to come out of your own juices . . . You have to work for this; empty your mind for it.[10]

There are no shortcuts to shamanic transformation.

Ordeal and fire

In addition to mastering out-of-body experiences that led to ecstasy and associated trance states, an initiated shaman might also understood to have mastered fire, which in archaic times was venerated as a supra-personal power. In fact, traditional archeological materials traceable from African and Siberian tribes indicate that originally, many of the great shamans, magicians, and spiritual rulers of various tribes were smiths. Because they physically worked with and handled fire, smiths were the first to be called masters of fire. In the Uakut religion, for example, K'daai Magisn, Chief Blacksmith of the Underworld and Temperer of Iron, is said to have caused shamans to be introduced into the world in the first place.[11] Girru, the Babylonian fire god, was both god of metalwork and the purifying element of fire that destroyed evil. Identified with fire in heaven, fire in the hearth, and the sacrificial alter fire, Girru, like winged Hermes, mediated between god and humankind.[12]

Connections between the image of the shaman and the image of the blacksmith are compelling. Both images connect with ideas about human creativity and the kind of intuitive intelligence that imagines the creation of meaningful forms out of elemental chaos and the raw materials of experience. More precisely, such meaningful forms were created using a form of energy that over the course of human history had only recently been domesticated: *fire*. All over the world, blacksmiths were regarded as shamanic because they mastered the mysterious and magical element that originally was the sole prerogative of the gods and had to be stolen for the benefit of humankind, as in the myth of Prometheus. Early human beings must have been awestruck, even terrified, by fires set by numinous actions of the gods, like lightning storms and volcanic eruptions. The later taming of such awesome energies by smiths, who somehow contained them, started them, stopped them, and used them to melt metal ores and create useful tools, weapons, and implements, must have been equally impressive. So, too, did a shaman learn to tame and use an inner fire of erupting autonomous energies (collective spirit powers that belonged only to the gods), demonstrating impressive capacities to his people. Uniquely, then, the images of blacksmith and shaman symbolize mediation between an outer and an inner world.

Culturally speaking, we can say that the image of the blacksmith symbolizes a point at which we human beings entered a new phase of civilization – the Copper Age, the Bronze Age, and, later, the Iron Age. I suggest that analogously, the image of the shaman stands at a similar inflection point in the development of the human imagination and a meaningfully accessible inner life that is heralded by the emergence of psyche as a new phenomenon in the world. I also suggest that a symbolic understanding of the image of the shaman allows us to trace the evolution of a human tendency toward a particular kind of ego formation, one that includes an individualized experience of something that we call psyche, and a depth of imagination that includes what Jung called the religious instinct.

Fire itself is, of course, much older than the smelting of metals, and far more elemental than its use by blacksmiths and its connection to shamanism. In the Christian tradition, an authentic God experience always 'burns' you, but it does not destroy you, just as the burning bush revealed the presence of God to Moses (Exodus 3:2–3). Writing about fire as divinity, philosopher Gaston Bachelard calls it 'ultra-living,' by which he means both intimate and universal: '[Fire] . . . lives in our heart. It lives in the sky. It rises from the depths of the substance and offers itself with the warmth of love. *Or it can go back down into the substance and hide there, latent and pent-up, like hate and vengeance*' (italics mine).[13] Among all phenomena, says Bachelard, fire is the only element to which we attribute the opposing values of good and evil: '[Fire] is gentleness and torture. It is cookery and it is apocalypse . . . it is wellbeing and it is respect. It is a tutelary and a terrible divinity, both good and bad. It can contradict itself.' In other words, fire shines in paradise and burns in hell. Such paradox summons possibilities of human experience that are more chthonic, shadowy, and dark than those we attribute to solar heroic journeys of light, conquest, and triumphantly established victory.

Fire is also seen as magico-religious power: 'The Buddha is burning,' states the *Dhammapada*. As a symbol of extraordinary energy, fire burns away dross, making whatever endures its heat – or is *set* in it – incandescent, like itself. As a central symbol of divine love, or ultimate union in mystical literature, fire is thought to consume and transform the soul. Inner and outer pain are implicit as impurities burn away, but implicit also are heat, warmth, and union. Expressing longing to be consumed by such a fire, mystics use the image of a moth drawn helplessly to flame. Hidden in the hem of his overcoat so that he would never be separated from it, Pascal's note to himself read simply, 'From about half past ten in the evening till about half an hour after midnight, FIRE' and then, he added, 'Tears . . . tears of joy!'[14]

Akin to the image of Buddha burning, tantric texts describe kundalini awakening as an experience of intense burning or light, radiating from aroused chakras that course up and down the spinal column throughout the body. Both yogic and tantric disciplines employ techniques of breath control and transmutations of sexual energy to induce such heat. The great resistance to cold often displayed by shamans of the arctic or by Buddhist adepts of Tibet even today verifies this bodily capacity for transformation.

Eliade wrote of shamans as the 'hot' ones. Already heated to an extreme degree by the excitation and ardor of a terrifying sacred initiation, shamanic furor only increased inner heat, flooding the shaman with a mysterious, irresistible force that could reach a frenzy of magical intensity that plumbed the depths of a shaman's very being. Images of fire also move into images of light: among Inuit shamans, clairvoyance is thought to be the result of *qaumeneq*, which means lightning or illumination - a mysterious light that a shaman suddenly feels in the body, inside their head, and in theor brain (not unlike the rise of kundalini in the Indian *yogin*) that enables them literally and figuratively to see in the dark even with closed eyes, perceiving that which is hidden from others. With *qaumeneq* come feelings of ascension, distant vision, foreknowledge of the future, and sometimes the perception of invisible entities.[15] Andreas Lommel writes,

> Every real shaman has to feel an illumination in his body, in the inside of his head or in his brain something that gleams like fire, that gives him the power to see with closed eyes in darkness, into the hidden things or into the future, or into the secrets of another man.[16]

Historically speaking, both literal and symbolic associations link fire and mystical heat with access to states of ecstasy. In the most archaic strata of humanly recorded magico-religious experience, fire itself – understood as the *desire to create* – originated Creation. More specifically, fire generates: when we fall in love, we 'burn' with desire. Medieval alchemists labored to learn the fine art of keeping just the right temperature under their transformative vessels: too little, and opposing elements could not combine; too much, and a fragile retort might break. For alchemists, a process of *calcinatio* symbolized the descent of human consciousness into an animal realm, where it underwent and endured the energies of fiery instinct. Sometimes a therapeutic relationship feels like an alchemical situation: too little heat and psyche seems to flee, drying up even as dreams recede; too much heat, and an emotional furor breaks out, threatening overspill and inundating necessary boundaries.

Fire and affect

Psychologically speaking, an encounter with fire refers to the ordeal of experiencing and enduring intense affect. This fact was brought home to me by vivid dreams that I had at the beginning of my training. After three years in a wasteland of dreamless oblivion that I alluded to in the Introduction, and before the capacity for feeling my feelings returned to my bodily senses, I dreamed that I was

> *standing alone on a low hill in a bare, seemingly empty landscape. It is evening, and the bleak landscape I overlook dissolves into an almost utterly dark, starless sky. I have been waiting for a very long time. Suddenly in the distant sky I see what looks like a moving light, bright red-orange and yellow. I see that it is an enormous being of light, entirely made of flame. A fiery angel alights on the hill beside me, feathers of flame falling from it, scattering over the dark ground, and I am filled with awe. The flaming angel is hermaphroditic, an enormous woman with great flaming wings and flaring garments, yet with a penis. The angel wraps me in its arms, folding us in together with its wings, and its penis penetrates me. Finally, I am warm again, all the way through, inside and out, and I talk and talk, telling the angel everything.*

Surely the dark, emotionally barren landscape represented my lifeless life with unreachable, 'un-feelable' feelings, for which I had, indeed, 'waited for a very long time.' Filled first with awe and then with an extraordinary sensation of opening to feeling and a bodily sense of myself, I felt literally embraced, penetrated, warmed, and wrapped in the all-embracing wings of this Great Being, whereupon I began to freely speak, 'talking and talking, telling the angel everything,' unburdening my heart.

At the time I had few dream associations, but one story of my early life came to mind. When I was two or three years old, before my father was sent to the Pacific front in World War II, he reportedly carried me in the crook of his arm up and down a steep mountain trail called Robin's Trail at our family compound high in the Sierra Nevada mountains. I was told that as he walked with me on his arm, I chattered incessantly, about anything and everything, as if I never wanted to stop. Loss of my father was sudden, and lasted four years. When he returned, he had been physically wounded and traumatized. I am sure I 'waited for a long time' indeed: I never really resumed that kind of conversation with him or perhaps with anyone. The earlier dream I quoted in the Introduction also came to mind, wherein huge wheels of golden light wheeled across the walls of a dark basement. Even then, I wondered whether those wheels of golden light had become personified into this angel of fire. Sometimes, as imagery fills with emotional and sensate intensity, the most abstract symbols imaginable become slowly humanized. The fact that such things happen moves me almost as deeply as the dream did.

A second, related fire dream happened about halfway through my process. In this dream, a large gray granite stone burst into flame all along one side, as if 'stoniness' itself were to ignite. Occurring later, this fire spoke to an entirely different aspect of affect, the potentially consuming and destructive effect that negative feelings and affects have and the need to be able to stand one's ground in the face of them. If in the face of destructive feelings of anger and rage we maintain ourselves with integrity, such an ordeal has a refining, consolidating effect. Forging a capacity to emerge from a such a refining and consolidating ordeal was probably one reason for the archaic shaman's initiatory trial, which often generated intense anxiety. In this dream, an image of relative invulnerability to fire seemed to point to a growing immunity to identification with raw affect, for much of the stone did not burn. In the mythic Old Testament story, Shadrach, Meshach, and Abednego, emerge from a fiery furnace unscathed by Nebuchadnezzar's rage: perhaps psyche was reaching toward a time when I could look back over feeling 'tested' in the fire of archetypal affects, reaching for a more psychological perspective. A few months later, I dreamed that I leaned into (embraced?) the rough, warm bark of a towering California redwood tree whose trunk was clearly scarred by fire, but still this tree stood tall. In this dream, my right eye felt 'marked' by a sparking pool of liquid fire, as if a spark were caught there, but as I gazed into a sunset behind the tree, the spark or the glow moved out of my eye (and being?) to merge with the colors of the sky.

Throughout further ordeals of intense affect that I underwent both in and out of training, that dream-image of my fire-scarred redwood tree stayed with me, offering a reassuring marker of growing resilience and affect tolerance. The dream accompanied knowledge I (as a native Californian) had gleaned from firsthand experience of living with (and fearing) the California wildfires of the California forests. Although a California redwood may char and smoke, it is not consumed by fire because redwood usually doesn't burn, whereas the wood of other trees burns easily.

In Jungian language, the growth of affective competency or emotional literacy points to shadow integration, which Jung defined as the psychological integration of aspects of life that haven't been consciously lived. The slow integration of a shaman's own fiery affects and shadowy impulses probably gave an archaic shaman authority over previously unconscious libido, too, and a shaman's subsequent training, *tempered* by repeated plunges into the molten magma of a spirit world, would have become a secret aspect of the shaman's authority and charisma in the tribe. Today's therapeutic communities acknowledge similar integration and humanization of archetypal affect in those who complete the arduous process of psychoanalytic training, since 'trainees' spend many hours diving deep into the unconscious in the interest of integrating personal contents. They have had to learn how to apply self-knowledge to their clinical work with other people, and these aspects of training have been closely supervised by modern-day initiation masters.

In most mythologies the price of integration and an ability to relate to the magico-religious power of fire required sacrifice, and a frequent sign of such a sacrifice was a debilitating wound. Consider the disabled Hephaestus, Greek god of artistic creation, who was also a smith and a master of fire. Despite his extraordinary creative power and his marriage to Aphrodite, Hephaestus was never successful in love, and he was often a laughingstock of the other gods. Or remember Prometheus, who stole fire from the gods for the benefit of humankind and was punished by being chained to a rock while every night his liver was eaten by an eagle. Agni, the Hindu god of fire, was also disabled and known as 'Footless' – perhaps as an allusion to how flame seems to dance without touching ground, flickering above that which it consumes. Wayland the Smith, a Norse god, was hamstrung, imprisoned on an island, and said to 'taste misery among snakes.'

Images of disabled or wounded gods amplify our image of a 'broken' or 'wounded' shamanic ego that – while exposed to collective energies within and without – has been able to witness (relate) and learn from them. Because they were unconsciously related to erupting images of the collective psyche in ways a more heroically developing ego would not have been, probably the more conscious an archaic shaman became, the more they suffered. For an historic shaman, to be 'chosen' by the gods meant to be 'chosen' to experience an extraordinarily full range of affect with an extraordinary degree of intensity: to be plunged into fear anger, resentment, anxiety, elation, joy, terror, despair, desire, and exaltation and to experience the fullest range of emotions imaginable. If an archaic shaman were to mediate and negotiate between the gods and others, they first had to survive – and learn to contain – overwhelming experience. If a shaman was successful, they – already known as a master of ecstasy – earned yet another title: master of fire – and this title indicated that the shaman had become more or less impervious to *compulsive identification* with intense affect, if not to affect itself.

The shaman and the soul

As a prototype of an individual who is separated from others because of inner necessity (an imperative from the gods), the image of the shaman sets a kind of psychological evolutionary pattern for our individuality too. Doesn't a lot of this sound like psychoanalytic training? The development of an archaic shaman demonstrates a pattern for anyone who outwardly separates themselves from *participation mystique* with others and inwardly separates their ego (disidentifies) from collective powers. Out of solitude and difference, and in the name of a (divine?) calling, an archaic shaman sought first to save their own soul and then to influence others toward the well-being of a group, thereby becoming a mediator and model for anyone who fully lives the human condition 'between the worlds.' This difficult navigation – between the Scylla of feelings of powerlessness (victimization) and the Charybdis of ego-aggrandizing power over others – easily goes off the rails in the direction of power over others on one hand, or melodramatic feelings of victimization, on the other. In those of us who flourish where we perceive affliction (suffering) and difference as signs of distinction, it is seductively easy to exchange human affliction and loneliness for social power and magical influence, but unconscious identification with the figure of the ancient shaman is no joke: speaking psychologically, it can be lethal.

Someone who has repeatedly experienced ascent to the sky (elation) and descent to an underworld (fear, anxiety, anguish) has firsthand knowledge of the extremes of excitement and depression, inflation and deflation, archetypal dimensions of the unconscious and its affect images. Let's say that as a master of ecstasy, a shaman in training became well acquainted with techniques of dissociation and extreme introversion (trance). Within a forge of personal experience, these psychological states transform into seeds of voluntary detachment and access to interiority. Secure in the possession of such powers, an archaic shaman was also presumed to have developed immunity to intense emotion, to magical heat, to burning, intense desire or anger, and to fear or the flames of ecstasy itself. Relatively immune to the influence of passion (a shaman's own, or that of another), an archaic shaman could live as if the approval or disapproval of others were irrelevant. Today, such an attitude betrays a lack of heart, as well as wisdom, within therapy or without.

Remember that for people who possess shamanistic magic, mythological and magical levels of the psyche are here and now. An archaic shaman had immediate access to what we call dream time, a background of dreamlike reality that for others of their time was crusted over and inaccessible; their 'active imagination' meant daily communication with the spirits. Such access gave shamans their healing efficacy. But the end of a shaman's initiation was not – as it is for the hero – a return to the social group: the end result of a shaman's initiation led instead to an extra-social vocation that was relatively independent of collective compulsion or agency, yet it was still somewhat contained by their group and its traditions.

The archaic shaman was believed to represent a human ability to influence the powers that be, and ideally, this influence would be beneficent. Through pre-initiatory and initiatory experience, a shaman came to know of the soul's precarious existence as a psychic unit, the soul's instability, and the soul's inclination to forsake the body, thus becoming easy prey for demons and sorcerers. Considered to be a specialist on the human soul, a shaman was believed to be able to *see* the soul, *know* the soul's destiny, and either to cure the soul or accompany it to the realm of the shades. This knowledge made the archaic shaman an image of our first spiritual guide and psycho-pomp incarnate, and it also makes the shaman our first psychotherapist.

Eliade suggests that shamanism *per se* may be one of the oldest and best examples we know of *theurgy*, a conceptualization that characterizes any mysticism that endorses supernatural powers generally, any mystical system that works marvels using either black or white magic, or any behavior that seeks unconsciously to influence the unconscious of others. Perhaps theurgy held sway in early shamanism, but today it needs to be worked through and de-literalized by any modern person who is struggling through their analytic training. In the interest of our own humanity, I see our real work today as graduating from unconscious identification with both the creative and the destructive powers of the psyche. This will entail suffering a cultivation of reflective self-awareness and a capacity to witness: it also means a painfully slow accrual of wisdom, and it means learning how to live what Jung meant by a symbolic life.

In the final analysis, the implicit theology and the implicit philosophy of an archaic shaman depended on the *spiritual value* that they accorded to ecstasy, and ecstasy itself was valued because it 'released' the shaman from purely personal identifications for a larger life. Freedom and transcendence were attained through ascent, flight, invisibility, and an experience of the incombustibility of the body – even in the face of fire.[17] But as I suggested earlier, shamanic acts of unconscious transcendence that attempt to transmute our human, limited, and corporeal modality of being alive into the spirit's modality can be dangerous today, particularly when they threaten a human integrity of personhood. Perhaps protection of that precarious, human integrity informs the value of the psyche itself, in that the *psyche as soul* relates us to issues that are constellated by spirit in our time in ways that we as individuals cannot do, sparing us from endless cycles of repetitive enactments and pain for ourselves and others.

Eliade suggested that in a fearful world, the shaman's central role in the defense of the psychic integrity of the shaman's community depended on assuring the tribe that they were not alone in a foreign world surrounded by demons and forces of evil. On a more personal level, however, a shaman needed their fellow beings to know that despite all the gods and other supernatural beings to whom prayers and sacrifices had to be addressed, a shaman was human, just like the others. Despite being able to see the spirits, go up into the sky and meet the gods, or descend to the underworld to fight demons, a shaman was simply a specialist of the sacred, able to mediate the world of spirit powers, sickness, and death, on soul's behalf.

Today this translates into something that is hard to describe. For me, it is a 'something' that seems to be uniquely available in an experience of personality development that can occur within the matrix of depth psychology and its various training programs. My personally creative expression of transformative suffering eventually led to this book, and I continue to hope that my experience of making unconscious suffering conscious – sufficiently worked through and personalized within this profession – will help others who suffer similarly. I anchor this hope in my trust in therapeutic training and practice, and in my trust of the worth of creative disciplines (like writing or painting, or dance). I also trust that my perpetual struggle to practice not just consciousness (mind) but conscious *awareness* (mind and body) is worthwhile, and I trust in many simple, human activities that I value far more than the any transport of ecstasy, whether drug induced or not.

Mythic parallels to a shamanic ordeal

Our ancestors didn't *read* myths, as we do, or even think about them. Then as now, myth was gradually derived from experience rather than the other way around. Our ancestors *enacted* myths, vividly, and myth had all the force and impact of something fully experienced by anyone who participated in their enactment. The mythic figure of Wotan, for example, personified an actual state of possession.

Such personification was not arbitrarily conceived of but emerged as, from, and about the psyche's repeated experience of a daemonic spiritual factor that consolidated enough in one individual at some point in the collective psyche to form an image, rather than simply possessing that person, or tearing them apart. The knowledge that this basic insight conveys makes up the core of my evolutionary understanding that the psyche gradually evolves from collective tendencies toward instinctively behavioral enactment into an individualizing internalization of 'affects-upwelling-into-images-into-dreams.' Gaston Bachelard's generous definition of an archetype helps us here, because it includes affect *inhering* in affect images that complex the psyche. For Bachelard, images generate affect, which is to say, *images are not 'things' in themselves*. An archetypal image, says Bachelard, indicates the presence of a 'reserve of enthusiasm which helps us to believe in the world, to love the world, to create the world.'[18]

To balance an evolutionary understanding of the psyche with a symbolic understanding means to recognize that the psyche also dissociates, particularly under the impact of trauma, as if to say that when trauma occurs, an evolutionary chain of psyche's instinctively natural development is broken *within* a dreaming individual. Affect and image are then blocked from union. Bachelard's 'reserve of enthusiasm' can't reach the ego, let's say, or can't find a mode of expression, let alone awareness. What we then see in dreams is code not only for contents that are unknown to us, but unknown to the dreamer's mind as well. As therapists, however, we have to assume that such material resides within the somatic unconscious.

In our attempts to understand ego development and the phenomenon of conscious experience today, we've developed our vertical understandings of psyche: height and depth, up and down, presence and absence, and lost and found. A vertical understanding complements our older, horizontal understanding through a current of linear time, in which we reside when we speak of developmental psychology for individuals, or shared (collective) biological and cultural evolution. The intersection of horizontal and vertical understanding gave Jung the psychological space he needed to experience the spirit of the times and the spirit of the depths crossing paths (as in 'the imperishable world erupts into this transitory one,' to use Jung words in *Memories, Dreams, Reflections*). Jung used a symbolic, cruciform lens of shamanic perception to clarify his personal, affective experience of this intersection.

The major reason myth made ancient people feel so alive was because it constellated a full spectrum of emotions. Greek tragedies were realistically mimed and ritually enacted, as were the dramatic rites of death and rebirth in the Egyptian cult of Osiris. To the collective soul of Egypt, for example, red symbolized death and resurrection, the color of passion reborn into a higher order.[19] An archaic shaman's dismemberment ordeal has distinct parallels with the mythic story of Osiris's dismemberment at the hands of Set, and a renewal of the shaman's blood and organs echoes the importance Egyptian mythology placed on the ritual preservation of the organs after death. Shamans wove an archaic oral tradition in telling stories to their tribe, just as ancient Egyptians sought to preserve their culture by weaving their myths into funeral shrouds, as if blankets of culture could shelter their bones. (Perhaps those small, culture-wrapped mummies resting in glassed-in cases at The New York Museum of Natural History find comfort even today, I thought, surrounded as they are by stories of home.)

Archaic shamans preceded Egyptian culture by thousands of years, but in the same way that Osiris suffered the agonies of transformation *alone* until he was blessed by Horus, his son (symbolized by an image of hawk or falcon), so would a shaman 'suffer' dismemberment and death alone before being reborn with the power of magical flight. (No one rescued a shaman.) Not until then was he or she entitled to carry a bird-staff like the one we see in the Lascaux Cave, because not until then would a staff truly testify to the ritual, hard-won presence of a shaman's tutelary spirit – as if the psychoid realm itself entered the picture. Jung comments that in the life of early peoples, the spontaneous unfolding of the unconscious and its archetypal images must have intruded everywhere (CW9i:260), for to an archaic mind, the mythical world of the ancestors was a reality equal if not superior to the material world. Before psyche became conscious it was slowly evolving out of nature, like a flipper or a fin. Our present understanding of psyche *per se* was unimagined. Now we take it for granted that archetypal imagery proceeds not so much from physical fact as it does from how the psyche *experiences* physical fact, and we recognize that the psyche can behave so autonomously (or autocratically) that it can literally deny tangible reality or make statements that fly in the face of it. Thus early descriptions of initiatory experience may strike us as vivid, compelling, and extraordinary, but we need to remember that early minds were not sheltered by the recognitions we use.

Only in recent years have contemporary Inuit shamans admitted (when pressed) that, of course, they speak of inner experience, but the experience is of such intensity that there is no way they can express it other than to objectify it in the world.[20] Archaic tribes accepted a shaman's experience with spirit as a fact of life, not as a fact of the psyche. Here is a recent example from *Autdaruta*:

> Some time afterwards, he (the initiator) took me on a journey again, and this time it was so that I myself might be eaten by the bear; this was necessary if I wished to attain to any good. We rowed off and came to the cave; the old man told me to take my clothes off. . . . I was somewhat uncomfortable at the thought of being devoured alive. I had not been lying there long before I heard the bear coming. It attacked me and crunched me up, limb by limb, joint by joint, but strangely enough it did not hurt at all; it was only when it bit me in the heart that it did hurt frightfully.[21]

The ritual death of a shaman like this one appears metaphoric to our understanding, but it vividly describes an affective experience to a depth that is not ordinarily apparent in our contemporary ego world. For early peoples, a shaman was simply someone who began their professional life by falling into the power of the demons: the person who pulled out of dark places could become a shaman, and the person who remained became sick or died.

Bones and X-ray vision: the transformative power of initiation

In the shamanic tradition, contemplation of one's own skeleton was a rite designed to prepare a neophyte for spiritual revelation. Eliade suggests that the X-ray drawings found in Paleolithic caves reflect a widespread belief that the shaman's soul is located in the skeleton, and an ability to see oneself as a skeleton certainly suggests an ability to pass beyond the profane human condition.[22] Reduction of familiar flesh to dry and hidden bones symbolizes a reduction of personality to its essential structure. Even today, an analytic reduction of personality is meant to cast aside the ego's ways and bring about a subjective experience of bleakness and mortification. Relentlessly reductive analytic interpretations can reduce one's sense of psychic reality to its archetypal bones and/or stimulate early, regressive material: thus a psychological experience of reduction may bring feeling states that medieval alchemists would have assigned to processes of *mortification*. Present-day analysands can be glad that most depth psychotherapies never consist *solely* of rigorous analytic reduction.

As a basic, inner structure of the body that supports us, the skeleton is the body's least destructible aspect over time, for relatively speaking, our bones survive the dissolution of our flesh. Because skeletons manifests endurance, bones were regarded as the most enduring and immortal aspect of a person. Symbolically speaking, bones refer to the residence of the animal soul. The belief that preservation of the bones is necessary for resurrection is rooted in peoples older than *Homo sapiens,* for bones colored with ochre and preserved in their natural order have been found in the remains of prehistoric peoples.[23] Perhaps we can say that the skeleton is to the manifest body what the archetypal field of the Anthropos behind self-imagery is to the manifest ego: a structural core about which a body grows and within which a soul comes into being.

Just as we become part of the manifold essence of the world through our bodies, we become part of the manifold essence of an inner world through our souls (see Jung's *The Redbook*, 264). When something goes bone deep, we know we've been touched to the core, to the level of animal self. This level was well-known to the archaic shaman. Similarly, when I say I know, or feel something, in the 'marrow of my bones,' I have an indisputable, undeniable recognition in the deepest center of my being. The Igluik shaman Angutingmarik's song about an initiatory vision of a bear spirit that reduced him to a skeleton goes like this:

> Earth, earth.
> Great earth.
> Round about on earth
> There are bones, bones, bones,

> Which are bleached by the great Sila
> By the weather, the sun, the air,
> So that all the flesh disappears.[24]

All around, only bones: today we might translate this shaman's experience of being reduced to bleached bone by the great Sila as being thrown into the depths of the archetypal psyche, overtaken by spirit itself. In the past thousand years, Sila (or Silla, one of the oldest Inuit deities) was supplanted by Sedna, Mother of the Sea, and when caribou became a major food source, by Caribou Mother. But Sila is still a potent spiritual factor in the background. Thought to be formless, and seldom if ever depicted, Sila is, to the Inuit, a spirit of the sky, wind, and weather. As *Silap Inua* (The Wind Indweller), Sila is also the substance souls are made of, a concept that is somewhat akin to the Hindu idea of *Paramatman,* or Emerson's idea of the great Over-Soul. 'Indwellers' were also understood to be ideas with which the mind could think, so it occurs to me that *in the old stories of Sila, The Wind Indweller, we can discern an ancient 'outline' or presentiment of ideas about psyche itself.* Pressed to state whether he truly believed in any of the powers he told about, a Nunivak shaman answered Rasmussen like this:

> Yes, a power which we call Sila, one which cannot be explained in so many words. A strong spirit, the upholder of the universe, of the weather, in fact all life on earth – so mighty that his speech to man comes not through ordinary words, but through storms, snow-fall, rain showers, the tempests of the sea, through all the forces that man fears, or through sunshine calm seas or small, innocent, playing children who understand nothing.[25]

And, when told of the power in the air (The Wind Indweller) at Icy Cape, Rasmussen continues:

> The shaman does not get the power from the animal (spirit), but from a mysterious 'power' in the air' at the same time as it is near to them, it is so infinitely remote that it cannot be described. It is a power in the air, in the land, in the sea, far away and around them . . . only a shaman knows about this power, he is the medium. He works on the mind and thoughts as much as he can.[26]

In this conception, suggests Daniel Merkur, shamanic power is clearly obtained from The Wind Indweller, and shamanic power is something quite different from the power of the animal spirits that function as the shaman's helpers. In addition, Inuit shamans are aware that shamanic power consists of mastering their own thoughts.[27] In this way, we can imagine shamans as ancestors of our modern meditation masters.

More will be said about indwellers and spirits in the chapter on helping spirits. Here let me simply suggest that given certain psychological conditions, any of us can be reduced to feeling as if we are 'animal,' or have an animal soul. When I was a child who played What Kind of Animal Are You? with other children,

I once answered that I had trouble enough being the animal that I was, let alone pretending to be another. Some felt that I spoiled the game, but 'I meant' what I said, even if I didn't realize what *that* might 'mean.' If an archaic shaman-to-be survived being dismembered and fit together again, no wonder a return to earth felt like transformation.

In the Old Testament, inundated by prophetic visions and personal dismemberment, Ezekiel prophesied for Israel dismemberment for an entire people, mandated thus by Yahweh: *Desolation, and a scattering throughout the Valley of the Dry Bones*. Christian mystics have been eloquent about the soul's 'dark night,' and a visionary image of the World Tree in Carl Jung's *The Redbook* is titled 'The Dark Night of the Soul.' Beneath this image, Jung wrote, 'He sees the tree of life, whose roots reach into Hell and whose top touches Heaven.'[28] Like the later prophet and psychologist, the archaic shaman who was gripped by Sila was torn from ordinary life by the tremendous impersonality of an awesome otherness – the sheer intensity of a spirit world. Also like a prophet, a shaman undergoing initiation experienced *themselves* as an agonized, mediating link between the old and the new – between a common, everyday world and the sudden revelation of a sacred dimension of reality: between an old, odd feeling of containment in a group and a new, raw, individual status that was demanded by developing evolutionary needs of others.

I mentioned earlier that both Western and Chinese alchemists have written about processes of mortification, dismemberment and death that accompany a 'decomposition of the elements.' Torments that formed aspects of an alchemist's experiential procedure belonged to a state alchemists called the *iterum mori*, or reiterated death, described in the *Rosarium* as the 'cutting up of the limbs' or being divided into smaller and smaller parts, the mortification of these parts, and the changing of these small parts into the nature that is in the stone. This aspect of the opus refers to a psychologically transformative experience in which the ego of one's personality suffers the sea change of being 'cooked and smelted,' as it were, or taken apart and welded together again.[29] I also suggested that the relationship of *mortificatio* to dismemberment and flaying pertains specifically to the birth and revelation of an inner human being, the Anthropos. This alchemical processes entails a complete and painful disorientation of one's entire psychological world, including the loss of one's conscious point of view, the loss of all on which that dominant of consciousness had been based, and the loss of one's primary modes of coming to grips with life in the world. Processes referred to by this change in consciousness are so extreme and radical that the ego experiences them as 'death,' either as repeated death (see *iterum mori* earlier) or as a prolonged, unrelenting process of dying.

The shaman and the goddess

Shamanic initiation was also a prototype for initiation into later mystery religions established once the Goddess as 'elemental feminine' had been differentiated from the all-encompassing flow of undifferentiated existence. From every age, Goddesses symbolize the ambivalent powers of wilderness or wild nature – deleterious and beneficial, destructive and creative, terrifying and nutritive. In later cultures, the Goddess ruled in imaged guises of the mystery religions: at Sumer, she was Innana; in Assyria, she was Ishtar; at Ephesus, she was Artemis or Cybele. In Cyprus, she was Aphrodite, our lady of the animals. Egyptian Isis, revealer to humankind, was known in Hellespont as Mystes, our lady of the mysteries. Shamans tell their own version of serving the Goddess in the Siberian tale of Sedna, the Sea-Bear, Mother of the Sea, and Mother of Beasts, somewhat as follows:

> Once a pretty Inuit girl, Sedna was loved and pursued by a bird spirit. She tried to escape in a boat with her father, but the spirit caused a storm. To appease the spirit, Sedna's father threw his daughter overboard. When Sedna clung to the side of the boat, her father chopped off her fingers, which became the seals, walruses, and whales in the sea. Sedna herself sank to the bottom of the ocean where she became Queen of the Underwater Realm. Now she keeps her creatures at home with her until hungry people above demonstrate reverence for life. In this shamanic tale, Sedna functions as a mythic representative of the Great Mother or unconscious forces of nature. In Inuit lore, shamans become supplicants to Sedna, visiting her and appeasing her by combing out her long, seaweed hair. They sing to her, courting her favor until Sedna releases her seals and walruses for food for people in the world above.[30]

For a long time, we have made easy distinctions between nature and culture, overlooking an original unity. But I suggest that in simply having a dream life today, we all become supplicants to Sedna, attending to her Underwater Realm. Beyond this, as shamanic personalities, every time a creative impulse moves us, we visit raw nature now *assuming* form, begging sustenance from Sedna, Queen of the Underwater Realm. Perhaps shamans were the first to penetrate nature so deeply that it becomes spirit, and when shamans returned to tell their stories they began what we now recognize as a long, slow process of applying thin veneers of human culture onto nature in the raw. In *Becoming Half Hidden*, Daniel Merkur proposes that in Inuit shamanic initiation, individuals are confronted similarly. In some fashion, he tells us, Inuit shamans appreciate that their visions ultimately depend on the light of the Sun Woman's lamp, meaning plain, unassuming, natural light. Their inner light, which they obtain from the Moon Man, is at best derivative. A pre-cultural world of nature is knowledge communicated to every initiate but kept secret, for it is feared that 'unmitigated nature' would reduce us all to beasts.

Merkur reminds us that when a shaman looked upon Sedna's chopped-off fingers as the food – seals and walruses on which her peoples' lives depended - or when the shaman reported a conversation with The Wind Indweller as a visitation, nature was indeed being celebrated, but the very process of the shaman's celebration simultaneously claimed nature for a world of culture. Animal ceremonialism that accords seals dignity comparable to that accorded

> to humans, or intercourse with The Wind Indweller in various forms – these acts in themselves impose what we call culture on phenomena that otherwise belongs to what we simply take for granted, if we notice it at all.

Like it or not, we human beings are culture bearers, and it is our nature to acculturate. When we desire to make things, formulate things, sing things, paint things, we are obeying a primary human urge to elaborate nature in human form. Probably we have always celebrated nature, but *our very process of celebrating nature claims nature for a world of culture* too.[31] In other words, from early on, the shamanic profession has coevolved with cultural images. Thus shamanic personalities cultivate the imagination, simultaneously grounding themselves in various ways that link back to utterly mysterious powers released in any precipitous separation *from* and simultaneous immersion *in* greater depth. Shamanic personalities belong to all shamanic professions skirting the edges of wilderness, whether of inner or outer worlds.

For example, only in the past 150 years have we been able to see nature as *deep*. Finally, we have begun to recognize that we are not *in* nature but *of* nature. Creative impulses pouring through a shamanic personality, or the shamanic aspects of any person today, are simply individual versions of combing Sedna's hair. Like Inuit shamans, we seek to learn the ways of The Wind Indweller, courting inner and outer weather, inner and outer wild. Rilke's ninth 'Sonnet to Orpheus' celebrates this transformation beautifully, and I italicize the shamanic imagery:

> Only you, who dare to *lift the lyre*
> *inside the inner labyrinth and maze*,
> will find the *pathway back into the light*
> of endless gratefulness and praise.
> Only you, who on *death's bitter flowers*
> have *slept and fed*,
> will *sing a living song*
> to what was *given up for dead.*
> What *shimmers on the pane between the worlds*
> will quickly slip away:
> *internalize what you behold.*
> When *born of these two realms*
> *our words and ways*
> *become more valuable than gold.*[32]

In short, Rilke's sonnet is about loving this world. Orpheus, to (and about) whom Rilke wrote his poem, sought and lost his beloved Eurydice in the Underworld. In Rilke's sonnet, Orpheus and Rilke together instruct us in how to dwell within soul.

In this book, the 'two realms,' the 'two worlds,' are about our experiences of life and death: if we *internalize* our experiences of these 'two realms,' feeling our way into the heights and depths of deaths both large and small, we may find joy again, and praise, learning to value human brokenness into a gold that mends and heals our broken pots. We learn how to complete ourselves, humming like Rilke's 'bees of the invisible,' singing invisible human energies into material form – words and symbols for psyche and food for soul.

Notes

1 Merkur, Daniel: *Becoming Half Hidden: Shamanism and Initiation Among the Inuit.* New York and London: Routledge. 1992. 3. Among the secret languages of West and East Greenland shamans, circumlocutions for 'shaman' are 'he who holds himself hidden,' and 'he who is half hidden.'
2 ibid. 8.
3 Dodds, E. R.: *The Greeks and the Irrational.* Berkeley, CA: University of California Press. 1968. 71–88.
4 Ferguson, John: *An Illustrated Encyclopedia of Mysticism and the Mystery Religions.* London: Thames & Hudson. 1976. 17.
5 Quinan, Clarence: 'The American Medicine Man and the Asiatic Shaman: A Comparison,' in *The Annals of Medical History.* New Series. Volume 10. New York: Harper and Brothers. 1938. 509–530.
6 Funk and Wagnall's: *Standard Dictionary of Folklore, Mythology and Legend.* Edited by Maria Leach. New York: Funk and Wagnall's. 1972. 155.
7 Muller, F. Max: *Introduction to the Science of Religion,* as quoted in Briffault: *The Mothers: A Study of the Origins of Sentiments and Institutions.* Volume 2. New York: The MacMillan Company. 1972. 59.
8 Funk and Wagnall's: op. cit. 925.
9 Von Franz, Marie-Louise: *The Feminine in Fairytales.* New York: Spring Publications. 1972. 94–101.
10 Fire, John (Lame Deer), and Richard Erdoes: *Lame Deer, Seeker of Visions.* New York: Simon and Schuster. 1972. 64–65.
11 Funk and Wagnall's: op. cit. 573.
12 Briffault, Robert: op. cit. 536.
13 Bachelard, Gaston: *The Psychoanalysis of Fire.* Translated by Alan C. M. Ross. New York: Beacon Press. 1964. 7.
14 Oxenhandler, Noelle: 'Pascal's Jacket,' in *Parabola.* Fall 1994. Also Ferguson, John: op. cit. 141.
15 Ferguson, John: op. cit. 106.
16 Lommell, Andreas: *The World of the Early Hunters.* Translated by Michael Bullock. London, England: Evelyn, Adams and Mackay, Ltd. 1967. 60.
17 Eliade, Mircea: *Birth and Rebirth.* New York: Harper and Brothers. 1958. 95.
18 Bachelard, Gaston: 'La Poetique de la Reverie,' in *On Poetic Imagination and Reverie: Selections from Gaston Bachelard.* Translated by Colette Gandin. Dallas, TX: Spring Publications. 1987. 97–98.
19 Layard, John W.: 'Shamanism: An Analysis Based on Comparison with the Flying Trickster of the Malekula;' also, 'Malekula: Flying Tricksters, Ghosts, Gods, and Epileptics,' in *The Journal of the Royal Anthropological Institute of Great Britain and Ireland.* Volume 60. 517.
20 ibid.
21 Merkur, Daniel: op. cit. 245.
22 Eliade, Mircea: op. cit. 59–63.
23 Funk and Wagnall's: op. cit. 155.

24 Merkur, Daniel: op. cit. 295.
25 ibid. 314.
26 ibid. 314–315.
27 ibid. 315–316.
28 Jung, C. G.: *Liber Novus*. From *The Redbook* by C. G. Jung, edited by Sonu Shandasani. Copyright 2009 by The Foundation of the Works of C. G. Jung, Fig. 45 in Healy, Nan Savage: *Toni Wolff and C. G. Jung: A Collaboration*. Los Angeles: Tiberius. 2017. 132.
29 Eliade, Mircea: op. cit. 17–18.
30 Eliot, Alexander: *Myths*. Maidenhead, England: McGraw-Hill Book Co., Ltd. 1976. 172.
31 Merkur, Daniel: op. cit. 337.
32 Rilke, Rainer Maria: 'Sonnets to Orpheus, No. 9.' Translated and rendered by Chris Neufel-Erdman. Personal correspondence.

Chapter 3

The shaman and the vertical hierarchy of worlds

Images of the center and the axis mundi

When the archaic shaman returned after experiencing death and rebirth, they often described their journey in terms of magical flight up and down a vertical axis that centered the cosmos. Important archetypal imagery seems to form clusters throughout such narratives, like images of the center as the zone of the sacred, the axis mundi (an axis of the world), and the cosmic or world tree, a vertical dimension of experience primarily oriented by the idea of 'the North' and the North Star, and the motif of ascension as it relates to images of birds, wings, and flight. These powerful images are rooted in our common mind,

Mircea Eliade, in his seminal work, *The Sacred and the Profane*[1] tells us that for early religious people, space was not homogeneous but clearly divided between a sacred space where human beings lived (defining an ordered cosmos) and a profane space *outside* sacred space that represented a disorganized chaos occupied by foreigners, malevolent ghosts of the dead, and demons. Sacred space was defined *as such* by what Eliade calls a hierophany (from the Greek adjective *hieros* meaning 'holy,' and the verb *phainein*, meaning to 'reveal or bring to light.') Kin to *theophany* (the revelation of a god) but different, hierophany suggests a wider-ranging eruption of numinous contents from a spiritual world into a world of chaos and relativity. The specific location of a hierophany automatically became a sacred center of orientation, cohesion, and vitality for a community. Often it marked the founding of an encampment, alter, or village, places of sacred efficacy and power. Eruption of the *numinous* consecrated a particular spot as 'open' to a world above, simultaneously establishing a paradoxical point of passage from a horizontal mode of existence to a vertical mode of being. Over time, shamans learned to master such points of passage, transitioning between differing planes of reality in answer to needs of their own as well as needs of the tribe. During his painful, personal descent into the abyss, Jung made such a transit from the spirit of the times to an encounter with the spirit of the depths.

Eliade cites the following example from the Arunta, a nomadic Australian tribe of hunter-gatherers known as the Achilpa, reported by B. Spencer and F. J. Gillen in 1926:

> in mythical times the divine being *Numbakula* (their great ancestor) fashioned the sacred pole (*kauwa-auwa*) from the trunk of a gum tree and, after

> anointing it with blood [and establishing their culture and institutions], climbed it and disappeared into the sky. This pole represents a cosmic axis, for it is around the sacred pole that *territory becomes habitable, hence is transformed into a world.* The sacred pole consequently plays an important role ritually. During their wanderings the Achilpa always carry it with them and choose the direction they are to take by the direction toward which it bends. This allows them, while being continually on the move, to be always in 'their world' and, at the same time, in communication with the sky into which *Numbakula* vanished.
>
> (italics mine)[2]

Eliade makes it clear that the Achilpa believed that their ritual pole was the central organizing and sanctifying principle of tribal life and the only means by which they could communicate with the transcendent sky realm. Once when the pole broke the entire clan was in such consternation that they wandered about aimlessly for a time, and finally lay down on the ground together to wait for death to overtake them. In other words, for the Achilpa, life was not possible without an opening toward the transcendent. For early human societies, an eruption of the sacred, whether in the form of a special sign or a dramatic theophany from the gods, indicated that a breakthrough from plane to plane was effected, a breakthrough that connected 'this world' with an upper world on the one hand (the divine) and a lower world (an underworld, or a world of the dead) on the other. Vertical connections establish communication between these three cosmic dimensions, and in premodern cultures, such vertical connections gave rise to what Eliade called the *system* of the world. A vertical system of the world involved the following conceptions and cosmological images: a sacred place that constitutes a break in the homogeneity of space; an opening by which passage from one cosmic region to another is made; communication with heaven, that is expressed by one or another of certain images, all of which refer to the axis mundi – pillar (cf. *universalis columna*), ladder (cf. Jacob's ladder), mountain, tree, vine, and so on; and a world, meaning our world, that lies around this cosmic axis. Hence the axis mundi is located in the middle, as if the naval of the earth were the center of the world. Hence, the axis mundi is located in the middle, as if the naval of the earth were the center of the world.[3]

This was the sacralized world into which an archaic shaman was born, and their initial religious orientation was permeated by tribal assumptions and collective imagery. But a shaman differed from an ordinary tribesperson. For a shaman, initiatory death and rebirth involved the 'death' of such a collective, tribal understanding of the world and an individualized rebirth into a compellingly *internalized experience of the sacred.* Torn from normal participation in tribal culture by overpowering visions and/or an incapacitating illness, a shaman might report that while being taken apart and put back together again, they were actually climbing the world tree or were being carried by an eagle to fetch their soul again: a communally sanctioned outer axis mundi had become their *internal* axis, giving the shaman privileged access to more than one real world. Thereafter, as a master of flight,[4] a shaman had direct, personal access to the spirit world by way of self-induced trance, mediated experience of that trance for the benefit of the tribe. Further training with initiation masters along the path helped a shaman become a 'technician of ecstasy'[5] and a master of trance.

Images of the world tree

Our word 'tree' comes from Old English *treow*, which also means 'true.' Perhaps an early woman staring long and thoughtfully at a tree found herself enveloped in a vision of verticality that centralized spirit on earth. Perhaps she told her experience to her tribe, and maybe her individual experience of that particular tree somehow helped others feel more rooted in their lives, 'truer' to themselves and their surroundings. Who can say? In later mythologies, a world tree appears as a religious symbol all over the world, centering an archaic shaman's cosmology. In the shaman's overwhelming initiatory experience, a world tree embodied the *presence* of the *just-so-ness* of 'life in a particular moment,' its verticality and height opening to a world of spirit above and its tangled roots inhabiting a darkening world of ghosts and demons below.

Symbolically speaking, a horizontal dimension refers to collectivization and secularization, while a vertical dimension refers to individuation and sacralization. A shaman's imaginal passage up and down the tree's branches and leaves – first unwittingly and then with practiced skill – are analogous to what later-developing cultures differentiate as *dimensions of spirit* or a *hierarchy of worlds* and what in our time Erich Neumann called a system of reality planes.

The Yakuts, for example, believed that a shaman's soul was carried off by the Mother Bird of Prey and placed on a branch of a tree in the Underworld, while the shaman's body was cut into pieces and devoured by spirits of illness and death: hence, the first soul the archaic shaman learned how to recover was their own. In other regions, shamans made drums from branches of the world tree. The Mongols held that the shaman's steed was tethered to the world tree, just as Odin tethered Sleipnir to Yggdrasil.[6] Norse myths depict Odin himself 'tethered' to Yggdrasil, pierced in the side with a spear, and hanging upside down in a symbolic death that gave him mystical knowledge and allowed him to discover the Runes. Like shamans did, Odin extended his knowledge by communication with the dead, a clear allusion to secret or esoteric knowledge often associated with shamanic initiation. And like the Egyptian Horus, who lost an eye in a battle with Set, Odin is also one-eyed, having exchanged his second eye for a drink from *Mimir*'s Spring of Wisdom.

Because it forms a link between three great dimensions of reality – Underworld, Earth, and Sky – Yggdrasil is a guardian tree, affording both shelter and nourishment. Norse imagery pictures an eagle that sits on Yggdrasil's topmost bough, a great serpent or dragon that gnaws at its roots, and a squirrel who runs up and down the trunk, carrying insults from one end to the other.[7] As an expression of the psyche itself, the tree denotes the life of the cosmos – consistency, growth, proliferation, and generative and regenerative processes; it is a kind of summary of life's inexhaustibility. We often visualize Yggdrasil as a ladder stretching between Heaven and the Underworld, or a road between worlds, or a bridge between heaven and earth. Climbing a tree at the center of the world, a shaman gathered heavenly knowledge.

In the Babylonian Heaven, the Tree of Truth and the Tree of Life guard the Eastern Gates. Western culture (e.g., the book of Genesis) offers two trees, with symbolic implications that have been related to later processes of personality development: the Tree of Knowledge of Good and Evil, for example (the one we always choose), symbolizes the development of our Western ego, whereas the Tree of Life might stand for the primal self. New Testament writers joined these two trees with a third – Jesus's cross – a tree of death and rebirth. Raised on the hill at Calvary, the cross was believed to stand at the mid-point of the earth on the very spot in Eden that was once occupied by the fatal Tree of Knowledge of Good and Evil.[8] Immediately after his death on the cross, Jesus is said to have acted something like a shaman, descending into hell to recover the lost souls of Adam and Eve, the original man and woman. Some symbolism identifies the Third Tree with the Holy Spirit as an intermediate reality linking ego and self in a relationship referred to by Jung as an ego-self axis. For Erich Neumann and Edward Edinger, the ego-self axis forms both the psychological backbone of an individuating personality and the archaic shaman's axis mundi.

Perhaps Jung was the first to suggest that in terms of psychological symbolism, the image of the tree is the prototype of the self – a self that in turn symbolizes both the source and goal of individuation: from the Anthropos and *gnosis* is born the tree, says Jung, which is also called *gnosis* (CW13:459). For Jung, therefore, the tree stands for the still-unconscious core of a personality, the plantlike or vegetative nature of the image, indicating a state of deep unconsciousness. This image also clearly implies that the self has its roots in the body – indeed, in the chemical elements of the body (13:242) – just as a tree is rooted in, and fed by, chemical elements of the earth.

In Hindu cosmology, the World Tree symbolizes the human spine along which run the chakras – verticality again. The Hindu image reminds me of the Greek meaning of *aeon*, the spinal marrow, on the silver thread of which (according to ancient Jewish exegesis) someone's life – their *aeon* – depends. Those same scholars called the nerve system of the solar plexus 'the web of the sun,' and we call that same 'web of the sun' the sympathetic nervous system. Trees also figured in myths associated with the mysteries of Isis and Osiris. Originally known as an immanent tree spirit, Osiris's tree – the *Djed* Pillar – is both Osiris himself *and* a symbol of rebirth and transformation of the god as king of the earth.[9] Tree and pillar, mast pole and Egyptian Djed are images of the psyche and its central armature: the ego-self axis. Buddha found illumination under the Bodhi Tree.

Discussing how we can connect the image of the tree or the axis mundi with the idea of individuation, Marie-Louise von Franz writes,

> The process of individuation is a process of inner growth (*like a tree*) to which one is attached; one cannot get away from it. If one says no to it and does not accept it, then, since you are not in it, it grows against you, and then it is your own inner growth [that] kills you. . . . [This] means that if a person is completely infantile and has no other possibility, then not much will happen. But if the person has a greater personality within – that is, a possibility of growth – then a psychological disturbance will come, that is why we always say that a neurosis is a positive symptom in a way. It shows that something wants to grow; it shows that the person is not right in his or her present state and if the growth is not accepted then it grows against you, at your expense, and then there is what might be called a *negative individuation* . . . inner maturing and growth goes on unconsciously and ruins the personality instead of healing it. . . . There is no other choice. It is a destiny which has to be accepted.
>
> (italics mine)[10]

Von Franz is using early Jungian conceptions here, speaking early Jungian language that has been considerably refined by later clinical experience by several people. Notable among them is Donald Kalsched, who has developed an understanding of the survival defenses that in the aftermath of severe trauma become anti-individuation and anti-life forces. Such defenses can prevent the growth that von Franz references, turning against self-activation and self-actualization. When these defenses take hold in a personality, the trauma survivor is indeed 'not right in their present state.' But it is not growth that 'ruins the personality instead of healing it'; rather, a system of defenses that once saved the personality now conspires to prevent change, including the inner and outer growth that von Franz is talking about (personal communication).

Using the tree as an example of an archetypal image, Erich Neumann reminds us that whenever an encounter with the numinous takes place, ego is encompassed by non-ego, and the change that takes place in one's personality can range from a momentary trance to a lasting transformation. Change can take the form of an orderly process, or it can happen as a seemingly chaotic, directionless eruption that transforms or destroys a personality in a flash; it can manifest as a religious experience, as love, as an artistic creation or a great idea, or as a delusion. Neumann reminds us that whenever the mystical element is manifest, the hitherto acceptable rigidity of a world that revolves or is ordered around ego is shattered, while a 'dynamically changed and changing *world behind the world* is revealed.' 'Thus, for example,' says Neumann,

> one and the same tree may be revealed as the seat of the godhead or may as world tree symbolize the mystery of the psychological world; as a world of natural law it may fulfill a life of scientific effort, or it may reflect in poetry

> or art the *numen* that it is. All these are only diverse aspects of the numinous world-content 'tree,' which we designate as an archetype, because to encounter it is to be drawn into a mystical trance and metamorphosis. Experienced in this way, the whole world is numinous: every place, every thing, every situation and every living creature, for they are potential bearers of 'sparks,' as the Hasidim said, capable of kindling and illumining the human personality. The world and its contents are numinous, but this is true only because man is by nature a *Homo mysticus*.[11]

Neumann's words remind us that we evolve out of the context of an ensouled world, the anima mundi – a world that is alive *out there* – long before we become able to experience ourselves as people ensouled. Such a process of internalization and ensouling has its roots and origins in the shamanic personality itself.

Images of 'the North'

Just as the top of a pole or a tree is considered 'above,' so too when looking at the globe of the earth do we consider the top of the axis on which the earth spins to be the North Pole. Consequently, the image of the World Tree resonates with the image of the Cosmic Mountain whose peak culminates in Cosmic North, the point around which the earth revolves. Stress laid on the symbol of the pole is the same as that laid on the double constellation of The Great Bear and the Pole Star: while The Great Bear or Big Dipper aptly helps us get our 'bearings,' the zenith becomes a primordial image of the center around which the mystic inwardly revolves, in line with the Pole Star – the North Star – as a cosmic symbol of the reality of the inner life. For the mystic and the shaman, ascent leads toward a Cosmic North chosen as a point of orientation. In shamanic lore, the heavenly pole or the top of the tree is so far off that it is the threshold of 'Beyond,' and that is thought to be where shamans were born and initiated.

Henri Corbin emphasizes how important 'the North' and the northern dimension is to that 'dimension beyond,' which *as symbol* is alone capable of providing Western humans with a cosmic orientation:

> [This primordial image is] . . . the heavenly pole situated on the *vertical* of human existence, the cosmic north [appears as] the 'midnight sun' . . . in many rituals of the mystery religions. . . . Later Iranian Sufi masters refer to the Night of light, the dark Noontide, the black Light.
>
> Preceding all empirical data, the archetype-Images are the organs of meditation, of the active Imagination; they effect the transmutation of these data by giving them their *meaning* and precisely in so doing make known the manner of being of a specific human presence and fundamental *orientation* inherent in it. Taking its bearings by the heavenly pole . . . this presence then allows a world other than that of geographical, physical, astronomical space to open before it; it is the ascent out of cartographical dimensions, the discovery of

> the inner world that secretes its own light, which is the world of light; it is an innerness of light as opposed to the spatiality of the outer world.[12]

Within the analytic process, dreams of 'the North' or of the North Star can suggest an orienting center that may be emerging in a patient's life. Sometimes a loss of orientation can be seen in chaos among the stars or in an injury incurred from a falling star. Near the end of my analytic process, as the corresponding struggle to reorient myself with the help of analysis and others ensued, early memories of deep wounding began to surface in a dream that revealed my own devastating loss of orientation. I dreamed that I was 'working' with another woman whose body I saw splayed out against the night sky, outlined as if it were a constellation. The woman had been split from chin to pubis by a falling star, and I realized that this woman had to be an aspect of myself.

In the following chapter, I name this dream the Dream of the Night Sky Woman and discuss it as an illustration of the reality of the psyche. Here let me simply say that when I first dreamed of her, the image of the night sky woman alarmed me, because it suggested, among other things, how 'cosmic' had been my early wounding, how 'dis-astrous' it had been, as 'disaster' (from 'dis-,' to separate, and 'aster,' meaning star) means to become separated from one's guiding star. It would take a long time to find my compass again, to find an 'inner light' or North Star by which to orient myself.

Images of birds, ascension, and flight

Paralleling the motif of the bird atop the World Tree are multiple associations of the shaman's trance with the ascending flight of a bird, particularly a hawk, eagle, gander, or duck. Remember the Mother Bird of Prey who sequesters the shaman's soul? Sometimes a shaman used a *quena*, a duct flute made of bird bone, to capture the keening sounds of wind and high air in magical performance.[13] During the Sun Dance, Indigenous Peoples of the Great Plains of today use flutes made from eagle bone, and myths concerning the origin of the shaman posit direct intervention of a god or god's representative, the eagle, as the Bird of the Sun. In India's *Avesta*, an eagle lives in the mythical all-healing tree.[14] Hoofbeats of the shaman's steed can be heard through drumbeats, but the pounding rhythm also brings to mind beating wings of spiritual transport that simultaneously elevates the shaman's soul and conjures up familiars.

In the tale of *Amor and Psyche*, an eagle brings Psyche a cup so that she can obtain lifegiving water from a great ever-circling river that simultaneously feeds the depths of the underworld and issues forth from the highest crag of a huge world mountain. Without the help of Eagle (spirit in a helpful form), Psyche couldn't perform her third task: to drink from the torrent of living waters, meaning to take her small portion of the living stream of life and give it form, without being overwhelmed and destroyed.[15] An image of an eagle offering Psyche a cup brings to mind images of eagles holding the shaman aloft, an eagle flying away with Ganymede, or even Zeus in swan form, raping Leda: each mythic image outpictures individual human bodies that serve as containers of psyche and soul, bodies that are dis-membered and re-membered, anew.

Generally, wings symbolize spirituality, imagination, and thought. Jung suggests that a winged foot or wings on the heels of a deity (as in Mercurius/Hermes) indicate the power of spiritual evolution. We also find wings emblazoned on the helmets of heroes, on the caduceus, and on thunderbolts, expressing more spiritual qualities of the symbol. Greek artists portrayed both Love and Victory as winged figures, while winged animals seem to depict the sublimation of the symbolic qualities usually ascribed to each animal. The wings of Pegasus, for example, symbolize mobility in the aerial dimension as well as on earth. Jung writes,

> Birds are thoughts and flights of the mind . . . the eagle denotes the heights . . . a well-known alchemical symbol. Even the *lapis*, the *rebus* (the Philosopher's Stone), made out of two parts, and thus often hermaphroditic, as a coalescence of Sol and Luna, is frequently represented with wings, in this way standing for premonition and intuition. All these symbols in the last analysis depict that state of affairs that we call the Self, in its role of transcending consciousness.[16]

In many cultures, birds are thought to be spiritual messengers, and the soul itself is depicted as a bird (remember the bird-pole and the shaman in the Caves of Lascaux). In folktales, language spoken by the birds is a medium of warning, advice, and prophecy. We still say, 'a little bird told me.' Bird-headed creatures have been around for a long time. The Egyptian god of earth, Geb, was goose headed,[17] and one of the three great gods of the Ostyaks of Siberia was a Goose God who lived in the mountains in a special nest under the care of the shaman.[18] Hindu mythology gives us Garuda – a form of the sun and a vehicle of Vishnu – who has the head of a bird, the wings of a bird, and the body of a man. Garuda is also the implacable enemy of serpents: as such, he recalls the eternal shamanic warfare between the Bird and the Serpent (one at the head, the other at the foot of the World Tree) egged on by the squirrel. Harold Bayley's *The Lost Language of Symbolism* suggests that the word 'goose' is allied to *goost*, the ancient form of 'ghost,' or spirit, from the Anglo-Saxon word *gos*, meaning a ghost or spirit. Perhaps the original sanctity of the goose accounts for our expression 'silly goose,' since the word 'silly' was originally of pious derivation and meant 'happy,' 'blessed,' 'innocent,' and 'gentle.'

Shamanic lore also includes images of the Raven. In many mythologies, the Raven was originally white. In North American Indigenous and Arctic Polar stories, for example, the Raven is the Great Light Bringer, a promethean figure who brings light and fire to humankind and is burned black in the process.[19] The Great Raven, Gahgagoowa, leader of the Iroquois Society of Mystic Animals, is involved in the creation of curing songs. An image of dark and light together, the Raven becomes a culture hero, agent of transformation, and the trickster figure of the cycle of tales from the Indigenous Peoples living in what is now the North Pacific Coast from Alaska to British Columbia and of the Inuit in Western Alaska.[20] According to the Inuit (the Apatac of the Noatak River), Tulungersag, or Father Raven, was the origin of everything and the creator of all life. A holy life power that originally began in the shape of a human being, Tulungersag changed into a raven so that he could explore the abyss (later named 'earth') when he left heaven. This myth describes the beginning of the world as an awakening into consciousness.[21]

Odin had two ravens, Hugin (Thought) and Munin (Memory), who sat on his shoulders and whispered news of the world into his ears. In alchemical lore, either the black raven or a raven with a white head signifies the light that emerges from darkness in the process of blackening, or *nigredo*. In my descent into the *nigredo* and gradual emergence over the course of an analysis with Edward Edinger, I had the following dream: 'A white seabird is flying over the ocean, each wing marked with a band of black and a voiceover says, 'She's earned her stripes.' Needless to say, this dream was reassuring.

The shaman's resurrection as a bird helps us imagine what it is like to be reborn as a soul, imagery that is paralleled in the story of Osiris reanimated by the Ba-Bird (a bird with a human face and head) after his death at the hands of Set.[22] In this story, the animating symbol is the eye of Osiris's son Horus, *transferred* to Osiris in the underworld to assure his everlasting life. In later Egyptian mysteries, Horus is a hawk deity. Representing the rising and setting sun, the image of Horus representing the cyclical nature of time.[23] Such an image helps remind us that, today, personality transformation happens only over time, dream after dream, hour by hour, and day by day.

As the end of my analytic process neared – week by week and year by year – and I attained a greater orientation to a 'north' of my personal life – I had another dream: A great brown bird (a falcon or a hawk), its head turned to the side, gazes over its folded, bejeweled wings, and each wing is outlined in shining, multi-colored, precious stones. I see this majestic bird from behind. A voice says, 'There is a change in the order of things.' This dream brought me an image of a beautiful bird, a messenger between two worlds with attributes both of heaven and earth – wings as bejeweled as a heavenly garment, yet earthy red-brown plumage. My analyst thought that perhaps the bird symbolized a capacity for intuitive flight and keen-eyed vision 'coming to earth' and becoming more grounded psychologically; I simply felt deeply honored, visited somehow by a royal messenger, or gifted with a transformative glimpse of another world. As in Rumi's poem *The Seed Market*, a 'perfect falcon' became part of my world, 'for no reason.'[24]

Perhaps 'a change in the order of things' referred to what Erich Neumann (Neumann, 1968) called a change in reality planes. In this dream, the wings of an ordinary falcon – a bird as common to the natural world as matter, body, soul, and affect – are elevated, uplifted, and bejeweled. It also felt propitious because it so resonated with mythic images of the falcon-headed Egyptian god Horus, one of our earliest symbols of the wholeness of life resurrected in the wake of painful dismemberment and crucifixion. I felt as privileged to return as Horus must have felt, from death at the hands of his brother Set.

Other birds associated with spiritual ascent and descent include the dove, often used to depict the Holy Spirit, inspiring to both prophets and people of action. A dove descended on Jesus at baptism, and Jesus himself promised the gift of spirit in the form of the Holy Ghost. Considered to be both a source of wisdom and the power of life, the Holy Ghost manifests itself through ecstatic utterance or by an experience of unusual powers. At Pentecost, ecstatic disciples still experience the coming of the spirit

And what happens with angels? Over the centuries, bird imagery has modified into various imagery of angelic beings. To us today, angels are age-old symbols of beings whose hidden operations bring wisdom and protection, or – as with fallen angels – the dangers of being possessed by the dark side of such powers. Angels personify powers and intelligence at the roots of Being under both creative and destructive aspects. Even if we understand them as the power and intelligence behind the archetypes, our psychological and emotional relation to angels can never be simply a matter of an attitude toward a principle, however, because actually meeting an angel is always visceral experience – a unique meeting with the unconscious through a specific image that personifies powers and intelligence that reach us from the primordial origins of our individual lives.

We find attendant bird imagery in the motif of the feather, an image that is also charged with spiritual symbolism (see earlier reference to my image of a flaming angel). Because of its beauty, fragility, and scarcity, bird plumage has mana that grants spiritual power to the one who wears it. Worn by shamans, feathered headdresses served as material manifestations of a spiritual energy centrally located in the head, not unlike the significance of the halos depicted in Christian and Buddhist iconography. Feathers can also symbolize blessings and prayers, as if a feather's fragile filaments could express the most potent of forces. We also find the symbolic importance of delicacy and lightness in the Egyptian belief that after death, the soul itself is judged by the goddess Ma'at, who weighs the soul's heart on a balance-scale against the Feather of Truth: if the heart is pure, the scale will balance; if the heart is heavier than a feather, it is burdened with 'sin,' and – in Egyptian belief – consigned to the Underworld.

Birds and flight; feathers and wings; and the motif of ascension are variations on core imagery that plays an essential role in shamanic initiation. Trees and pole-climbing rites, myths of ascent or magical flight, or ecstatic experiences of levitation and mystical journeys to the heavens (the other side of the 'night sea' journey) are all images that point toward a shamanic calling. From earliest times, mystical powers of flight were attributed to Asiatic shamans who, in early stages of initiation, were sometimes found entranced among the treetops.[25]

Marie-Louise von Franz writes of a story she once heard that illustrates how such instinctive behavior still breaks through in raw form even today: a young boy, going through a period of mental stress, was sent to the country to work with his uncle on a farm. Instead of working, the boy climbed a tree where he made a nest. His uncle left him alone except to give him food. The boy remained in the tree for a month and then came down, quite reasonably. Von Franz comments that the boy instinctively saved himself by borrowing from the unconscious (the shaman instinct) and that he had the good luck not to be prevented from doing so. We could say that the boy went through a shamanic initiation. Probably he had an experience of the collective unconscious while he was up there, but rather than avoiding the threat of such experience, he entrusted himself to it. Sitting in a tree means to retreat from reality and retiring into what is threatening: the boy had just enough instinct to cure himself and keep himself from madness. The danger, of course, is a complete loss of connection to reality; the advantage is that threatening content may, with acceptance, become a second womb – a nest in a tree – out of which rebirth can (and does) take place.[26] The environmental artist Andy Goldsworthy's latest film, *Leaning Into The Wind* (2018), offers a beautiful example of a shamanic personality in action. Goldsworthy ends this film by depicting himself (barely visible) perched high in one of the trees that line a fog-enshrouded British expressway, mostly unseen by passing motorists. I could hardly believe my eyes.

Psychologically speaking, imagery of flight and ascension tend to express identification with intelligence, with secret, intuitive, or premonitory things or with metaphysical truths. A winged horse and a shaman's steed and ascent and flight symbolize energy suddenly freed from its entrapment in a complex or in bondage to the imprisoning aspect of the Great Mother or nature itself: they also signify the birth of spirituality and the possibility of transcendence. Essentially, magical flight expresses both ecstasy and the soul's autonomy. Perhaps the image in Lascaux of the shaman who is bird-masked and entranced before the unconscious (depicted as a mortally wounded animal, the bird-pole fallen nearby) is one of the earliest graphic descriptions of this kind of experience. Entranced, their mind like the flight of the bird or feathered arrow, the shaman catapulted from an earthly state to meet directly the *mysterium tremendum* of the unknown. To be deemed a lord of magical flight meant that others also recognized the shaman's ability to enter a state of ecstatic ascension, to endure the experience, and to return safely to earth for another journey, at another time.

Notes

1 Eliade, Mircea: *The Sacred & The Profane: The Nature of Religion: The Significance of Religious Myth, Symbolism, and Ritual within Life and Culture*. Translated from the French by Willard R. Trask. New York: Harcourt Brace & World, Inc. 1959.
2 ibid. 33.
3 ibid. 37.
4 Eliade, Mircea: *Shamanism: Archaic Techniques of Ecstasy*. Translated from the French by Willard R. Trask. Bollingen Series LXXVI. New York: Bollingen Foundation. 1964. Pantheon Books.
5 ibid.
6 Davidson, H. R. Ellis: *Gods and Myths of Northern Europe*. Baltimore: Penguin Books, Inc. 1964. 145.

7 Funk and Wagnall: *Standard Dictionary of Folklore, Mythology and Legend*. Edited by Maria Leach. New York: Funk and Wagnall's. 1972. 193.
8 ibid. 96.
9 Nagel, Georges, 'The Mysteries of Osiris in Ancient Egypt,' in *The Mysteries*. Bollingen Series XXX. Volume 2. Princeton, NJ: Princeton University Press. 1968. 119, 126–127.
10 von Franz, Marie Louise: *The Problem of the Puer Aeternus*. New York: Spring Publications. 1970. 10–11.
11 Neumann, Erich: 'Mystical Man,' in *The Mysteries*. Bollingen Series XXX. Volume 2. Princeton, NJ: Princeton University Press. 1968. 384–385.
12 Corbin, Henri: *The Man of Light in Iranian Sufism*. Translated by N. Pearson. New Lebanon and New York: Omega Publications. 1994.
13 Funk and Wagnall's: op. cit. 915.
14 ibid. 33.
15 Neumann, Erich: *Amor and Psyche*. New York: Harper & Row. 1956. 105–106.
16 Jung, C. G.: *Integration of the Personality*. New York and Toronto: Farrer and Reinhart. 1939. 189.
17 Funk and Wagnall's: op. cit. 505.
18 ibid. 250.
19 von Franz, Marie Louise: *The Feminine in Fairytales*. New York: Spring Publications. 1972. 32.
20 Funk and Wagnall's: op. cit. 928.
21 von Franz, Marie Louise: *Creation Myths*. Zurich: Spring Publications. 1972. 21–22.
22 Funk and Wagnall's: op. cit. 100.
23 ibid. 505.
24 *Rumi: A Year With Rumi: Daily Readings*. Translated by Coleman Barks, with John Joyne, Nevit Ergan, A.J. Arberry, Reynold Nicolson, and others. February 16. New York: HarperOne. 2006. 62.
25 Ferguson, John. *Illustrated Encyclopedia*. 18.
26 Von Franz, Marie Louise: *The Feminine in Fairytales*. New York: Spring Publications. 1972. 133–134.

Chapter 4

Journey and the helping spirits

Accessing another world

As we have seen, the shaman's experience of vocational call involved an involuntary, initiatory journey into an underworld, or another world – a world 'beyond.' The shaman's odyssey penetrated what Erich Neumann calls the psyche's different reality planes, including archaic levels in which the psyche's symbol-forming powers originate, giving birth to, or complexing, undifferentiated energy from primordial levels of the psyche. These powers confronted the shaman with 'beings' or 'presences' – usually animals – one of whom would become a shaman's individual soul animal and helping spirit. The part-human, part-animal images of later cultures proceeded out of the same originative planes of reality: from these levels of the unconscious, culture and civilizations themselves originate, build, continue, and change over time. In many ways, it is the animal world that has made being human imaginable.

Generally speaking, the primary way we human beings seem to deal with all-encompassing chaos is to break it up, splitting it into two different elements or essences. Recorded experiences of archaic shamans are the earliest attempts we see of dividing the environment into visible matter (bodily, physical being) and invisible spirit (soul, spiritual being) in an attempt to achieve what amounted to overall orientation and spiritual efficacy. Here also we find a point of departure from our earliest speculations concerning voluntary abandonment of the body, the omnipotence of intelligence, and the immortality of the human soul. Archaic shamans attempted to make capital of the separation between body and soul and matter and spirit, whether they merely desired that separation or recognized it as a fait accompli.

Importantly, shamans do not create the cosmology, mythology, or theology of a group; shamans *internalize* it, thereby transforming cosmo-theological concepts into a concrete mystical experience and an experiential itinerary for a journey into personal ecstasy. Thus internalized, the tribe's cosmology, mythology, or theology became part of a shaman's personality. What for the rest of the community would remain a cosmological ideogram – the site of the center of the world, for example, identifiable 'out there' by a remarkable stone, a building, an altar, or a tree – became an internalized place of beginning for a shaman's inner journey.

Any manifestation of the sacred implies both a breakthrough in subjective experience and the opening of Neumann's reality planes of the objective psyche, never only one or the other. Black Elk, the visionary Oglala holy man, describing his mystical perception of the Hoop of the World spread out before him as he stood alone on the summit of Harney Peak, found these words for 'both/and' *and* for 'something more':

> Then I was standing on the highest mountain of them all, and round about beneath me was the whole hoop of the world and while I stood there *I saw more than I can tell* and *I understood more than I saw*, for I was seeing in a sacred manner *the shapes of things in the spirit*, and *the shape of all shapes* as they must live together like one being.
>
> (italics mine)[1]

In other words, as the spirit world opened Black Elk's perceptions, it simultaneously *opened itself to* him in a deeply subjective experience of multiple worlds. Similarly, Maria Sabina, a Mazatec shaman from Mesoamerica reports,

> There is *a world beyond ours*, a world that is *far away, nearby and invisible.* And there is where God lives, where the dead live, the spirits and the saints, a world where *everything has already happened and everything is known.* That world talks. It has a language of its own. I report what it says.
>
> (italics mine)[2]

Journey as story

Perhaps the shaman's soul journey interiorized an experience of humanity's deep memory of the travels and adventures of a mythical hero of long ago. Whether the world to which this journey was made was thought of as heaven or hell, or an extraterrestrial paradise or a mysterious land at the bottom of the sea, and whether it was accomplished by a ship's voyage to an island or by the scrambling ascent of a mountain, a quest was undertaken, sights were seen, and a safe return was stressed. The fact that the archaic shaman's story of a journey into an underworld or an upper world is the earliest story we know that claims to be experience based makes it relevant to us in terms of common humanity and our collective identity.

Today we imagine that such imagery relates to the psychological adventures of the unfolding personality. We suggest that a shamanic personality, 'chosen by the gods,' is someone who has been touched by archetypal experience. Out of a group's unconsciously evolving psychological development, shamanic personalities function as a kind of mouthpiece for individual and collective explorations, and although an archaic shaman certainly would have lacked what we call ego consciousness with which to reflect on their experience, a shaman's journey is our earliest recording of an ongoing, evolutionary thrust within the objective psyche toward individual consciousness. We understand that a successful response to a vocational summons by someone so 'chosen' displays an intensification of potential ego potency in the face of profound brokenness, when such a person feels completely at the mercy of overwhelming forces of nature or the gods. That shamanic person's 'initiation' and subsequent training then elaborates and strengthens a subjective sense of self, resulting in the acquisition of increased psychological strength. This strength continues to accrue as the shaman in training learns the lore of a profession and moves into practice, and much of this potency comes from the reintegration of the shaman's experience of another world. Unlike the hero's journey, the archaic shaman seems to have undertaken their journey in search of something crucial to their own future *and* the future of the tribe. It may be that all the shaman knew then was that a piece of themselves was missing, captured by the spirit world, but that was enough to make the shaman our first sojourner in quest of lost souls – initially their own and then the souls of others.

According to William Reed (1978), the phenomenon of journey proceeds out of four major ideas, attitudes, notions, and beliefs that go on to make up a kind of 'natural' spiritual tradition. Originally, individual shamans would have embodied and enacted this tradition, but the same ideas persist in many contemporary spiritual traditions today, where they form a kind of vital core consisting of four notions:

1 All true wisdom is found far from human beings out in great solitude and can be acquired only by suffering. Only privation and suffering open one's mind to that which is hidden from others.
2 One is not called by self-wish: one is chosen.
3 Taboos exist between nature (the goddess) and human beings: someone must mediate, and one who does so becomes a shaman.
4 The soul gives each living thing the particular appearance it has: the soul of a human being is a tiny human being (the homunculus, the child – remember how Jung's soul appears to him as a girl in *The Redbook*), the soul of a reindeer is a tiny deer, and so forth. All things have souls, and spiritual forces exist everywhere.

Like Reed's articulation of the early notion of shamanic initiation and power in Chapter 1,[3] this list indicates something of what an archaic shaman stood for, what they experienced individually, and what the idea of a shaman symbolized for a tribe. In the far past, the idea of what it meant to individualize oneself out of a collective group could be articulated in no other way: individual shamans 'came into being' to mediate individuality itself. If *someone* had to do it, the archaic shaman *became* it, 'it' meaning someone who embodies individual life.

Then as now, experiences that the archaic shaman had in trance states were expressed in images from the real world – images of trees and the earth, images of mountains that must be climbed and animals that must be confronted or befriended, images of the sky above and stones beneath – imagery that is similar the world over. Culture after culture speaks of journeys into the 'beyond' and/or a descent into psychic depths (journeys to the dead or an underworld) that pacify existential anxieties in a people, increasing collective certainty and confidence by turning chaos into cosmos. Procedurally developed images of a pilgrimage, a way, the Buddhist Eight-Fold Path, the *Via Contemplativa*, a pilgrim's progress, or the symbolic Quest for the Grail are cultural articulations rooted in the original experience of an archaic shaman. The common thread of otherworld journey accounts is *story* itself, and today we consider otherworld journeys as *works of narrative imagination*, conveyed in language that is shaped by universal laws of symbolic experience and the local and transitory mores of a given culture. In Siberia and among the Ainu of Japan, shamans were believed to have created writing,[4] and in more classic times, Mercury (like Odin) was believed to have discovered or created runic letters.[5]

Our earliest literary narratives of descent to the underworld include the story of Innana, the Sumerian goddess of fertility, the story of Demeter and Persephone, and the Mesopotamian tale of Gilgamesh, the legendary ruler of the city-state of Uruk, and his comrade Enkidu (Zaleski, 7). The story of Gilgamesh and Enkidu deserves special mention because it *does not* equate an experience of journey to another world (here, an underworld) with nascent ideas of death and rebirth or life after death and some form of salvation following a return. Over time, most stories speak of a return to this world and usually develop into early *morality* tales, interwoven with ideas about salvation, immortality, or everlasting life. But Gilgamesh fails in his bid for immortality: both Gilgamesh and Enkidu die, and the whole idea of journey ends. But the story of Gilgamesh is our earliest *mortality* play, and the shock of failure brings home to a psychologically informed listener today (as it unconsciously implied to ancient listeners around camp fires) the possibility of life's singularity and death's finality, including the terrifying possibility that initiatory death might not be survived. On the other hand, if initiatory death *were* survived, 'new life' that followed originated in an 'other' dimension of reality that was entirely different from the sense of an everyday world.

Now, following Jung, we call this 'other' dimension of non-ordinary reality the unconscious, and we understand that the unconscious seems to extend into the psychoidal depths of cosmos itself. We also understand that it *is* possible to 'die' in these depths and never return (psychosis), and we understand that *if* we return – like a successful shaman – any emerging 'new life' has little to do with ego effort and is more a matter of the 'grace of the gods.' New life that is experienced in such a vivid encounter with the reality of the psyche does restore meaning.

A personal example may illustrate what I'm trying to convey. In my early thirties, having suffered my way through the various calamities that led to the psychological 'breakdown-breakthrough' that I described in the Introduction, I indeed felt as if I had 'died' to my previous ego identity and that I no longer knew who I was. I felt as if the root of my being had been severed, and this feeling was so inchoate that I began a series of unconsciously destructive behaviors (such as walking numb and unseeing into Manhattan cross-street traffic) that came perilously close to endangering my life. As I began talking with someone, these unconscious behaviors ended. Around three years later, toward the end of my analytic work as I began my own clinical practice, the unconscious 'imaged' the kind of wound that could initiate such morbid suffering. My dream pictured an 'initiatory portal' into my new calling, and I subsequently named this portal The Dream of the Night Sky Woman (see Chapter 3).

> *I am working with a woman whom I see splayed out against the dark night sky, as if she were a constellation. She has a long scar from chin to pubis. She has been split from stem to stern by a falling star.*

This dream gave me a dramatic image for the cut I had felt 'to the root of my being' three years earlier after the birth of my son, but it also gave me a dramatic image for the chasm of self-doubt into which I had fallen – a chasm so deep that it stunned me in the moment and rendered me numb for at least three years. In the dream, the wound was clearly to a 'woman I am working with,' while just as clearly, this woman was myself. At the time of the dream, I understood it to mean that I needed to keep in mind (as I faced patient after patient from my analytic chair) that at bottom, meaning underneath it all, I was also working with my own personality. Then (at the time of the dream) the closest I came to actually 'feeling' the emotional contents of this dream with my analyst was to repeat in a puzzled, peculiar kind of way – once each hour over a period of about six months and usually as I was leaving his office – that I felt as if I couldn't stand up straight. I did stand up straight as I walked, but the sensation was something like that of having a ghost limb. What I felt emotionally was that I was doubled over in the middle as if to hide a gaping wound. I felt as if I had a terrible psychological cramp that covered a terrible void, a missing *something*.

Yes, my abdomen was crisscrossed with caesarian scars, but those were not the scars I felt: what I *meant* when I said, 'I feel as if I can't stand up straight' was something like, 'I feel as if I have been gutted, like a fish' or 'I feel as if something has been stolen, something is missing from my deep insides, from my inner being.' On one level, the Dream of the Night Sky Woman surely alluded to the embodied but deeply anesthetized physical experience of a badly bungled cesarean section three years earlier and the twelve days of lost time during which I had no contact with anyone, including my baby son. In psyche's language, I was alluding to something that I was trying to feel but could not put into words or conceptualize; in psyche's language, I was referring to a feeling I struggled to recover and experience consciously – a kind of psychic cramp, a cramp *in psyche*, a gap perhaps, a stretch, or some kind of breach in Being that I felt unable to reach across alone, and no one could breach it with me.

Now I imagine that gap as a gap in Being, a gap in time: a gap that also became a portal or a 'space' through which the deep imagination poured. This has always been so, and the shaman was the first to know it. Sometimes images visit from there, emerging, it seems, like creatures from the deep. Into that gap dreams flow, day and night, where they move like little boats between two shores, tracking the deeper currents that move beneath them. And from time to time, something like 'god' visits this space, sometimes greatly welcomed, sometimes greatly feared, and often both at once. In more everyday parlance, now this 'gap' has become soul space, or soul itself, about which I *may* think but about which much more often I feel. And these days – most of the time – I *can* stand up straight, and I've spent the following years occupying myself by filling in aspects of an emerging 'personhood,' even as I practice and write.

Usually we accept the position of stars in the sky something 'given,' and we create constellations by linking stars together and telling stories about what we see. In my dream, the constellated night sky woman's wound has healed and scarred over, but the fact that her wound was created by a falling star suggests that something fated – something profoundly impersonal, archetypal, ineluctable, and collective – occurred. The same occurrence – the woman taking her place as one among other 'fixed points' in a starry heaven – also suggests transpersonal dimensions of meaning that might slowly be acquired over the years it would take to work through an experience of such in-depth ego collapse. In any case, stories like my narrative of ego death and rebirth and others like it underscore the idea that a journey to another world might refer us to an utterly different realm of experience that is acquired within *this* world – an experience of *symbolic* death – and I understand this realization to be the seed of the completely new idea we have today about the symbolic dimension of human experience that has grown into our ideas about life in the unconscious and the reality of the psyche per se. Stories like my own, when understood symbolically, refer us to something we wrestle with in *this* life with *this*-life consequences rather than with life as it has been collectively envisioned, extending into a second ongoing realm resembling (for example) the Christian heaven, or life seen as a series of reincarnations, or life everlasting in an Islamic Garden of Paradise. Collective stories like these are analogous to early records of several nascent ideas that early humans created as they struggled with existential questions about life's impermanence and meaning and the finality of literal death.

Shamanic motifs of journey, dismemberment, transformation, and continuing life, as well as the presence of a storyteller or a singer of the journey, formed our legends in that the archaic shaman's journey between the sacred and the mundane was the primary bridge and battleground between two worlds. Images of journeying can range from the opening and closing of doors to boundaries crossed and barricades erected on the borders and frontiers of different countries; from expeditions to the tops of distant mountains to stories of sailing past the Clashing Rocks or *Symplegades*, as in the journey of Ulysses. Scholars have even traced back basic features of the Odyssey to the wanderings of the arctic shaman hero known among the Inuit as Koviok, who – like Ulysses – survived countless adventures, but unlike Ulysses, finally returned home to his parents. Like Koviok, however, Ulysses also journeyed to an underworld where shades were brought back to life by blood sacrifice.[6]

For an archaic tribe, the living connection between individuals and the 'ancestors' (levels of the psyche that carry tradition and memory) was necessary beyond question. Individually and at great personal cost, a shaman's initiatory journey could effectively restore a primordial, mythical time when communication between sky and earth was easier. To the world to which the shaman returned and within which they felt themselves recovered, the shaman re-presented experience of an archaic *state of being* – a condition of humanity at the dawn of time. Like all shamans, they gained intimacy with natural forces that would replenish the psyche, thereby reinvigorating and restoring all that was blocked by difficult life experience. Ecstatically returning again and again, they could mediate whatever communication was innately possible between heaven and earth, mind and body, and above and below. Thus, over time, the archaic shaman's image slowly evolved to symbolize the following burgeoning possibility: individual human beings can consciously relate to collectively unconscious mind.

Gifts lost and recovered

If a shaman lost their gift for frequenting the underworld and became incapable of making contact with the spirits, sometimes her poetic gift for creating songs, dances, and images might simply vanish, as if a shaman simply ran dry. But so important to the tribe was the shaman's connection to the 'other world' that if it broke – if the shaman 'failed,' say – sometimes the link was sought again *by the tribe* and regained. In a fascinating account of this kind of turnabout, Andreas Lommel[7] tells us that once the men of an Inuit tribe gathered to mediate for their shaman in hopes of reestablishing a link with their dead forefathers. People of the tribe rubbed the shaman and sang over him until he became entranced, freeing his soul to wander about until it found the ancestral spirits. Meanwhile, the spirits, wishing to reestablish relations with the living and missing the shaman as he missed them, also looked for the shaman. When the two met, the soul of the shaman told the ancestor spirit (often his father or grandfather) that he had lost his way to the underworld and couldn't find any more songs. Helpful spirits promised to send for him soon and the shaman emerged from trance. Days later, the shaman heard the 'call' and went back into trance for a week. Spirits came, tore his soul to pieces, put it together again in the underworld, showed him dances, and sang him songs. This time when the shaman returned, he could function again. That on occasion a tribe would serve as the shaman's bridge to restore an individual link to the 'other world' underscores the unique, dynamic reciprocity that inheres (even if seldom articulated) in shamanic individual-and-group interrelatedness.

Helping spirits

Sometimes shamanic journeys are made in the company of or on the backs of special animals. The image and story of white-winged Pegasus, steed of poets and a vehicle for flights of inspiration, resonates with these aspects. Or winged or unusual horses like Odin's eight-legged Sleipnir might be visualized as the mount of the shaman's soul as it set out on a journey to heaven. Odin, riding on Sleipnir like a shaman, discovered the secret of travel between the worlds. The !Kung Bushmen of the Kalahari say that

> God is the power that made people . . . like a person, with a person's body and covered with beautiful clothes. He has a horse on which he puts people who are just learning to trance and becoming healers. God will have the person in trance ride to where he is, so God can see the new healer and talk to him.[8]

(The !Kung phrase for 'dreams' literally means 'a gathering up of the spirits.')[9]

Today we interpret Odin on Sleipnir as a psychic expression of the idea of human and subordinated animal instinct, like Agni riding a ram, or Christ riding an ass into Jerusalem, or Mithras riding the bull. In a recent movie, *Avatar*, the protagonist undergoes a life-and-death struggle to master his own flying dragon, who then grants him the power to journey anywhere. An important purpose of a shaman's journey has always been to contact (among a throng of summoning spirits) a kind of 'animal mother' or origin animal, meaning one individual helping spirit that was independent of the shaman. In part, this helping animal would then be thought by the tribe to embody the shaman's visionary power or prophetic gift, extending into or penetrating both past and future.

Often an animal spirit appeared in a particular form into which a shaman might learn to transform himself. In other words, once a spirit had intruded into the shaman's world, it had to be completely embraced. Bears, wolves, stags, and all kinds of birds and snakes – *any* form of life – might become a helpful animal companion, and an archaic shaman often had more than one. An animal spirit functioned as a shaman's alter ego, like a new or second identity (twin?) or a double. The simple presence of an animal held to be a shaman's soul companion indicated a direct connection with the beyond and the world of nature, so much so that if a shaman's animal died, the shaman might die too.

In a wonderful study of the image of the bear in nature, myth, and literature, Paul Shepard and Barry Sanders ask, 'Is the bear simply a large hulk upon which the infantile mind projects the human figure, and are we to accept the myth of the Bear Mother as the simple confusion of personal ontogeny with human history?' Citing Carl Jung's answer, Shepard and Sanders return us to our bodies as the context of mind: no, says Jung. 'Each night in sleep we hibernate a little: our breathing and temperature are modified; ingestion and elimination are forgotten. The bear,' Jung says, 'is at the center of this excursion toward death's second self' (i.e., sleep).[10]

Shepard and Sanders also see the bear as 'feminine,' which suggests that a feminine principle of birth, growth, death, decay, and rebirth lies at the heart of veneration of the bear: 'the bear is the supreme model – and therefore the guiding spirit – of the theme of renewal.'[11] For an archaic shaman, friendship with animals and an ability to transform oneself into an animal indicated the successful integration of an initial shamanic call. Connection with an animal spirit not only caused initiation in the first place but – following transformation – became a goal of initiation as well.

All over the world, archeological records teem with hybrid images of human-animal combinations. Images of spirits etched into the walls of the great temples of India and ancient Egypt represent human beings with heads of jackals and elephants or birds and baboons. Outside the Great Pyramid rests the Sphinx. We know about mermaids, angels, centaurs, and satyrs, even if we've never seen them. Pictures of fabulous creatures reside in bestiaries and bibles, as well as in our dreams. Perhaps the oldest of all figurative images, the famous statue of a lion-headed man (see Warren Coleman's[12] extended meditation on this image) dates back forty thousand years to Aurignacian times, but a preoccupation with animals is not only Paleolithic. Intimate contact with animals also affects us today. Apparently, animal metaphor is one of the most important ways we've come up with for communicating beyond the essential privacy of individual subjective experience. How would we offer anything of our subjective selves without making metaphors? Not only is our anthropological literature on religion and folklore full of shapeshifting animal images and creature possessions, but vampires, monsters, Septapods, and flying dragons show up in films and literature, prowling the popular imagination every day: witness such current movies as *A Monster Calls*, *Avatar*, or *Arrival*, or read Philip Pullman's *His Dark Materials*, imaginatively providing us with armored bears and picturing each of us with an animal demon with whom we have been born, from whom we dare not separate.

In my own situation, I had dreams of animals to which I had to relate in some form or other. In an early dream, I placed my left hand on the head of a wild lioness; in a later dream, I was instructed to keep my distance from a caged, grieving mother bear. But no individual creature made itself known to me as an ally, and I did very little active imagination with animals. I presume that reconciliation with my animal self has taken place mostly in the unconscious through various forms of bodywork, like dance, yoga, and Pilates. However, I've always followed animal images in my dreams closely, and here's a dream of recent vintage wherein animal energies form a kind of living, holographic mandala in which I participate by moving in and out of palpable but invisible energy streams. This dream happened after I hauled my old shaman thesis manuscript out of the closet and began to imagine a rewrite:

> *I am entering and moving within living, invisible energy streams (like holographs) of three of four animal beings – upper left a dolphin, upper right a giraffe, lower right a snake, and lower left a lion and/or an eagle? Mostly I seem to be moving in and out of an invisible 'shadow' of the snake, which rises up, much taller than I am – in fact, Enormous. Dancing with snake-energy feels remarkable. I move in and out of other different streams of energy that are also made visible in palpable, feelable forms.*
>
> *Then the dream shifts, and I'm climbing down a ladder, a step or two from the ground. Next to me on her ladder, perhaps two steps higher than I, is a woman in a beautiful rose-madder-colored gown. She looks across to me and*

tells me that I should be studying the collective unconscious, but I reply that I thought I had come to work on something else (consciousness?).

In rewriting this book, I have in fact moved from an amplificatory, collective, associative form to a much more personal account of encountering the shaman, grounded in my story and my dream material. Perhaps it is significant that all the animals in this quadrated structure are able to move with ease through at least two elements, or two worlds: the giraffe lives both on earth but stretches to the sky, the dolphin lives both underwater and breathes the air, the snake is at home both on the earth and under it, and the lion/eagle live on land and in or beneath the sky. In the dream, both conscious and unconscious points of view are represented both verbally and through animal metaphor, the two points of view that thread throughout these pages. And to conclude this chapter, I am going to amplify two specific animals: each in its own way is crucial to the phenomenology of shamanism, and each in its own way has played a part in my story.

Bear

Probably a shamanic genealogy could be written for all the animals that were familiar to ancient peoples, but the bear seems appropriate to trace here in detail not only because of Sedna the Sea-Bear – she whom the arctic shaman learns to propitiate – but because the bear has always seemed to symbolize a kind of tutelary 'bestower' of the curing power of medicine. Above all other animals, the bear is thought to be the supreme physician of the woods, bringing insight and healing out of darkness. Ceremonially buried skulls of cave bears have been found in caves in the high Alps that date from the time of the Neanderthals, while other sacrificial offerings of the head, skull, and (other) bones of bears indicate the continuation of a bear cult that existed right up to the Upper Paleolithic period. Apparently, a bear cult also existed in the North, persisting in the circumpolar cultures of Europe and Asia from the Lapps and Inuit across to the Ainu of the northern-most island of Japan.[13] The Ainu and the Gilyaks of Siberia practiced a bear cult of their own as late as the beginnings of the twentieth century.

Shamans of several Indigenous Peoples in what is now called California impersonated bears or were thought to be transformed into bears, because the bear was the powerful spirit helper from whom vision seekers obtained their supernatural powers.[14] Patron of Keresan, Tewan, Sioux, and Zuni Curing Societies, the bear was paramount in other places in North America too, as the Sioux considered the bear to be the patron of wisdom, medicine, and magic. During a bear dance performed for curative purposes, shamans impersonating and 'calling' the bear were believed to transform into bears, and benevolence from an animal so ill-tempered took on a particularly powerful significance.[15]

In essence, a shaman's garment – though not always a literal bearskin – was also an animal disguise. Thought by some to be the oldest portrayal of a shaman we have, the sorcerer of the Trois Freres Caves of Lascaux in Southern France shows us a human figure fully disguised as an animal. The engraving pictures a shaman wearing antlers and who has a startled look. One can see through the animal 'mask' to his human surprise, so perhaps this is also our first portrait of the 'human.' Entered by spirit, this shaman would have behaved outwardly like the animal he inwardly 'portrayed,' thereby establishing a link with the spirit world and the collective unconscious. Like wearing antlers of a deer, putting on the bearskin implied going so deeply into one's animal nature as to be taken over completely, thereby finding a source of new energy and a way to rebirth.

In both Greek and Latin, the bear was considered feminine, and ancient religions emphasized the bear's positive, motherly qualities, particularly the ethical side of maternity, or motherly concern and care. Extraordinarily meticulous with her cubs, a mother bear could be more attentive and self-sacrificing than human mothers. Pythagoras called the she-bear 'the hands of the goddess Rhea,' referring to the formative skill of mother nature who – like a mother bear – leads undeveloped, imperfect form to beauty and perfection.[16] Callisto, the companion of Artemis, turns into a bear, lifted into the sky as Ursa Major by Zeus to save her from being hunted down, and Virgil uses the image of the bear when he refers to spiritual birth, where attitudes of devotion, perseverance and self-sacrifice are foremost.

For us, conjoined human/animal images remind us that we live in life-long tension between what we think of as our humanity and our animal nature. The animal in us holds us to what is present, to *who we are* at the moment, not to who we have been, who we might become, or how our ways of living – our social distinctions – might describe us. The tough challenge to modern people – to embody full, individual personhood – means to learn to pay attention to one's own animal nature and bodily context of mind, without which we cannot and do not function. To live close to the animal self means to pay attention to one's own particular individual body with its particular sexuality; its individual, concrete, and personal life; its individual and personal history; and its individual and personal death. Long identified with spiritual well-being and physical health and healing, the bear has become an animal of beginnings and re-beginnings, too, worthily symbolic of recovery from spiritual and physical illness and revival from death.

According to Sy Montgomery,[17] author of *The Soul of an Octopus: A Surprising Exploration into the Wonder of Consciousness*, many Native American peoples say that the bear taught them how to use native herbs and plants as medicines. Montgomery adds that an Alaskan hunting guide watched, puzzled, as a grizzly methodically stripped the bark from a willow shrub, which bears don't normally eat. After shooting the bear, the guide noticed that the bear had an abscessed tooth, around which was packed willow bark, the source of salicylic acid and the active ingredient in aspirin (19). Montgomery also notes that while in a Native American tradition, the bear may be said to have taught the tribe how to use medicinal herbs, in some Far-East Asian traditions, the bear *is* the medicine: bear blood is believed to cure nervousness in children, and the bones are said to treat rheumatism.

Furthermore, bear fat is prescribed to cure baldness, remove pimples, treat colds, darken hair, sharpen wits, and prevent hunger. Eating a bear paw is said to ward off colds, cure beriberi, and generally revitalize the body, especially the hands, while the gallbladder is the part most prized (29).

Jackal

We can understand the jackal as embodying a transformative process of death and rebirth that is remarkably similar to the shaman's dismemberment and return. Like the shaman, the Egyptian jackal-headed god Anubis figured as psycho-pomp and a leader of souls through the realms of the Egyptian underworld. Like Wotan, Anubis was thought to be the god of the dead, because like Wotan's Bears and Wolves (named Ravener and Greed), Anubis digested the slain. According to one account, after Set overthrew Osiris, Thoth and Anubis remained faithful to Isis, and while Set occupied the throne, Anubis swallowed Osiris, holding and protecting him until Isis could reassemble him.[18] This made Anubis an avatar between the worlds. The Greeks identified Anubis with Hermes, their major mediator between the realms of the gods and humankind.[19]

Robert Lawler and Deborah Lawler discuss how the Egyptians might have seen the jackal: tearing the flesh of its prey into pieces, a jackal buries them, and does not eat them until they rot. As a symbolic incarnation of certain characteristics, functions, and processes of nature, a jackal-headed god represents a vital function that is incarnated in a particular animal. Whether Egyptians saw the jackal symbolically or not, the image of the jackal emerges as a symbol out of the psyche's collectively accumulated experience of observed behavior; after all, swallowing and taking in the dead is a process that is both physical and psychological, one of several universal processes that are undergone by all forms born into nature. Other processes such as growth, assimilation, coagulation, decomposition, and transformation are well-known to alchemy. Like a shaman, Anubis led the souls of the deceased into the first stages of the lower realms of the World of Transformation. We can understand the image of Anubis as a symbol of discriminating judgment that occurred in the early stages of the Egyptian death-rebirth process, because while the jackal is eating, he performs a precise, innate process of discrimination, separating out elements capable of transformation from elements that are untransmutable (Lawler, 14).

Our analytic minds can be jackal-like in function. Just as digestion can be understood as a destructive process, the process of psychoanalysis – sometimes imagined as 'learning to metabolize unconscious experience' – can feel destructive too. Essentially, a process of digestion breaks down forms into their constituent elements; just so, the psychoanalytic process breaks down or reduces unconscious material or behavioral patterns into constituent elements that are interpretable as part of personal history. Not only can reductive psychoanalysis *feel* destructive as it analyzes symbols and behavior into more elementary forms, but it can also *be* destructive and feel as if it is decomposing life itself, especially when we are seeking greater integration and coherence. Here it can help to remember that the analytic procedure is happening under the auspices of a presiding 'god,' like the jackal. Jung was clear that within the overall process, psycho-synthesis must follow the reductive process of psychoanalysis. Within the jackal's domain, digestion and disintegration are early aspects of a two-stage process that leads to new integration, including a return. One hopes that one's analysis does the same.

When the archaic shaman returned from their dismembered state, they brought soul with them, wrestled out of the land of the dead from among the broken shards of a fragmented self. Just so, the shamanic process serves the soul. As Edward Edinger reminds us,[20] the word 'psychotherapy' is a product of two root words: *psyche*, which means soul or life spirit, and *therapeuein*, which originally meant 'to tend or render service to the gods in their temples.' The etymology implies that service to the soul and service to psyche are not just secular affairs that minister to the analytic mind. Service to soul and service to psyche have transpersonal dimensions: rebirth into new life results in life newly ensouled. Gold has begun to rim the broken places.

Just as Lord Jackal Anubis determines the time of death and decomposition, he determines the time of transformation and rebirth too. If a shaman had the jackal as an ally, they could be assumed to have firsthand knowledge of the depths of death and rebirth from the inside out, because ultimately, the shaman was one who had contact with spirit wherever spirit was to be found. Then as now (and, importantly, in psychotherapy), shamanic mediation may be necessary before real intimacy with all that is animal in us returns. Indeed, an archaic shaman may have journeyed far and wide, but with the help of their animal spirit, the end of the journey always brought them home.

Reflections on the animal and the World Soul

The last two hundred years of patriarchal dominance and what Jerome Bernstein calls the hegemony of the Western ego led to the slaughter of millions upon millions of animals and contributed to the tragic extinction of species after species at a bewildering rate. A patriarchal attitude simply tends to subjugate the animal to being a 'lesser' creature over which humans dominate. Correspondingly, and unfortunately, the field of psychoanalysis tends to understand 'the animal' in us similarly, as instinct to be subordinated to human ego desire and intention. Freud's famous dictum 'where it was, there ego shall be' is emblematic of a one-sided dominance of human over animal nature, but hopefully this will change as it begins to dawn on us that we are simply one animal species among many. The fact that animals are what they are, and nothing other, makes them excellent representatives of a mysterious ground of being with an attendant wisdom and a sense of permanence that underlies change, that undergirds the human psyche. For us, animal images represent the archetypal basis of an instinctive life, a life that symbolizes an essential integrity of instinct within the entirety of the self.

In Jung's later years, he tried to balance the one-sidedness of his own patriarchal attitude. Reminding us of age-old unconscious wisdom stored up in animal nature, Jung points out that when we let intellect take too big a place, intellect itself makes 'darkness.'[21] He even goes on to say,

> Consciousness discriminates, judges, analyzes, and emphasizes the contradictions. It's necessary work up to a point. But analysis kills, and synthesis brings to life. We must find out how to get everything back into connection with everything else. We must resist the vice of intellectualism, and get it understood that we *cannot only understand.*
>
> (italics mine)[22]

The shaman's sense of kinship with animal nature and capacity for linking spirit and matter helps us hold the necessary tension between comprehending Jung's two 'understandings,' the first meaning taking in and acceptance, and the second meaning embracing a realization that understanding goes only so far. Underlying wisdom and the instinctively deep integrity of every animal that inhabits it is imperiled in this warming world.

Carl Safina gives a wonderful portrait of interspecies communication at levels of being that we can barely imagine, let alone understand. In his latest book, *Beyond Words: What Animals Think and Feel* (2015), Safina quotes a moving and compassionate description, told to him by Lyall Watson, about an extraordinarily poignant encounter that Watson had as he watched a whale on the seacoast of South Africa. Even when the whale submerged, Watson tells us, he continued to feel the air reverberate in a strange rhythm that seemed to come from behind him now – from the land itself. Then, as Watson looked across a gorge, he saw standing in the shade of a tree a female elephant whom he recognized (from a broken tusk), an elephant who was not only a matriarch but the last of her Knysna tribe. It occurred to Watson that she must have come to the edge of the ocean to hear the under-rumble of the surf, the nearest and most powerful source of infrasound, because she was lonely and no longer had kin to talk to in the forest. Watson imagined that the sound of the surf would comfort her, accustomed as she was to being surrounded by the life sounds of her herd. Then suddenly, Watson felt the throbbing back in the air. He realized, to his astonishment, that the blue whale had surfaced again, pointing inshore, with blowhole clearly visible, and that the matriarch was there for the whale! In his own words, Watson says,

> The largest animal in the ocean and the largest living land animal were no more than a hundred yards apart, and I was convinced that they were communicating! In infrasound, in concert, sharing big brains and long lives, understanding the pain of high investment in a few precious offspring, aware of the importance and the pleasure of complex sociality, these rare and lovely great ladies were commiserating over the back fence of this rocky Cape shore, woman to woman, matriarch to matriarch, almost the

> last of their kind. . . . I turned, blinking away tears, and left them to it. This was no place for a mere man.
>
> (96)[23]

Watson's capacity to feel the heartache and tears in this story helps connect us with our common animal heritage: what alchemists thought of as the anima mundi and what Carl Jung thought of as the World Soul. It is an animal soul in us that best communicates within our own species, and it communicates between species too. The animal soul interconnects our life in an inner world and the life of the world itself, and these are the levels of interconnection on which the shaman operates. Watson's recognition that 'this was no place for a mere man' underscores his own animal sensitivity. After all, animals, as Henry Beston reminds us,

> shall not be measured by man. In a world older and more complete than ours, they move finished and complete, gifted with the extension of the senses we have lost or never attained. They are not brethren, they are not underlings: they are other nations, caught with ourselves in the net of life and time, fellow prisoners of the splendor and travail of the earth.
>
> (2003)

Notes

1 Neihardt, John G. (Flaming Rainbow): *Black Elk Speaks: Being the Life Story of a Holy Man of the Oglala Sioux*. Lincoln: University of Nebraska Press. 1961. 43.
2 Halifax, Joan. *Shamanic Voices: A Survey of Visionary Narratives*. New York: E. P. Dutton. 1979. 130.
3 Reed, William: 'Shamanist Principles of Initiation and Power,' in *The Shaman from Elko*. San Francisco: C. G. Jung Institute of San Francisco. 1978. 47.
4 Eliot, Alexander: *Myths*. Maidenhead, England: McGraw-Hill Book Co., Ltd. 1976. 122.
5 Davidson, H. R. Ellis: *Gods and Myths of Northern Europe*. Baltimore: Penguin Books, Inc. 1964. 141.
6 Lommel, Andreas: *The World of the Early Hunters*. Translated by Michael Bullock. London, England: Evelyn, Adams and Mackay, Ltd. 1967. 43.
7 ibid. 139.
8 Shostak, Marjorie: Nisa: *The Life and Words of a !Kung Woman*. Cambridge, MA: Harvard University Press. 1971. 300.
9 ibid. 327n.
10 Shepard, Paul, and Barry Sanders: *The Sacred Paw*: *The Bear in Nature, Myth and Literature*. New York: Viking Press. 1985. 70.
11 ibid. 106.
12 Coleman, Warren: *From Act to Image: The Emergence of Symbolic Imagination*. New Orleans, Louisiana: Spring Journal, Inc. 2016.
13 ibid. 188.
14 Funk and Wagnall's: *Standard Dictionary of Folklore, Mythology and Legend*. Edited by Maria Leach. New York: Funk and Wagnall's. 1972. 124.
15 ibid. 126–127.
16 Zeller, Max: 'The Way of the Bear,' in *The Dream – The Vision of the Night*. Edited by Janet Dallett. Los Angeles: The Analytical Psychology Club of Los Angeles and the C. G. Jung Institute of Los Angeles. 1975. 107–126.

17 Montgomery, Sy: *The Search for the Golden Moon Bear*. White River Junction, VT: Chelsea Green Publishing. 2002. 19.
18 Nagel, George, 'The 'Mysteries' of Osiris in Ancient Egypt,' in *The Mysteries*. Bollingen Series XXX. Volume 2. Princeton, NJ: Princeton University Press. 1968. 120.
19 Schwaller de Lubicz, R. A.: *Symbol and the Symbolic*. Translated by Robert and Deborah Lawler. Brookline: Autumn Press. 1978. 66.
20 Edinger, Edward: 'The Vocation of Depth Psychotherapy,' in *Science of the Soul: A Jungian Perspective*. Edited by D. Sharp and J.G. Sparks. 2002, Toronto: Inner City Books. 2002. 83.
21 Jung, C. G.: 'The 2,000,000-Year-Old-Man,' in *C. G. Jung Speaking: Interviews and Encounters*. Edited by William McGuire and R. F. C. Hull. Princeton, NJ: Princeton University Press. 1977. 89: also 'On the Frontiers of Knowledge,' 420.
22 ibid. 420.
23 Safina, Carl: *Beyond Words: What Animals Think and Feel*. New York: Henry Holt and Company. 2015. 95–96.

Chapter 5

The shaman and solitude

The shaman and religious solitude

William James defined religion in his 1902 Guifford Lectures in Scotland as the feelings, acts, and experiences of individuals in their solitude, insofar as they apprehend themselves standing in relation to whatever they consider divine. The philosopher Alfred North Whitehead added to James's definition by stating that religion is what an individual *does* with their solitariness: therefore, if one is never solitary, one is never 'religious.' In this chapter, I reflect on a particular *quality of solitude* that I imagine the archaic shaman was the first to undergo in discovering a spirit world. Today, we experience that quality of solitude as we discover an inner world. All of the shaman's gifts and talents lay in their discovery of this kind of solitude, and so do ours.

Separated by definition, within a tribe the shaman was marked by an earlier experience that set them apart. In early tribal societies, separation from the tribe usually implied exile, abandonment, and sometimes literal death. But the archaic shaman was different. They actually sought solitude and retained a functional tribal membership, mediating to others the tribe's unconscious mind. Bridging a second world, a spirit world, with the world of everyday life was the early shaman's solitary form of being religious. Unconscious forces had formed and conditioned their sensibility over time, as if the psyche's thrust toward individuality had been shaped by an electric current to conduct that very current, like a lightning strike making its own path. Thus, the historical shaman's existential situation gives us a phenomenological map for current ideas about individuality that require psychological differentiation of an individual from the group, and it also underlies Jung's idea of the ongoing process of individuation.

The *symbol* of the shaman eloquently expresses a subjective experience, in solitude, of a *peculiar quality of wholeness* into which any of us can stumble. There can be a rare felicity of aloneness and its deep insights. Usually, creative ideas come to an individual when alone, and most works of art are developed in a sharp awareness of solitude. But we can grow into 'strange shapes' if we are too much alone.

All of us are subject to crises, illness, and accidents, and the realities of life and death also open us to such experiences of solitude. Here's an example of an isolated insight I had as an early adolescent when I overheard my aunt Lucy tell someone else about a dream. My grandfather, slowly diminishing from Parkinson's disease and old age and to the growing distress of his children, had taken to bed in a silent confinement that went on for many years. One day, I heard Lucy, his daughter, lament (as did others, I'm sure), 'Why can't Papa just die? Why does this have to go on and on?' That night, Lucy dreamed as follows, and the next day I overheard her tell her dream:

> *I am shown a large, beautifully colored, woven carpet, much like those that furnished Amistad (her early home), but this carpet has a long thread lying loose at the very top. A voice said, 'the pattern of your father's life is not yet complete.'*

Overhearing Lucy's dream was an early moment of soul for me, a kindness of the psyche, as if her dream 'shamaned' me too: Lucy's dream felt relevant to a whole situation, so that I understood something not easily apparent: why my very ill grandfather was still alive. Perhaps, I wondered, even my grandfather felt eased by his daughter's dream, his unapproachable solitude contained in a dreamscape that was larger than both of them. I also – a wide-eyed, silently listening adolescent who hadn't spoken with her grandfather for a long time – felt the sense of wholeness that Lucy's dream portrayed. I caught an intuitive glimpse of how life can complete itself with meaning beyond our understanding. Each of the three of us were somehow united in our solitudes by Lucy's telling of her dream. I give this small example to show how from time to time, memory itself shamans us, as if in these pages, personal memories and I together scry patterns of soul larger than I alone can see.

Lonely in his own time, Carl Jung suggested that simply *attaining consciousness of the present* makes each of us into a solitary being: every step we take toward fuller consciousness removes us further from the 'maternal womb of unconsciousness in which the mass of men dwell' (CW10:150). Later, having become fully conscious of the depth of his solitude, Jung also suggested that we need to become decently unconscious again in order to rejoin the human race, but the point I want to make here is that from a psychological point of view, contemporary individuality and personhood are forged out of both departure from unconsciousness and return.[1] Furthermore, this pattern echoes and reverberates with a shaman's classically vertical pattern of journey from the heights of the World Tree to the depths of the Underworld and home again, mediating their soul's return to human embodiment.

As our understanding of the mind-body synthesis has become more finely tuned, we no longer imagine the human brain as an intricate but ultimately simplifyable mass of electronic circuitry governed by wiring diagrams. Now we presume that our brains fundamentally consist of endocrine tissue in which the essential reactions and the internal traffic of nerve impulses are determined by biochemical activators and their suppressors. If we align our current understanding of the human brain alongside the paradigm of the shaman's initiatory experience, what I have referred to as a 'shaman instinct' may appear in modern individuals as a kind of 'shamanic quotient' that is probably chemically determined. As if a genetically determined quality of individuality were an elemental aspect of the warp and woof of personality, DNA may blueprint a tendency toward shamanic solitude into an entire personality. If this is so, the archetypally shamanic quality of individuality can never be reduced to, or simply explained away by, understanding early developmental experience, traumatic or otherwise.

In keeping with collective wisdom, we generally assume even today that artistic talent is innately unique. In the last century, in fact, an artistic personality was thought to have been 'elected.' Most of us feel that artists are born, not made, at least to some degree, and most of us think that the development of creative talent consists of more than matters of environmental resources and training. Artists themselves usually imagine themselves 'alone.' For example, poet and critic Paul Zweig (who died in 1984) imagined himself a solitary figure sealed inside a transparent globe, floating serenely above a world painted by Hieronymus Bosh: this figure, says Zweig in his memoir, 'possesses everything and also nothing. He has been offered a key to the myth, but the vehicle of his vision is also his prison' (Zweig, 1976). Paul Elouard expressed his solitude as the discovery of 'another world' *in this one*, and acknowledging the intimate connection between solitude and brokenness, Yeats's Crazy Jane sings that 'nothing can be sole or whole, till it has been rent.'

Zweig's, Elouard's, and Yeats's respective poetic visions intimate the experience of shamanic solitude that underlies the subjective *quality of wholeness* that one discovers along the path as psyche leads the wanderer toward an experience of what Jung meant by the alchemical image of the orphan. In the orphan experience, brokenness and wholeness interfold: the 'neglected' or 'exiled' one is the one to whom angels reveal themselves and animals speak. And when stripped of the shelter of previously unconscious identifications, Jung's image of the orphan opens into Erich Neumann's image of *Homo religiosus*, 'sole and whole,' poised on the brink of previously unimaginable self-discovery: solitude and brokenness, solitude and wholeness, echoing broken pots and mending gold.

In a class I attended in Zurich, Marie-Louise von Franz told us of a young boy who was sent to live with relatives because he was acting strangely. Upon arrival, the child climbed high into a large tree where he stayed alone for several days, and when he finally came down, he acted normally and was sane again. Marie-Louise von Franz commented that the child must have 'reached into a collective archetypal pool' to find a healing pattern of energy and behavior. Seen through the lens of the shaman complex, this boy's pattern of behavior resembles a shaman's journey up and down the World Tree. We could say that his solitary tree experience enabled him to rebalance his world. Perhaps he felt as another young man felt, more recently caught building tree houses in Central Park, New York, who said of his work, ‘I like to be in trees. I like to be up, away from everything. I like the solitude.’

Living with activated archetypes: a solitary pursuit

Jung once said, ‘Whenever an archetype appears things become critical, and it is impossible to foresee what turn they will take. As a rule, this depends on the way consciousness reacts to the situation’ (CW10:461). The shaman archetype is no exception, and clearly there are different ways to live it out. One way is to live ‘with’ the archetype, immersed in shamanic patterns of energy and behavior, like the boy and the young man above, solitary in their respective trees, but without awareness of what they were enacting. Both moved beyond a temporary seizure by the archetype when it had served its purpose. Another, often taken by those who call themselves shamans today, is to identify with the archetype and find a lifestyle and source of meaning in its imagery and ways. A third way is to actively cultivate the archetype as one spirit among many in hopes of learning as much from it as possible without making it life defining. This third way entails a quality of consciousness that this book hopes to cultivate in its readers.

All of us both suffer and benefit from the archetypal forces that flow through our personal lives, and if we try to repress these forces, they can become dangerous. A repressed shaman instinct can become autonomous and crazy in someone who is hallucinating its imagery and tormented by its energies. An instinct to mediate turns back on itself if it has no one to mediate to and no context in which to mediate (Moore, 170–171). Black Elk shared his big dreams with his people so that he would *not* become ill. Similarly, many artistic personalities feel that they *must* do the work to which they feel called; otherwise, they will die.

Artists, mystics and poets are free to share dreams and creative expressions with the social and cultural worlds in which they live, and this somewhat ameliorates their isolation. But psychotherapists have the additional task of receiving and being affected by such creative energies without immediately discharging them into the cultural milieu. The reason for this is to protect a therapeutic vessel of transformation, which requires extensive training and maintaining shamanic solitude. The shape and calling of their profession determine that therapists work within proximity to the shaman complex most of their days, finding ways to let shamanic energies and images pass through their lives without personally identifying with them. In Jung’s personal plunge into the unconscious, he acknowledged archetypal energies but tried not to identify with them, and we therapists must follow suit: on the one hand, we struggle to bring shamanic energies into consciousness because they form and inform our work, and on the other hand, we differentiate and cultivate our personal lives so that the energies of the shaman complex ‘use’ us and pass through us, forming and informing the psyche before they recede. There’s an ‘art of living’ to this two-handed awareness, an art of letting things happen in the psyche that Jung named an *art of the psyche* (italics mine), about which most of us know very little (CW13:20).

The collective desire to appear chic these days by appearing to be a creative person is seldom accompanied by any comprehension of how staggering it is to have been dealt a shamanic hand in life. When the idea of being an artist is idealized, it is usually with no comprehension of either the solitary burden of such a fate or the inevitable cost that this fate implies for one's chance of having a personal life. In modern imaginative and psychological literature, writings about the archaic shaman abound. Books on shamanic voices and visions appear, and weekend workshops advertise how to be a shaman, while sophisticated museums exhibit vast arrays of shamanic art and artifacts. Gurus and guides call themselves 'shamans' the world over, so clearly does the shaman's image fascinate us. All this is to say that raw shamaning proliferates in varying degrees of literal enactment everywhere I look, but rarely do I see the psychological significance of such enactment discerned.

Beyond this contemporary fascination with all things shamanic may lie a collective impulse that urges us into differentiating what the image of the archaic shaman symbolizes. In this chapter, I describe that urge rising in recognition of a *quality of psychological solitude*. Because the core, felt meaning of the instinct to shaman in an individual is to differentiate from a group, the deeper meaning of the complex seems to be a collectively instinctive (spiritual) call toward the psychological integrity, or the wholeness, of shamanic solitude. I say this because without psychological understanding, being overtaken by the shaman complex means to undergo a literal enactment of separation, alienation, and exile, and many artists allude to such an experience. 'In every single story I write,' says Canadian storyteller Sharyn MacCrumb, 'there is someone who feels like a stranger.' Stan Dragland, the Newfoundland writer, titled his ongoing series of essays *Strangers & Others: Newfoundland Essays*, and a third friend, painter Frank Lapointe, described how he treks alone through island landscapes every winter to find inner and outer inspiration for his gorgeous, weatherly watercolors. 'Do you ever take a friend along?' I ask. 'No,' Frank replies, 'I'd be too concerned about how that other person is feeling.' An excerpt from Frank's diary reads, 'This metamorphosis of nature into imagery will meet me everywhere I turn, just like the vision that always appears from the edge of somewhere, just when I think I am alone.' In other words, Frank needs his solitude.

The urge toward shamanic solitude

Every creative activity involves a torment of loneliness that sets an individual apart from others, but the instinctive urge to achieve a shamanic state of solitude lies deeper. The compulsive seeking of shamanic solitude corresponds to *an inborn longing to accomplish a deeply individual and self-reflective grasp of personal experience of inner and outer reality*. This longing has a religious quality, as if psyche itself longs to re-link consciousness to its origins. In someone whose basic instinct is toward self-knowledge, the urge toward shamanic solitude appears to be indispensable, acting as a neurological imperative. Jung writes about it this way:

> The development of personality from the germ-state to full consciousness is at once a charisma and a curse, because its first fruit is the conscious and unavoidable segregation of the single individual from the undifferentiated and unconscious herd. This means isolation, and there is no more comforting word for it. Neither family nor society nor position can save him from this fate, nor yet the most successful adaptation to his environment, however smoothly he fits in. The development of personality is a favor that must be paid for dearly . . . only acute necessity is able to rouse it. The developing personality obeys no caprice, no command, no insights, only brute necessities; it needs the motivating force of inner or outer fatalities.
>
> (17:293, 294)

In fairytales, a period of solitude often brings about a turning point in the story, transforming the hero's situation. In *The Handless Maiden*, for example, after the hero's hands are cut off by her father and her loving king gives her silver hands, she spends seven years alone with her son Sorrowful in a cabin in the forest before she grows real hands again. In this tale, solitude indicates a time of introversion, a long, lonely state of being left to one's own resources that directs us again toward the archetypal image of Jung's orphan. Sometimes – as in this fairytale – a transcendent aspect, something autonomous from another world, an angel, or a helpful animal enters the story to link even deep levels of nature before a healing resolution happens.

Mystics like Julian of Norwich often have a paradoxical experience of solitude. Thought to be the first woman ever to write a book in English, Julian spent twenty years in an anchor-hold (a kind of little cell) built into the side of a church in England, struggling to find a language for her inner experience that the larger church could understand. During that time, it might have looked as if she were alone, but she tells us that the case was exactly the opposite: she experienced delight, freedom, intimacy, and cosmic hope.[2] In my relatively small (seven-year) time of solitude spent living alone in New York City, I was immersed in an eight-year analytic training situation, so I felt accompanied by a training community of fellow trainees: thus, I included them as healing aspects of the 'alchemical gold' that slowly began to mend my sense of 'brokenness.' Something of Sorrowful was there for me, as in the fairytale, but so too were glimpses of Julian's freedom, hope, intimacy, and rare delight.

Through a mythic lens, periods of solitude mark experiences of psychological transformation and transmutation, times of undergoing inner experience that are remarkably similar to the shaman's initiation. Prophets assume theological overtones, translating the voice of a voiceless god. Jonah, for example, was swallowed by a big fish and taken where he didn't want to go. Spit up on a new shore to prophesize in spite of his earlier desire, Jonah's story is a fine metaphor for any experience of death and rebirth. Job's sufferings, about which Jung wrote in depth, are also understandable as a prolonged period of initiation in solitude. Now as then, we do not enter willingly into the belly of the beast. Only in looking back did I understand my own initiation in ways that I explored and elaborated on during subsequent years of analytic training in Zurich and New York. And though I've never been able to pinpoint exactly when the image of the archaic shaman first hove into my view, misty outlines of the complex clearly inhabited my psyche long before I fell headfirst into the archetypal field. Had I known what to look for earlier, a few dreams might have alerted me, but dreams need pondering over time – time I had yet to live through. Seldom does consciousness change on the spot. Only the intimate and heartfelt *experience of the reality of the psyche* that accompanied me over time enabled me to make real, personal sense of what I was experiencing; only over time could I anchor a personal experience of psychological depth into the amplified outlines of a psychological complex. In my situation, it was as if Jung's transcendent function activated the archetypal unconscious to neutralize chaos and imbalance. Not until that happened was my renewed sense of a personalized ego able to relate to a renewed sense of shared reality. It was as if transcendence itself *moved instinctively by way of psyche's symbolic process*, worked its way through the shaman complex, and welcomed soul home.

So let's say that in a modern person, the urge toward introversion often characterizes an activated shaman complex. When that is happening, withdrawal into solitude (expressed symbolically in fairytales) becomes a conscious choice to come to terms with one's inner world. This awesome task (also known as individuation) is what works to regenerate a damaged ability to act, or simply *to be*, in the world. And individuation plays itself out in a personal life, but personal life doesn't come about only in a therapeutic milieu, as if introversion were a precinct sacred to psychology alone. The memoirs of a friend of mine, a former Catholic priest, demonstrate that a process of individuation occurs over the course of a lifetime.

Nick was born in Ireland into a family constellation that appointed him to represent the family as a priest in the Catholic Church. Nick loved sports and did well at them, particularly hurling, but eventually he came to love reading too, and he developed a life of the mind. After he took his priestly vows, Nick worked in parishes in Africa and Newfoundland. When Nick's call to solitude came, he was still within the church, so he founded a hermitage, literalizing his introversion into the solitary life of a hermit potter. Eventually, for all kinds of inner and outer reasons, Nick left his hermitage behind to live the life of an ordinary citizen. Now happily married, Nick's highly creative, spiritually expressive disciplines include meditation and writing his memoirs.

Nick's writing tracks his experience of inner urgency toward forming a meaningfully personal stance vis-à-vis the collective traditional religious container (his church) that formed and held most of his earlier life. To paraphrase his words, Nick tells us that he progressed from experiencing authority 'out there' to discovering an inner authority of personal experience. He moved from identifying himself as 'Catholic' to finding a truly Catholic embrace of the mystical underpinnings of all religious traditions. Nick also moved from an early definition of spiritual life as a life that belonged to the Church to an understanding that a spiritual life is quintessentially human. Nick underwent a brief period of therapy to 'discern the spirit' of his journey's trajectory while he was still living under the auspices of the Church, but the most solitary aspect of his individuation process happened within a religious tradition rather than a psychological discipline, since Nick lived out his time of literal solitude as a hermit in Newfoundland's lovely Codroy Valley.

Another religious person of my acquaintance lived her solitude outside the religious container in which she began. Joan, a former nun, found her way out of her traditional role after she dreamed that she successfully rolled up the black tarmac of a 'straight and narrow highway' so that she could carry it under her arm as she set off on her own two feet through a beautifully flowering meadow (Joan's somewhat domineering father had been a highway engineer). 'One or two profound, mystical experiences I had in my dreamlife became enough to last me a lifetime,' Joan once told me; 'I loved teaching medieval literature, and I loved living with my sisters, but I simply didn't need to be a nun anymore.' Nick's and Joan's respective experiences show how the psychological solitude I'm describing can be a crucial aspect of psychological individuation, whether or not it separates us from collective or traditionally meaningful containers

Embodied manifestations of a shamanic irruption

Jung was convinced that the development of individuality is an evolutionary phenomenon, and I have speculated that shamanic individuals with an inborn, instinctive urgency toward self-knowledge emerge out of collective necessity. Both Sigmund Freud and Carl Jung thought of themselves as 'alienists.' They worked with people who were subject to intrusions from a second world they called the unconscious, and they themselves were frequently disturbed by such intrusions. Shamanic energy lent fire to their sudden, collaborative friendship, as well as the ashy remains of the sudden, inexplicable estrangement that neither man was able to grieve to the depths of repair. Sometimes I'm convinced that the entire field of psychotherapy has emerged, shamanic, in Western civilization just over a hundred years ago, out of sheer collective necessity. How else would an awareness of something like the psyche's symbolic process and a 'symbolic life' seep into possibility? That inner quality, that reaching for the most uniquely individual stance available to a person in the present moment, is a shamanic indicator. When a solitude-oriented pursuit of an individual standpoint has been activated in a modern personality leading to a full-blown eruption of the shaman complex, watch out: most of us do not achieve psychological solitude without undergoing a crisis – meaning without experiencing actual isolation – and to most of us, solitude still feels like an extreme and unbalanced psychological situation.

Different cultures understand and interpret solitude in different ways, and some Indigenous societies have made more room for it. An Indigenous child in what is now the United States, for example, who is recognized by the tribe as 'marked,' may be sent on a vision quest. Analogously, Nick, described earlier, felt drawn as a young teenager to the Catholic priesthood. He did not understand why but trusted that intuition and the position of celibate faith leader that it implied. On occasion, however, such collective beliefs also block psychological development. In the contemporary film *Whale Rider*, a young Maori girl, 'called' to the depths of her being, is locked in an impasse with everyone else in her society, in that her cultural tradition decrees that only males may inherit the position to which she feels called. Her lonely, life-threatening, but eventually successful journey to claim proper standing vis-à-vis her people engages forces beyond those of her cultural time and place: even the Great Whales summon themselves to assist her.

From a subjective point of view, in individuation, I am always 'my own problem,' so my body and my physical being is always the 'place' (i.e., psyche's symbolic 'space') of psychologically transformative experience. Maybe that's why indications of an activated shaman complex are often so visceral. Visionary experience permeates bodies, not just minds; even dreams wake us up in physically felt terror or ecstasy. Kundalini energy runs up and down human backbones, human spines. Paul fell off his horse on the way to Damascus and couldn't see for three days. Theresa of Avila as portrayed by Bernini melts with the penetrating energies of physical union with her beloved. When we are gripped by an archetypal pattern, it is as if some part of it must be literally enacted – as though we have to *do* whatever is necessary to be disoriented enough and unrelated enough to whoever else is around and whatever else is happening – ultimately, *alone* enough – to forge, take hold of, and maintain an individual take on inner reality. Then – of course – that individualizing realization has to be hauled aboveboard into individual consciousness, like a thrashing fish. Nascent individuality dawning within one small personality reverberates within that personality physically, bodily, as if chiming in with tremors of a World Soul, tumbling through sprawling civilizations seeking balance and redress.

Individuality versus personhood

From a cultural point of view, the shaman starts out as the oddball, the person who is 'different,' the one who 'doesn't fit in': in this sense, a person who is an individual, perhaps, but not yet a person. I felt like the 'black sheep' of my family before I discovered my personhood, and this discovery entailed a battle with inner forces as well as outer ones. Somehow riding psyche's evolutionary wave on whatever surfboard of awareness I was able to muster, I found myself pitted against psyche's autonomous dynamics and defenses. Only slowly did this struggle become soulful, since wherever there is shaman, there is soul. Had Jung not argued with the autonomous urgencies that greeted him from the unconscious, he would never have become as ensouled a personality as he seems to have become by the end of his life. Even though the psyche is the matrix of personality development, psychological solitude is so against our nature that we seldom achieve it unless we are 'thrown' into it. A psychological equation decrees that if we can't make an inner situation conscious, it will constellate outside of us as fate. As the unconsciously soul-seeking moderns that most of us are, we repeatedly act on unconscious imperatives, neurotic or otherwise, that will bring about such 'fateful' crises, engineering actual solitude rather than psychological solitude over and over again.

To put this in clinical language, it is as if when we remain psychologically unconscious of our inner contradictions, the outer world 'acts out' our conflicts and is torn apart. We are torn apart with it. Relationships break. Accidents happen. War begins, and war continues. Physicist Wolfgang Pauli thought of it this way: from an inner center, the psyche moves outward (in the sense of extroversion) into the physical world. If the psyche cannot be related to, understood, or recognized symbolically – and this happens only with ego consciousness – the psyche will be used by the self for its own ends and live itself out in the world as fate. And a person whose ego is unconscious of what is happening will likely be sacrificed to the self's unconscious designs.[3]

Let me offer a personal example: when I am able to maintain awareness of my mediating tendency and make a conscious choice about when it is appropriate and when it is not, I have less need for literal solitude or isolation in order to maintain my individual point of view. An unconscious compulsion toward outer life crises that formerly led me toward literal solitude is relatively defused. Solitude does not necessarily mean living apart from others but rather *not* living apart from oneself; it's about being fully present to ourselves, whether or not we are with others. In another scenario, when I am in conflict with someone, if I have enough ego consciousness to hang onto my sense of personal reality, I find it far easier to maintain my individual standpoint without either concretizing it (e.g., isolating myself and leaving the scene) or feeling as if I have succumbed to persuasion by outer forces.

What I am trying to get at in these two recent examples is a potential that we moderns have to actualize *psychological solitude* as distinct from shamanic enactments of concrete isolation. Sometimes a capacity for psychological solitude ignites and develops in therapy. British psychoanalyst D. W. Winnicott trenchantly observed that for all of us, the true ability to be alone begins with an experience of being alone in the presence of the mother. Winnicott's example pictures a playing child, impervious to a nearby mother who – despite the child's obliviousness – provides the enabling, unobtrusive environment in which the child can simply be. Therapeutic relationships offer a similar situation: the presence of a mediating, unobtrusive person in an environment within which one's sense of psychological solitude and potential personhood can safely develop. Whether such a precious opportunity for developing personhood is given by fortune or experienced in therapy, every experience of psychological solitude supplies a growing ego with cohesion and strength. At the other end of the spectrum, unfortunate or unexpected hospitalizations concretize solitude, while shock treatments, psychosurgery, and even drug experience can bring about the most terrible kinds of solitude imaginable.

Provided a certain degree of personality development, then, the ensouled personhood that can occur in solitude no longer necessarily depends on actual solitude. If consciously or unconsciously we persist in concretizing alienation or enacting solitude through neurotic behavior, we fall victim to shamanic isolation and seclusion. No *rubedo* is possible. Any innate potential we might have realized, any capacity to live passionately among others as ensouled people, slips away. Someone in this fix can express great concern for humanity at large (usually in lectures, books, and ideas), but there is apt to be short-circuits in behavior and 'everyday,' run-of-the-mill intimacy with other people.

In Jungian circles, there is a rumor, almost a myth, that only inner work is necessary in order to be whole-heartedly alive and true to oneself and one's inner forces. A companioning assumption is that each of us is wholly responsible for our own problems, and to heal, we need change only ourselves. Lying at the root of many modern therapeutic movements, this rumor has value as a corrective to the familiar, cruelly repetitive illusion that all individual problems are caused by environmental factors and other people. However, once we progress beyond illusory blame, this rumor helps create the one-sided assumption that every individual is a self-sufficient unit. Some thinkers, like Spinoza, imagine us as 'monads,' sealed singular beings without windows. Such a view not only denies the reality of a psyche that Jung tells us 'always consists of an I and a you' but also aborts any deep understanding of a self that in a profound reality consists not only of my individual self, but of other selves as well.

Encountered in psychological development, a tendency toward self-sufficient isolation can be dangerous and needs to be questioned: is it highlighting an unconscious need to literally enact shamanic solitude? Feeling like a misfit isolates you no matter what the reasons, but it also can lead to entrenched psychopathology. Yes, an archaic shaman's need for isolation may have been central, but the shaman's isolation was maintained from an unconscious need for self-protection, because a shaman maintained their individuality by necessity rather than by choice. If the archaic shaman's magical powers failed in the eyes of others, they might become a scapegoat, a sacrificial victim to the tribe. For an archaic shaman, sacrificing solitude would have meant giving up a sense of identity that had been framed in an unconscious call to vocation, so the shaman lived alone.

Solitude becomes a shamanic precinct when separation feels absolutely essential, and lack of solitude threatens fragmentation. However, every archetypal pattern is bivalent, and the shamanic pattern is always one of venturing into solitude only to rejoin the human race: departure and return. We really can't escape the archetypal necessity of going through the shaman complex in order to come out the other side. In modern people, relief from compulsive urges toward solitude happens when we become conscious of what we've been unconsciously enacting.

One danger of the solitary shaman and his calling is the tendency for spiritual inflation. Any of us can be 'touched' by spirit beliefs or seduced by the Powers, and the tendency toward isolation is one of these. But so is the idea that anything approaching a truly spiritual life requires a radical separation from the demands of the day. A similar conviction, less extreme but perhaps more insidious because it is more hidden, is the belief in the existence of an 'elite,' or a special group of people, or the felt-necessity to become a member of 'the chosen ones.' Yes, the archaic shaman had to be instructed in all kinds of secrets that were held away from his fellow tribesmen, and we, too, can achieve extreme concentration by being purposely unrelated to others, but this is a tendency that leads toward isolated *individualism*, not toward ensouled personhood. I don't believe it is possible to 'have a soul' and believe that one is better than other people, or, conversely, that other people are somehow better than you. This kind of judgment simply doesn't hold, and it implies the lack of psychological relatedness that undergirds the collective individualism and narcissism of our time. To become an ensouled person means to fully develop one's individual personality and this does not stop with unrelatedness to others: in the psychological trajectory of developing personhood, collective individualism, egoism and egocentrism are simply stages of development along the way.

French Catholic priest and philosopher Teilhard de Chardin writes about it like this:

> One must not confuse individuality with personality. The goal of ourselves, the acme of our originality, is not our individuality but our person. In trying to separate itself as much as possible from others, the element individualizes itself, diminishes itself, and loses itself. To be fully ourselves it is in the opposite direction, in the direction of convergence with all the rest, that we must advance – toward the 'other.' The true ego grows in inverse proportion to egoism. But for human particles to become really personalized under the creative influence of union, they must not join up any which way. Since it is a question of achieving a synthesis of centers, it is center to center that they must make contact, and not otherwise.[4]

Teilhard says that we must develop a center in order to relate authentically. I've made sense of Teilhard's statement by observing that for me, to develop a center means to develop one's feeling values, one's 'heart.' It means to become a person who lives within that relational, unifying field, that matrix or ocean or ether that buoys everything we know. It means, in Annie Dillard's lovely words, to experience 'our complex and inexplicable caring' for each other and for life, unearned and simply given. Apostle Paul called it 'love, that beareth all things,' and Buddhists call it The Great Compassion. In a Sufi world, the Fair Witness appears, and nothing can feel more amazing.

Paul and the Buddha are telling us that to become awakened, we must undergo an inward 'turn' or a 'turning' that returns us to something we have always known. Both of them point the way toward a *personal awakening* that ego consciousness undergoes, an awakening that always feels like a reawakening. This metanoia (beyond mind) of awakened return *feels like* a homecoming. It amplifies our understanding of what Carl Jung and Edward Edinger have told us about the psyche's religious function (*re-ligio*, to re-link). It deepens our understanding of any shamanic story of 'finding soul.' A personal capacity for human relatedness is hard-won, and true relatedness to what's in here and what's out there is a rare and precious development of the psyche: accomplishing this is up to conscious human beings.

Two dreams about the importance of psychological relatedness

At some time during my immersion in shamanic depths of the unconscious, I became more aware of how impoverished my life was in terms of relationships in the world. Overall, it had been a desolate and solitary time. Yet I began to feel some encouraging growth, as if tender green shoots were sprouting somewhere. I began to have occasional luncheon dates.

Two important mandala-like dreams announced and re-announced the urgency I began to sense toward feeling-relatedness out there, in the world. Both dreams offered deeply organic images of relationship, as if the unconscious held a profound intuition of exactly the kind of relatedness I lacked. Even though they happened two years apart and occurred during work with two different analysts, the two dreams belong together in that both urged me to carry my 'shamanic solitude' out into the world. Perhaps we can think of them as marking different stages of symbolic healing.

Artichoke Dream:

> *An enormous green artichoke fills my vision. Each enfolded artichoke leaf is overlaid, or engraved, as intricately as a Chinese ivory carving. Each carved leaf depicts a different human relationship – images of mother-child, lover-beloved, old-young, father-son, friend-foe. Actually, I realize that each leaf depicts aspects and forms of loving and hating, with all gradations in between.*

It seemed important that although the dream image depicted human forms of relationship, I knew in the dream that it really portrayed affects-in-relationships. Emotional literacy had never been a strong point in my family of origin, nor had it been given much attention in the highly intellectual cultures of my schooling and professional life. Unbeknownst to me at the time, fully feeling my affects in relation to other people lay ahead.

Of course, I came up with all kinds of associations to this image. First, the artichoke was the bud of the fruit of the plant, and were it left to bloom, it would flower into a giant purple thistle. The bud itself, when cooked to eat, held a bit of thistle nestled in the core; my mother had taught me how to remove the prickly center with a spoon. And I remembered visiting a museum of Asian art in San

Francisco, where I'd seen a breathtakingly intricate, round (like the artichoke bud), two- or three-foot-high Chinese ivory carving that depicted an entire world in miniature. But the color of the dream struck me most, more deeply than the image itself. My first thought was of Hildegard of Bingen's *benedicta viriditas*, her 'blessed greenness,' a time when the world feels blessed with grace. New York analyst Ann Ulanov's understanding of 'greenness' that seems to be emerging in our time is that it portrays the unfolding of a strikingly feminine 'mode of being,' a mode that has the capacity to personally receive, embody, and relate to the mystery of God.[5] Philosopher Arne Naess contrasts what he calls a skin-encapsulated ego with a greening self in our time, an ecological self with a wider construct of identity that is beginning to emerge: an ecological self feels coextensive with other beings and the life of our planet.

Ulanov and Naess expressed a bit of what I glimpsed in my experience of this dream, but in recognizing the full, implicit affect that underlies the color green, this passage from Jung spoke directly to what also felt like a dream harbinger of hidden stirrings with still-unconscious emotional implications:

> The state of imperfect transformation . . . hoped for and waited for, does not seem to be one of torment only, but of positive, if hidden, happiness. It is the state of someone who, in his wanderings among the mazes of his psychic transformation, comes upon a secret happiness, which reconciles him to his apparent loneliness. In communing with himself he finds not deadly boredom and melancholy but an inner partner; more than that, a relationship that seems like the happiness of a secret love, or like a hidden springtime, when the green seed sprouts from the barren earth, holding out the promise of future harvests. It is the alchemical *benedicta viriditas*, the blessed greenness, signifying on the one hand the 'leprosy of the metals' (*verdigris*), but on the other the secret immanence of the divine spirit of life in all things. . . . Green signifies hope and the future. . . . *Therefore this virtue of generation and the preservation of things might be called the Soul of the World.*
>
> (CW14:623–624)

In my personal life at this time, there were beginning to be intimations of hope and a future.

Peter Bishop (1998, 197) reminds us that the color green inheres in a deep stratum of reality known in alchemy as the vegetable soul.

> Weaving their way through the idea of the vegetable soul are ideas about the body and nervous system, nourishment, digestion, circulation, and reproduction; a fundamental substratum of consciousness; a repose that takes us back to childhood, to the beginnings of things; an anima involvement in the sensual world; an all-pervading cosmic life energy, and so on . . . but also profound melancholy, returning us downward into our own root concerns, and to the vegetative tragedy facing us today in the world.

Plants bridge the mineral and animal kingdoms, and images from the plant world express the mystery of life as it emerges from the elements. The vegetable soul connects us with a dark downwardness that we associate with melancholy, dirt, and depression. Old alchemists worked to create not only the Philosopher's Stone, but also a Vegetable Stone, a *lapis vegetabilis*, a *quinta essential*. The idea of a vegetable soul draws us into a twilight zone in which we can separate soul and body, psyche and soma, mind and matter only imaginatively, because after the mineral world, the vegetable level of the psyche represents the deepest realm of unconscious life. Thus, descent into the deepest levels of the unconscious symbolizes an increasing engagement with the body, in the depths of which a profound, fundamental life energy originates at the roots of the self (van Löben Sels, 2003, 78).

Rose Dream

As if to repeat the Artichoke Dream in a different dimension, the Rose Dream occurred two years later, underscoring the same message as the Artichoke Dream with an image of a different plant and a different color, unfolding the possibility, as it were, of an entirely new emotional register:

> *An enormous dark red rose fills my vision. Each petal is carved or engraved with a version of human relatedness – friend-friend, friend-enemy, brother-sister, mother-child, father-child, lover-beloved, husband-wife, neighbor-stranger, etc. The petals are so vivid that they tremble, as if each petal were formed from the blood of life itself, liquid, brimming, about to spill over the rim of itself.*

'The fire and the rose are one,' sings T. S. Eliot in 'Little Gidding,' mingling heart and heat, passion and love in mystical prose. In Jung's amplifications, the blood red rose is a representation of Mary, or the birthplace of Christ, and analogous to the eastern lotus. Jung finds a direct analogy to the Buddha in the 'Lotus in the Amitabha Land' (Jung, 1938, 36, 103). 'Mary' is represented as a sea flower in one hymn, and Christ as the sea bird that rests in her. This is exactly the eastern motif of the lotus (ETH 116); Jung continues, 'we find the chief parallel to the lotus in the hymnology of Mary, where she is called the flower of Heaven, the noble rose of Heaven, the rose without thorn; she is also greeted as the sweet rose, etc.' (ETH 3 March 1939). Associations easily flooded Jung's imagination, psyche spilling over the rim of his mind.

My initial associations were prosaic. I knew and loved roses. My mother and I, and both my grandmothers, tended rose gardens, but there were no roses around my little third-floor walkup Manhattan cubicle, nor had I grown roses for a long time. 'My Love Is Like a Red, Red Rose,' goes the song by the Scottish poet Robert Burns, but neither love nor roses were immediately at hand. 'What have you been up to?' asked my analyst, and I obediently offered up whatever associations I could pull together. Nor did I remember the earlier Artichoke Dream until several years later. But when I did remember, and when I placed these two dreams side by side, it seemed to me that the Rose Dream clearly portrayed a progression, a movement from the green beginnings of the alchemical opus that was suggested by the Artichoke Dream to something nearing the ruddy glow of the 'final' alchemical stage of the *rubedo*, when life opens to being lived passionately and fully in relationship, in the world.

From a psychotherapeutic point of view, the alchemical stage of *rubedo* indicates a process during which patients become able to bring insights and capacities gained in psychological solitude back into life in the world, and this had begun to happen with me. My dream rose – a full mandala, symbolic of totality and an image of the center – landed me smack into the middle of an imaginative experience of Eros, by which I mean an archetypal experience of love and an undefended heart. As a symbol of the heart, the rose blooms at the heart of any matter whenever love is at issue – not love in the abstract but love experienced in a related context.

I've always felt that the Rose Dream heralded the emergence of a growing capacity for an all-out, no-holds-barred way of experiencing myself and life in the world in a way that encompassed all the unconscious emotional experience I had found intolerable. A much fuller range of emotions became available to me, from tears so plentiful that they threatened extinction to a quiet joy that felt as if it healed the pains of body and soul themselves – everything, and every emotion that had not been fully metabolized within the 'body' of my incarnate life. The image of the rose was numinous. It moved my heart and mind together, and I began to imagine that possibly my life might grow into something more than the existentially 'blighted bud' of existence I had known. Out of my 'blooming' individual consciousness (albeit in a dream) and increasing personal awareness began to flower not more solitude and self-absorption but rather feelings of union with God and the world that felt mystical and eternal in a way that other unions I had known – whether of mind or body – had never been.

Jung gives us a cautionary reminder here (CW 16:454): although an experience of wholeness fully depends on the relationship of one person with another, essentially *the principle of self-other awareness or wholeness is the product of an intrapsychic process*, and this experience can be hard to integrate into conscious life. Surely psychoanalytic relationships pave the way for individuation, but in themselves, therapeutic relationships neither cause nor give proof of the psyche's transformative movement toward healing. Nor is the transformation implied by therapeutic relationships necessarily conscious. I could understand the Rose Dream only as a prolegomena to a sometimes-painful, sometimes-joyful retrieval of a soul into my body, because for me, neither healing nor transformation would ever occur outside of soul. Yes, these two dreams were mandala-like images of wholeness, but Artichoke and Rose bespeak plant-world wholeness, not human-world wholeness. Above all, these dreams suggest that the psyche is an organic source of human relatedness, the fullness of which no individual person can possibly embrace alone.

These two dreams were about healing my capacity to love; they did not announce the full arrival of love-in-the-world. Upon reflection, I ponder my being drawn to the colors rather than the structure of Artichoke and Rose, so that I didn't even notice the mandala structure until later. I responded to what I felt more than to what I saw – to what I perceived, than to what I thought, which may be fine in a dream, but reality requires much more. Jung wrote that the 'shimmering symbol expresses the *processes of the psyche*' more trenchantly and clearly than the clearest concept, in that symbols not only convey visualizations of the process but *bring about a re-experiencing of it* – bring about a re-experiencing of a twilight that we understand through 'inoffensive empathy' but that too much clarity dispels (CW13:199). My focus on the color of these dream images was an instinctive move made on the part of my whole being toward what my *embodied perceptions made me feel*, fishing perhaps for whatever would heal the enormous dissociation between body and mind that I had experienced years ago.

Notes

1 Edith Weigert (*The Courage to Love: Selected Papers of Edith Weigert*. 1970) writes about loneliness and solitude per se; Anthony Storr (*Solitude: A Return to the Self*. New York: Random House, Inc. 1988) addresses the importance of solitude in the lives of creatively fulfilled individuals.
2 McColman, Carl: *Christian Mystics: 108 Seers, Saints, and Sages*. New York: Hampton Roads. 2016. xix.
3 See Jung, C. G., and Wolfgang Pauli: *The Interpretation of Nature and the Psyche*. Bollingen Series LI. Princeton, NJ: Princeton University Press. 1955. 175.
4 De Chardin, Teilhard: *The Phenomenon of Man*. New York: Harper and Brothers. 1969. 263.
5 Ulanov, Ann: *The Feminine in Jungian Psychology and in Christian Theology*. Evanston, IL: Northwestern University Press. 1971; Ulanov, Ann: *Receiving Woman: Studies in the Psychology and Theology of the Feminine*. Philadelphia: Westminster Press. 1981.

Chapter 6

The shamanic personality and the profession of depth psychotherapy

Shamanic roots of depth psychotherapy

In a seminal essay called 'The Vocation of Depth Psychotherapy' (Edinger, 2002), Edward Edinger makes the claim that the vocation of depth psychotherapy constitutes a momentous empirical discovery in the early years of the twentieth century – a discovery that is on par with the discovery of subatomic reality and nuclear physics, which occurred at roughly the same time. Before this, what we now accept as the reality of the psyche and its archetypal contents (commonly referred to as the unconscious) was projected into the mysteries of the world as spirits or gods, related to there as the Great Beings of religious tradition and the other world of spiritual reality. And this was the cosmological world into which an archaic shaman was born.

Although the practice of depth psychotherapy is a new and unique occupation for the human race, it does have historical antecedents, and Edinger outlines three essential roots or tributaries of this new profession:

1. The physician-healer of the early Greek and Roman city-states.
2. The philosopher-scientist of the Platonic academy.
3. The priest-hierophant of ancient Israel and the early Christian Church.

Each of these traditions makes a unique contribution to the modern practice of depth psychotherapy, and from each tradition, we derive a certain attitude toward our work. From the physician-healer, for example, our profession derives an ethical concern for the welfare of a suffering patient. That is the understanding written into the Hippocratic oath: to respect confidentiality and do no harm. From the philosopher-scientist, the new vocation derives an emphasis on self-knowledge ('know thyself') and a Socratic method of dialogue in which truth is expected to emerge from within a patient through a process of carefully posed questions by the analyst/philosopher. And from the religious legacy of the priest-hierophant, depth psychotherapy derives an understanding that a patient who comes for psychotherapy feeling alienated and out of alignment with 'higher powers' requires mediation to those powers, whether that mediation comes in the form of 'confessing' to a priest/analyst or whether it comes through a therapist's mediation of the numinous realities of the transpersonal psyche by working with dreams, visionary experiences, inner voices, or part personalities.

Also like a priest-hierophant, a shamanic personality *shares* the experience of vocational calling, and (at least in the Jungian tradition) their 'calling' often happens in the form of a theophany, meaning a direct experience of the *numinosum*. Unlike the priest-hierophant, however, a shaman's calling was singular and unique. A shaman's calling might involve a form of possession or illness, or loss of soul, and the call is often *not* into a religious tradition (as it is with a priest or prophet) but instead into shamanic solitude, where individual communion with powers and spirit guides is apt to be the main and lonely event: in other words, a shaman's call involves a compelling plunge into the inner world.

In addition to Edinger's outline of the historical antecedents of our vocation, depth psychology, other investigators provide excellent reviews of the history of healing in Western culture. In his monumental review of the history of Western healing practices, for example, Henri Ellenberger (1970) traces the ancestors and forerunners of our contemporary psychotherapies back to animal magnetism, mesmerism, demon possession, exorcism, and various forms of hypnotic trance induction. Ellenberger finds uninterrupted continuity between these early forms of primitive medicine and the methods of modern schools of dynamic and depth psychology, and he distinguishes these modern methods from more scientific medical therapies that have taken over so much of modern psychiatry. Ellenberger points out that, just like our primitive healing forbearers, a modern psychoanalyst's personality is their major therapeutic tool. He also points out that psychoanalytic training includes a long personal analysis aimed at working out a psychotherapist's own emotional problems and that this is incomparably more exacting and initiatory than training in most other specialties. Ellenberger also observes that – having produced a revival of psychosomatic medicine – modern psychotherapy has divided itself into a variety of schools, each with its own 'great ancestor' and its own doctrine, method of teaching, and initiatory mode of training.

From what we can gather of their personal lives, both Freud and Jung fit the profile of a primitive healer more closely than they did a profile of the scientific therapists of their day, although Freud might have objected to this characterization. Psychoanalysts practicing within their traditions function in a shamanic fashion whether they recognize it or not. Alone in a room, separated from other human beings and the common flow of everyday events, therapists have an intensely personal and (simultaneously) an objective and impersonal relationship, with each person they see. Like a shaman, a therapist meets with another person in specifically ritualized 'ways' that are marked by particular circumstances and timing, acceptable and customary modes of behavior, and payment. Like a shaman, a therapist 'waits in a cave' to make sense and meaning out of whatever emerges. Like the shaman, the modern depth psychoanalytic therapist has usually felt 'chosen' by their vocation, and they carry the depth of this personal understanding into contact with a patient. But *unlike* an archaic shaman, a modern depth psychotherapist has been trained to understand that the dreams, visions, and active imaginative forms that they work with are *products of the unconscious*, and they have been trained in how to understand and relate to products of the unconscious as they present themselves in the constellated field of depth psychotherapy.

Although Edinger and Ellenberger offered compelling historical background parallels between early Western forms of healing and modern psychotherapy, neither dealt extensively with what we might call the proto-psychological period of ancient history, before the reality of the psyche had been discovered as separate from religion. Jung was fond of saying that religion embodied the psyche before modern science made the psyche an object of empirical investigation, but while Edinger's three antecedent traditions go back as far as the healing practices of the priest-hierophant of ancient Israel, they cover only that period in which those established traditions prevailed. No doubt (and I think Edinger would have agreed with this), healing started much earlier: thousands of years earlier.

In addition to Edinger's three sources, we can think of shamanism as constituting a fourth root of our profession, and it is unquestionably the oldest. I am approaching shamanism as not just another tributary but the *main river* from which the other three branches derived. And I am suggesting that this main river or fourth root of our profession involves an evolutionary step in human consciousness that we can think of as *the coevolution of the modern ego and its emerging awareness of the reality of the psyche itself.* What I mean by the reality of the psyche is the reality of the *whole* psyche, including its conscious and unconscious dimensions – all that Ellenberger outlined as the discovery of the unconscious per se. This means not just the unconscious as the 'unknown' dimension of mind, but the unconscious as Carl Jung conceived of it: an autonomous reality with its own otherworldly (meaning mythopoetic) contents and its own 'ways of being' – a 'second world,' as it were. This kind of unconscious cannot be 'assumed,' nor can it be consumed, by a one-world mind. Even Freud fell short of this breadth of understanding, as do the scientific movements within our current preoccupation with 'effective techniques' in psychotherapy. The vocation of depth psychotherapy requires, and depends on, an experience of and a theoretical understanding of the unconscious as an autonomous, imaginal dimension of the psyche's depths. And the shaman was the first historical person we know of to *experience* the psyche as an encounter with the spirit world and then to *relate* to that world in forms of active dialogues with spirits on behalf of the soul and their fellow human beings.

This represents a major step in the development of *the kind of ego* that can witness the psyche as part of an inner world (the fundamental basis of any psychology), and it has taken thousands of years to evolve. As the group member who was most vulnerable to archetypal energies of the group itself, and thus most prone to enacting the collective unconscious, an archaic shaman was also a person who interiorized (meaning individually contained and experienced) aspects of reality that for others would remain 'exterior' in whatever collective forms held the mythology or cosmology of the tribe. We can say that a shaman became a mystic, while others of the tribe remained 'church-goers,' or literalists; where other members of the tribe might talk about the bear as an animal spirit, the shaman was that individual who *met* the bear; after all, it was a shaman who said, 'until the bear bit my heart, I could not die.'

Clearly a projection maker or image carrier, the archaic shaman was also a projection and image *maker* for a tribe. In answer to the needs of others for articulating a meaningful contact with spirits, shamans *enacted* imagery from the collective unconscious, reaching beyond themselves. In an act of forming images, *a shaman broadened themselves as if laying hold of the world*, and after assuming power over 'the unknown,' they told stories about it to others. That's why we imagine that shamans must have presided over cave ceremonies, providing steps by which a sense of individual identity moved from mastery of the body schema toward an increasingly complex awareness of a 'self' in a context of cosmos and culture.

Today, we experience our head (skull) as inner, interior space, full of dark, image-laden labyrinths of imagination, memories, and personal history. We also assume that mythology exists in our dreams, fantasies, and the life of the imagination. But actually, the iconic imagery of what we call a dream world symbolizes a *cultural internalization* of the very caves that our ancestors experienced in the earth of this world. Literal caves functioned for early peoples as unconscious *exteriorizations* of the head or skull and for a shaman as a temenos or rotundum. I've often noticed small caves depicted in the distant background of many early Christian paintings of saints and the virgin and child and wondered if the caves allude to the earthly beginnings of the religious instinct itself; some 'mothering' cave must have given birth to the earliest healing practices that we can imagine, the actual cave sheltering people from danger from without and the silent, contained darkness within embracing those archaic cave ceremonies that embodied an imaginative space of 'another world.'

So, from a broader point of view, I am tracing depth psychology's history as a vocation from its early incarnation in ancient shamanism through the development of various other tributaries of self-development and healing right up to its present manifestation in psychotherapy, psychoanalysis, and the various healing arts. In the history and image of the archaic shaman, we witness someone who is seized by what we now call the symbolic process – someone without either the ego capacity or the psychological resources necessary to contain or become conscious of what is happening. With the advent of the vocation of depth psychotherapy, this 'proto-symbolic' human capacity has developed and evolved over time, so that by the time of Freud and Jung, various techniques to consolidate the ego and intentionally open the unconscious had developed – techniques like transference analysis and free association for Freud and active imagination for Jung. As depth psychology (as we know it) emerged into history as a new calling and a new form of human relatedness, a new profession was born. This progression gives us an example of how the archetypal imagination operates through *culture* to actually create its mediators – its shamans, artists, prophets, and creative people – all of whom mediate (consciously or otherwise) archetypal experience and reality to their collective surroundings.

The coevolution of ego and psyche: the birth of the symbolic function

Perhaps the first intimations of a human ego came into being the moment our Ice Age minds slowly began to separate out of their animal origins. Lascaux, Peche Merle, and Altamira are Upper Paleolithic caves in southwestern France and Spain that hold vivid images of an early human recognition of animal forms – such as horses and bison – that flooded into our newly ignited, newly dawning collective imagination. The human mind could not have perceived these images as 'other'; it was peeling back from total immersion in (unconscious identification with) the animal world. It has taken eons for those early caves to become 'the modern mind.' This process of objectification gives us evidence of the earliest ego formation we can imagine, and I am suggesting that the archaic shaman spearheaded this development, just as I am suggesting that the shaman complex has been spearheading our explorations of the depths of the inner world today.

Archeologists have found the remains of small juniper twists, fuses that apparently served as wicks for hand lamps that lit cave walls. Correspondingly small flickers of consciousness – the wavering wicks of human imagination – must have lit up at the same time, as if flickering lights within and flickering lights without emerged into the world together. Alongside animal drawings cluster those human handprints: Were they signatures? Did they indicate ritual ceremony and movements? We will never really know the intentions of the makers of those prints. But *that* they meant something – *to* someone – is certain. As precious relics of human making today, they remind us of how deeply consciousness and the imagination are rooted in the human body (Jung, CW13:242). We can only imagine the origins of the psyche and the dark beginnings of our human mind, and the origins of complex thought and our dreams are even more mysterious. But still, the early shaman was human, and as such, they incarnate the first possible flickering of ego development in the West: the image of the shaman reveals the earliest roots of psyche too.

In a mythic meditation on the development of the early human imagination, poet Clayton Eshelman imagines that the first turn of the human mind toward the modern was a 'crisis of the human' that resulted in the original birth and the original 'fall' of all of us (Eshelman, 2003). Eshelman outlines a psychological underground of myth, psychology, and prehistory in one fell swoop. Essayist Eliot Weinburger suggests that from that moment on, human history 'spun out' from a repression of the animal within and to the current extinction of animals without, so that the same 'fall' away from the animal that resulted in the repression of matriarchy and the rise of patriarchy (as well as the denial of the feminine principle) includes the transformation of a fecund underworld into the hell of suffering that has risen to the surface of our earth in twentieth century places like Dachau and Hiroshima.[1] Only by way of culture could the specifically human phenomenon of consciousness and ego formation that led to the vocation of depth psychotherapy have evolved into a figure like that of the shaman, who started as an actual *individual*, active in the small archaic societies that produced the remarkable paintings on the walls of those caves and progressed through variations and differentiations until – in the kind of quantum leap that Carl Jung expressed in his psychological writings – we can suddenly observe the shaman's image and symbolic function as *a psychic factor and a dominant of human experience* that is traceable from the beginnings of human history until now.

This is exciting because historical documentations of the shaman's doings suggest that the shaman and the psyche coevolved. Through a phylogenetic lens, we can imagine that a deep impulse in the unconscious, evolving toward Jung's collective or objective psyche, created the archaic shaman in the first place. In these pages, I contend that the same impulse influences predominantly shamanic personalities today and that this impulse is inherently inseparable from an instinctively evolving drive toward personality formation that, throughout human history, led to the modern discipline of psychotherapy.

During the last century, our present knowledge of the unconscious (discovered theoretically by Paul Carus, Arthur Schopenhauer, and Heinz Hartmann and experimentally and experientially by Jean-Martin Charcot, Hippolyte Bernheim, Pierre Janet, Sigmund Freud, and Carl Jung) demonstrates that what we formerly thought to be external is *internal*, forming and informing what we think of as the magical and mythic dimensions of the psyche. From a Jungian and psycho-evolutionary perspective, this suggests that the dynamism of the self, operating in history, has dragged us through individually subjective experiences of an exponentially expanding inner reality that we previously imagined resided 'out there.'

In summary, the earliest stages in the evolution of consciousness and ego formation in Western culture seem to coincide with the long-ago emergence of shamanism. We can think of the image of the archaic shaman as the prototypical image of any individual human being who is collectively utilized to mediate between transpersonal and human realms. Observing the archaic shaman in their culture, and observing their function as a collectively sanctioned mediator between two worlds – if we then *interiorize* this function and this emergence – we can well imagine that speaking psychologically, *the shaman stands for, represents, and symbolizes the symbolic function itself.* Furthermore, an active awareness of the psyche's symbolic function and its subjective impact *as the apprehension of meaning* and *the experience of soul* are things we not only ought to cultivate ourselves but hope that our patients will likewise experience in modern depth psychotherapy and analysis.

This process of interiorization or internalization – by which I mean discovering an inner life (an ensouled life) and learning to read it symbolically to understand ourselves – is a wonder and treasure of depth psychology that has taken centuries and more to come into being. Meanwhile, in the collective depths of the modern psyche, the archaic shaman beats their drum, has their visions, and dances their dances – an unconscious harbinger of an inner symbolic world to come. Either male, female, or nonbinary, and frequently androgynous – a collective figure seized to perform a collective function – the image of the archaic shaman represents anyone of us who is unconsciously 'at one' with the symbolic process and therefore *unconsciously oriented by soul.* Their instinct to mediate contents from the collective unconscious to a group will be a product of that group's instinct to bring about a mouthpiece, meaning that that group's unconscious desire to evolve a mediator or a translator out of that group's undifferentiated wholeness. The collective function of the group mind precedes the evolution of individual consciousness, and the image of the archaic shaman – the way I understand them – simultaneously bridges these two evolutionary processes.

A good example of how a group brings about a shamanic mouthpiece is given by Los Angeles psychoanalyst Shelley Alhanati (2004): Alhanati's timidity and shyness marked her as an unusual but gifted child in a loud, extroverted Greek family. Shelley tells a poignant story about her first experience of feeling met on a soul level by another person. Her family had moved from New York City to Athens, Greece, and five-year-old Shelley had to leave settled life with a wonderfully attuned grandmother for a raucous, boisterous atmosphere in a new home and a new country. Shelley tells us that she went through a period of muteness, repeatedly hiding under a table or behind a potted plant in the living room, and most people dealt with her by trying to cajole her into talking, putting pressure on her that only made her isolation worse. In mute solitude, unusual for a five-year-old, Alhanati exhibited alienation and emotional disturbance, attendant on the family's up-rootedness and chaos, to which other members of the family appeared to be relatively impervious. One day, however, an uncle came over to meet Shelley for the first time, and he did something different. As usual, everything was loud and intense, and as usual, Shelley was hiding behind a tree on the balcony. The following is Shelley's report of this incident:

> My uncle came over, sat down near me, picked up a toy bird, played with it silently, and then went home without ever having said a word to me. For a long time after that, I would talk only to him. I instinctively knew, by the quality of his presence, that he would find me through the interior of his own heart. Paradoxically, the message I got by his silence was that he would value my words. So I felt safe to speak. Neither of us could have articulated what the problem was, why I wasn't talking, but on another level, in an invisible, silent way, we were understanding each other.
>
> (759)

Alhanati tells us that she considers this incident her first experience of analysis. And it is perhaps not surprising that she went on to *become* an analyst, serving as a shamanic guide for the inner soul life of many patients about whom she has written with great sensitivity.

The way I see it, in her childhood story, Alhanati carried 'the inner life,' meaning the unacknowledged soul life, of her family. Alienation and disturbance were her inner demons, and she wore their masks and performed their wordless roles, hiding behind everything in sight. Ahanati was a baby shaman for her family.

No one really read her message except one uncle, who was wonderfully able to feel Shelley's need for ensouled companionship. Baby shamans often shaman as mouthpieces for the underside of a family, expressing unacknowledged emotional turmoil or portraying a soulful underbelly for the 'tribe' in which they live. Sometimes a baby shaman is the family poet, performing 'a religious function' for her family. An analysand of mine (an analyst in his own right) stumblingly described himself as 'somewhat autistic,' as he remembered himself as a child, repeating the same words over and over again until he 'drove his parents crazy'; when I suggested that he might also see himself as a baby shaman, a child who could only dance around with his mantra and mediate a highly disturbed spirit world *in* his family *to* his family, he brightened considerably, seeing both past and present in a new light.

Commenting on Alhanati's little toy bird as an intermediate 'third' that joined two silent partners in a potential space without words, Santa Fe analyst Donald Kalsched (2014, 230) writes, 'In the psychoanalytic situation, sometimes the toy bird is a dream, sometimes a gesture, sometimes a sand-tray picture, a movie, or shared enthusiasm for an insight, a book or a poem.' Kalsched's clinical concern is with the value of the embodied presence of another without interpretation and with mythopoetic vehicles that carry soul in the analytic situation. But it is also appropriate here to recall our earlier discussion of that early image (17,300 BCE) of both shaman and soul in the Bird Man of Lascaux (Illustration 2). In Chapter 1, we suggested that the image of the bird portrayed here appears in both the shaman's mask and the bird-tipped wand that accompanied the shaman in trance. Might the bird represent the shaman's soul? Or does the bird perhaps represent an animal ally? Or maybe – even in those times – the image of the bird pictures the soul of someone else (another tribesperson, or even the Bird Goddess herself) in need of mediation?

Not only did Shelley Alhanati shaman within her family by serving as a carrier of unacknowledged turmoil; she was also 'met' by a shamanically attuned uncle who 'sensed' how to relate to her through silence rather than words. As I elaborate in a later chapter, little Shelley's experience of coming into being was 'lit from within' by a *shared experience of silence*, which – as one of the seven attributes to be explored (silence, sound, gesture & posture, rhythm, mask, respiration, and movement) – is hardly unknown to psychotherapeutic work. I see these seven attributes as imaginative pools of participatory being. All of us participate in these attributes, the attributes themselves overlap, all the time, and each attribute is easily activated by the stirrings of the Anthropos. Not only do we engage these seven participatory pools and have them in common; we also dwell within them from the beginning of life. I will say more about that in Part Two.

As we have seen, I regard the instinct to shaman as a quintessentially human factor, meaning that I've come to see the shaman instinct as an essential element of the archetypal organizing schema of human personality, rooted in the collective unconscious or objective psyche. And the experience that is most essential to a shamanic personality is an *experience of the sacred* – the numinous or magical levels of the psyche: those dimensions of the psyche that are indissolubly linked to the effort all of us make to construct a meaningful world. Contrary to popular opinion, we have not just evolved out of an age of the gods into our rational, secular age and happily given up our more primitive, early assumptions about the world. The longing for an experience of the numinous is an element of the structure of human consciousness, not just a breakthrough moment in the history of human consciousness or an incident of some kind – like Moses and the burning bush or the angel Gabriel's annunciation to Mary. At the core of human nature, all of us remain seekers, no matter how enlightened we become, and the shaman is active in the Lasceaux and Peche Merle-like depths of the modern psyche, even though we may not glimpse it except on the movie screens of Hollywood or in glamorous images of our advertising industry. Though we may pride ourselves on having entered an enlightened, secular world, if we lose 'an inner world,' we have no way to glimpse, find, or even approach what is sacred to us. We have lost, or forgotten, our souls.

But the shaman in us does *not* forget. Therefore, when we ask our patients, 'What fascinates you?' 'Where, in your days, do you feel excited?' or 'What awakened your interest this week?' I see us as engaged in 'fishing for the shaman' in the psyche: Where is the secret worship going on? What has ignited imagination? Where does the heart beat more quickly? When we do this, we try to constellate that 'space between two worlds.' To put this in Jungian language, in a contemporary person, an instinctive reaction to a numinous image and a vague apprehension of the relevance of one's reaction to something not yet understood activates a linking function between the ego and a wider personality that is in the process of unfolding into symbol-forming activity. In depth psychotherapy, this is the very activity that we try to awaken. As Jungians, we say we try to ignite an ego-self relationship because *movement along the ego-self axis is what potentiates the symbolic process*. We can imagine the ego-self axis as analogous to the World Tree that the shaman must negotiate: just as an ancient shaman goes up and down the World Tree, knitting together two worlds and communicating their journey to their tribe, so too do our patients (and ourselves) move back and forth between a dream world and a world of everyday reality, relating personal stories of the journey, hour after hour, in an analytic process. In this way – offering the reality of the psyche as a shield against the meaninglessness of sheer existence – the whole symbolic discipline of depth psychology manifests the shaman.

We know that as the matrix of conscious psychological life, the collective unconscious continually influences ego consciousness and our 'civilized modes' of existence. From the standpoint of depth psychology, dimensions of experience commonly attributed to early human beings are present in deeper levels of the psyche we know too: collective levels of 'group mind' link us to the instinctive heritage we share with remote ancestors. However elaborate our development of civilized consciousness becomes, at deep levels of the psyche, we remain archaic. While we distinguish ourselves from ancestral assumptions that the explanation of everything is magic, early human beings still fascinate us, and that very fascination can acquaint us with our primitive nature and mysteries at the center of Being, here and now. In modern personalities, beneath layers of historical, cultural, and psychological overlay, the instinct to shaman functions in the depths of that collective matrix.

Contemporary shamanic personalities have innate access to magical and mythic dimensions of the psyche, and these are the same psychic dimensions that the archaic shaman unconsciously narrated to their tribe as stories about their journey to another world. Modern people 'narrate' meaning in a shamanic fashion as they magically enact or mythically embody their compulsively symbolic lives. When a shamanic personality enters psychotherapy, they seldom realize that they've been swimming in a projective field of unconscious assumptions, images, and expectations, because unless we've done a lot of psychological work, we do not comprehend the narcissistic charisma that accrues to unconscious identifications, nor we can we imagine the often-painful work of making unconscious identifications conscious that lies ahead, as we disidentify from archetypal energies in a process of humanization and personalization. 'Head shrinking' is the colloquial term for these processes. Understanding the shaman complex, how and when it constellates, and how to work within it can help practitioners navigate the activated energies of this highly charged 'field,' inside the 'cave' and out.

The shaman and ego training: therapy as an evolutionary step in relatedness

Given that instinct survives in the archaic depths of the objective psyche as part of our human heritage, the shaman instinct may be activated at any time throughout a lifetime, sometimes more than once. The activation of the shaman instinct happens through the shaman complex as a phenomenon *of* the psyche, a*bout* the psyche, and ultimately – providing that our ego is adequately developed and companioned – *for* the psyche's sake. Like an archaic shaman, a modern ego has to learn how to serve the growth of inner life, and bringing one's inner life into consciousness has its source in springs of embodied affect. Awareness of embodied affect in turn enters being only through a relationship with another. So we can say that the shaman complex is active whenever and wherever transference or countertransference occurs, and what we call transference is a general phenomenon in human relatedness in general. We take it for granted that whenever some part of the self is projected, the ego-self axis sets into motion deep affective levels of the psyche, and the shaman is present. If the shaman is held in mind, a therapist's shaman helps a patient to make meaning of conscious and unconscious energies within a patient's personality, serving as a bridge: thus, deeply unconscious human feeling emerges to a level of meaningful articulation.

Early on, shamanic personalities were flooded with numinous experience that resembled what Erich Neumann describes as 'uroboric' or pleasurable dissolution of the ego. Today, initiatory 'ordeals' mandated by shamanic training instead lead into ego consolidation and strengthening, and this is what brings to mind the rigors of analytic training in depth psychological work. Now as then, ascetic rites and rigorous ethical attitudes like those that are required in analytic training involve extreme exertion, concentration, and focus. And then as now, ascetic rigor gradually reinforces what we call an ego seed, which develops to become part of a constant striving to follow what Neumann describes as 'an inward path with mounting manifestations of the numinous' (Neumann, 1968). An ego seed holds an evolving potential for developing ego consciousness and ego intent. When, as happens in therapy, the instinct to shaman is benevolently evoked and the complex contained, the image itself is a stepping stone on a path toward ego development and individuation.

Remember how the archaic shaman's unconscious apprehension of a numinous image always posits the existence of others – a family, group, tribe, or audience – to whom their reaction mattered. When an archaic shaman returned 'reborn,' they worked with initiation masters to learn appropriate techniques and attitudes toward their previously unconscious journey and the 'powers' they met. Today, shamanic personalities share a mediating function with artists, priests, entertainers, and prophets, all in the business of communicating an inner (spirit) world to an outer collective. In the past, this function required either a conscious or an unconscious sacrifice of an everyday sense of identity for a collectively sanctioned vocational role: sacrifice was lonely business for an archaic shaman, requiring ascetic isolation and solitude.

Today, a prophet's loss of identity happens within the larger container of religious revelation – for example, in the Bible, God told Noah to go out and build an arc, never mind that he didn't have the time or the inclination. A priest's loss of ordinary personal identity tends to happen in a religious institution with all its accouterments and prestige; actors lose their identities within roles, and hopefully they come to know the difference between being onstage and offstage. But for the person who follows the shaman's call to individuality, loss of identity feels different, because solitude and the archaic shaman go hand in hand (see Chapter 5).

In this regard, by common definition, the word 'shaman' comes from the Sanskrit *sramana*, originally meaning 'ascetic' (to exhaust, to fatigue), and from *samana*, meaning 'Buddhist monk.'[2] Sometimes the Buddha was given the name Chakmoni, a corruption of the word *chaman*, and the word *Chamanists*, or *Samaneans*, designates the followers of Buddha. The Chinese pronunciation is *sa-men*, *cha-men*, or *cha-men-na*. In the Indian language, this word signifies 'he who knows how to quench his passions.'[3] 'Shaman' is also related to the Greek word *asketikos*, meaning 'exercised,' from which we get the English word 'ascetic.' In the Tungusic language of Siberia, *Saman* denotes both 'conductor of the ecstatic séance' and storyteller, or teller of epic or legend.'[4]

Self-differentiation occurs in shamanic solitude, and an observing ego has a chance to develop and establish itself. In psychoanalytic language, a differentiated ego includes certain differentiated capacities, like a capacity for cognitive organization that is necessary to witness one's own affects, which means a capacity to identify unconscious imagery associated with an affect, for example, and disidentify from the compulsive aspect of one's original 'state of possession.' During individuation, where the ego essentially serves as an evaluating and discriminating agency, it is crucial to be able to hold on to a sense of yourself, as the archaic shaman did in their inner journey, for example, or as Jung did in the active imaginations that finally led to *The Redbook*. Jung encountered forces within the inner world, but he did not give himself over to them. Instead, he listened to them; he argued with them; he had dialogues with his inner figures. But Jung did not identify with them. And when one of his inner voices described his inner work as 'art,' Jung countered, 'No, it's nature,' by which Jung meant an *inner nature*, with which he tried to keep faith.

A struggle to maintain a sense of one's self, to be faithful to one's inner nature in the midst of an initiatory plunge, often feels challenged by outer and inner forces. During my psychoanalytic training, at the especially crucial threshold of final exams, I felt besieged by outer relationship expectations – by an interesting man who had invited me out for dinner, by my parents who wanted to visit me that weekend from another city, and by a friend who was emotionally troubled – and I felt torn. But – to hibernate in my apartment for a week and immerse myself in Jung's writings – I said no to all these expectations (my parents were astounded). Finally, having called a taxi to take me to my downtown exam appointment, on that Monday evening, I emerged from my 'sanctum': A Manhattan yellow cab pulled up in front of the door, and I saw – clearly printed beneath the handle of the taxi door – the single word 'robin' (with a small 'r') – which was my given name. I was amazed. This synchronous event united inner and outer worlds, and it also helped to confirm my earlier, difficult decisions to stay faithful to my inner calling and commitments. This small event – perhaps only coincidental from the outside – felt huge from 'the inside,' and it provided a counterpoint to a dream I had eight years earlier that depicted a young man standing in the middle of a river, his clothing linked by many lines leading elsewhere, as if he were fish-hooked by other people's needs and desires. It had taken a while for my life to 'become my own,' and I passed my exams.

With the help of our shamanic forebears, we hope to accomplish what Jung did in today's modern world, but with a companioning therapist, hour by hour, day after day, and dream after dream. The application of knowledge is a distinctive evolutionary achievement of our species, and only an ego can 'apply' knowledge: that's why I suggest that learning to witness and engage psychological products *as products of the imagination* is also a step forward in human evolution. We no longer adapt to our environment primarily through slow biological evolution but through cultural evolution, and we know that the psyche as an element in itself is relatively new to Western culture. I suggest that through a psychologically sophisticated, long-drawn process of in-gathering and ego consolidation, we are also increasing our ability to serve as our own vessels. This means that we learn how to contain raw psychic energy long enough to allow its transformation into personal information. This process happens in ourselves and in our patients, and this is what enables us to change. Over time, we become less driven to repetitively encode untransformed psychic energy into a kind of repercussive behavior in order to punish or reward someone in the outer world.

What gathers an infant's personality together from within seems to be instinctive, affectively acute experience, as if one's personal psyche first forms out of an imaginative elaboration of physical aliveness and feelings in the body. This is why, in the psychotherapeutic profession, differentiating one's own 'shaman' means actively cultivating a relationship with the realities of the body's inner world. Because one's inner world originates in instinctive experience and relates to a primary psychosomatic partnership, one's ego-related awareness of the body remains crucial. Bodies are what we all have in common. Psychoanalyst Melanie Klein proposed that all originally unconscious fantasies are body based – about our own bodies and body parts and the body and body parts of our mother. As a therapist, I assume that psyche is found wherever soma is alive. But only with later ego development do most of us become aware that our alive body, with personal boundaries and limits, its inside and its outside, really forms a core – a 'vessel' – for our deeply imaginative self. Inner growth beyond action-bound immediacy of unconscious affect and images happens only as a strengthened, consolidated ego becomes self-aware. In the Jungian world, for example, a therapist relates to shadow by way of their own bodily personification of shadow, and within a psychotherapy hour, there is no other way to remain aware on a moment-to-moment basis. If I am afraid of a patient, I need to feel my fear before I can 'know' fear; conversely, I can assume that whenever I am unaware of soma, psyche is somehow lost. My individual personality incarnates increasingly as my ego becomes progressively self-related by way of shadow integration. Slowly, autonomous aspects of psyche's enactments diminish.

In psychotherapeutic training, the shaman instinct is discovered as we discover in ourselves a multitude of prehistoric psychic structures in the form of drives, primeval images, archetypal symbols, pockets of dissociated memory, and primitive behavior patterns. Training gives us a language for these things and theories about them. Given that the shaman constellates automatically within the field of the Anthropos, the instinct toward self-healing also constellates within the analytic field. This field exists in the space between analytic partners like a fluid medium, full of projective energies; psychoanalysis refers to this field under the rubric of projective identification, but I prefer to imagine it as the shaman's domain, within which we glimpse a fleeting figure, darting and dodging through imaginal space between self and other.

A therapist who is familiar with what I call the various attributes that serve as vehicles for these projective energies can avoid identifying with them and meddling with their operation – staying, so to speak, out of the shaman's way. But only by cultivating a relationship with our inner, archaic Being does the capacity for such intrapsychic awareness and witnessing consciousness happen. This cultivation gives us a sense of solidarity with the whole human species and with history that is far beyond whatever may be acceptable to the particular social milieu in which we live.

The self-discipline that cultivating this sense of solidarity entails enables a therapist to read the psychic language of another, and it teaches a patient (aware of being taught or not) how to cultivate their own individual relationship to the unconscious. In other words, *with ego effort and conscious self-reflection, the shaman as symbolic process heals the shaman as enacted behavior*. Ultimately, the shaman's movement is toward *the development of the psyche*, constellated from within, leading the psyche from infantile to cultural levels and releasing unconscious energy into ego capacities for cultural or symbolic activities. When in therapeutic work we become conscious of the shaman and take responsibility for its compulsive, autonomous operation in our individual lives, a corresponding potential for self-healing also emerges. A capacity for symbolic understanding increases. We become better able to witness our own inner process, and compulsive behavior lessens. Dreams get deeper, and life gets richer. Relationships develop outside therapy: we emerge from psychotherapy 'different' and differently, into a same and different world.

Dark aspects of the shaman complex

In therapy, the transformation of the shaman complex occurs in mutually recognizing its necessity, process, occurrence, and interactive nature within the analytic container. Activation also brings danger, because both participants in a therapeutic dialogue are vulnerable to fascination with the pre-symbolic, affective energies of the constellated complex. One way to think 'about' this fascination is to recognize that a deep archetypal image has been activated: that of the Anthropos, or whole human being. Whenever we function symbolically for someone else, and or someone functions symbolically for us, the image of the shaman and the field of the Anthropos constellate, meaning that the potential wholeness of a situation is being apprehended but remains unknown. When such an apprehension happens, someone in whom the archaic shaman complex is operative is apt to *identify* with potential wholeness itself, feeling compelled to *mediate* it somehow – help bring it about. In this mode of the complex, there is no real psychological space for 'otherness,' let alone for a personal appreciation of 'otherness'; instead, a compulsive need to maintain the balance of the situation (any situation, it would seem) exists, by (so to speak) grabbing the other end of whatever 'broken' archetypal situation happens to be presented.

Needless to say, the field of the Anthropos is powerfully constellated in psychotherapeutic situations where 'brokenness' and 'wholeness' are defining characteristics of the entire enterprise, so in this field, analyst and patient function shamanically for each other. For example, an image of the analyst (an 'image' as an *unconscious symbol* of wholeness) initially engages the unconscious fantasy of the patient. As a 'material' representation of immaterial psychological qualities and functions, the image of the analyst objectifies for the patient highly subjective realities that are implicit in the patient as perceiver and subliminal in the nature of human relatedness in general. Whenever an image, a word, a sound, a gesture, or a look expresses significance through the affect it evokes, we can say that that 'expression' is functioning shamanically (*pre-symbolically*), and the same holds true for a patient's effect on the analyst. Unconscious shamaning is inevitably part of any psychotherapeutic enterprise where the attitudes and personality of the therapist cannot help but play a significant part in the form and intensity of the psychotherapeutic process. When – out of unwitting postures, false assumptions, blind spots, private needs, irrelevant attitudes and standards, and biases or moral prejudices – a therapist is incapable of empathetic companioning, their patient will develop intense emotional reactions, representing unconscious efforts on the patient's part to bridge a gap of unrelatedness, just as when in childhood a child responds to significant unempathetic people for whom they unconsciously compensate, balance psychologically, or heal. In such a situation, we, as patients, become baby shamans, shamaning for our therapist like we did in our original families.

This is simply to point out that the potential influence of a therapist on the unconscious of a patient can be hurtful and dangerous, and these effects need to be appreciated. In any case, enormous personal responsibility is attendant on anyone who makes a professional living from the 'brokenness' of other people, from traces of love's distortions or love's lack, and from the effects of sickness and isolation, poverty and pain, and difficulty and despair. Young therapists are as prone to inflation as any patient. In supervisory consultations with candidates in training, it is not uncommon to find a new initiate excited and fascinated by idealizations and infusions of transference love. Often my task has been to teach them to recognize inflation as indicative of an activated shaman complex, helping them realize that all this idealization and love is not about them personally and helping them disentangle themselves from projected, idealizing images in which they are caught.

Any primordial archetype erupts on many different levels. It makes itself known in dream images, or a vision, or through subjective feeling experiences, or objective behaviors. The depths to which we are wounded, or lacking in personal development, are of the same measure as the same depths to which we are prone to be opened by an activated shaman complex. The clinical equation is, the more vulnerable one is to raw 'shamaning,' the more transpersonal and compelling will be the archetypal contents revealed. An actual eruption of the core imagery around such a powerful pattern may express itself in several ways: as a transpersonal, apocalyptic experience or as an intense emotional catharsis accompanied by imagery revelatory of mysteries, secrets, and synchronistic experiences. As an analyst, I may be confronted with an ego so overwhelmed that only 'the shaman' can speak its language; if this is the case, it helps if I also speak this language. Perhaps I have been through a similar experience, or – if that's not the case – at least I know how not to meddle with it or how not to take it personally. When this layer of transpersonal transference is activated, a great deal of harm can be done by a careless or psychologically predatory attitude. In fact, to take something personally when it is not meant to be personal is what I mean by a predatory attitude.

There are other indications of an activated shaman complex: as *unconscious shamans*, we will be fascinated by someone else's unconscious pain, for example, and be drawn to mediate it; the same can be said of someone's unconscious beauty or creativity. *Unconscious shamaning* involves us in a compelling, unconscious desire to complete 'the wholeness' of a situation and/or of another person. This desire itself signifies inflation, but when it is made conscious, it holds the promise of releasing constructive healing energies that may serve a patient's integration and healing. Whatever is in another's personality of which the other is unaware, or whatever exists that the conscious ego of that person seems unrelated to, attracts the shaman in us. This is to say that we head for fugitive or dissociated feelings instinctively, or we 'claim' whatever is lost or activate whatever is missing, underdeveloped, repressed, unlived, unrelated to, or unintegrated. When we 'find' the shaman in projection – in a role, perhaps, or a persona – the projection indicates where some vital influence is coming from – where unconscious worship resides. In that we usually sense taboo and fascination together, this projection tells us that something or someone has become sacramentalized.

Perhaps such a projection occurs in an important relationship with a friend or lover. Perhaps it occurs with parents or with children. Certainly, it often happens with a psychotherapist. Unconscious sacramentalization exists wherever our compulsive involvement is engaged – the love or hate, the 'foam around the edges' of our normal emotions, the seeming inability to either deal with something or leave it alone. To use a shaman's language, we behave as if we were seeking the missing or wounded aspect of a soul. Yet the field of the Anthropos (wholeness) from which such a compulsion springs has little to do with personal reality on either side of the equation, and for the *unconsciously shamanic personality*, such behavior brings about an exhausting, tumultuous, impersonal kind of life.

Learning to understand the ambivalent, compulsive power of projection is a crucial element in training. When an analyst is being idealized, an ability to differentiate such projections from accurate perceptions of one's own personality is a crucial part of 'shadow' work. Disidentifying from such projections depends on a corresponding awareness of what it means to have become sacramentalized; in turn, this awareness alerts us to the presence of the archaic shaman in the therapeutic field. Opportunity and danger both exist because sacramental energy consists of the ability to heal or harm – precisely those ambivalent powers that were accorded an archaic shaman by his tribe.

Like a shaman, alone and marked by 'difference,' therapists are constantly invited to accrue influence. And because the instinct to name the unknown, to make something conscious and 'whole,' is in itself religious, therapists inevitably invite transpersonal (mostly idealized) projections from their patients. Because of the unique attention Jungian theory gives to the archetypal psyche and the numinous images and experiences that characterize the collective unconscious, this is especially true in Jungian analysis. Edward Edinger makes the following important point about the positive and negative implications of these projections:

> There is a powerful tendency for the archetypal psyche to be inductively constellated by the analyst. This is often quite favorable and promotes the depth

> work that we try to do, but sometimes it is not in the best interest of the patient. Borderline patients, for example, may be in real danger working with those analysts who have a tendency, not really within their conscious control, to constellate the archetypal psyche. That is something to keep in mind. More than once, when I have had occasion to interview a potential patient, or when an analysis has gone wrong for some reason or another, I have referred that person to someone I know who does not constellate the archetypal psyche and is therefore relatively safe for that patient to work with.
>
> ('Science of the Soul,' 92–93)

Like other unconscious elements, as long as core archetypal contents symbolized by the image of the shaman remain unconscious, their uncanny power to influence others remains. When this happens, the shaman complex is apt to be lived out, enacted through the complex by an ego unconsciously entangled in identifications and projections and at the mercy of positive and negative inflations. Under such conditions, the issue of personal reality is utterly out of the picture. Like all instinct in primitive form, the raw instinct to shaman is indifferent to personal circumstances. We've all seen or known people whose lives seem to be consumed by an intense, compulsively lived destiny, lives that seem pulled like the proverbial moth to a flame. Someone caught up in an unconscious shaman complex seems unable to adjust to anything but a specially arranged environment; their adaptive capacities seem severely limited, including the capacity for personal relatedness. When someone is that deeply at the mercy of shamanically compulsive, unconscious behavior, they are victimized by the necessity for resultant shamanic isolation too.

When this happens, our relationship to reality is compromised. In order for any symbol to function, there must be a gap or a synapse over which (what Jung called) the transcendent function operates – like a bridge. In raw shamaning, there is no gap. Depth psychotherapy aims to restore this gap, restore what Ogden (1994) recently describes as a reflective function. After all, consciousness always takes two individuals: it takes two individuals to see through the mutual projections to the reality of any relational situation, and to me, *repairing our relationship to reality is what psychotherapy is all about.*

Thus, to accept the reality of the psyche also means to accept the fact that there is not necessarily a one-to-one correspondence between reality and our experience. The mind as such deals only with ideas: our minds do not relate to anything other than ideas. By working together in an analytic partnership, we can become acutely aware of our tendencies to 'mistake the map for the territory' of existence, so to speak; we see how we literalize, how we concretize, how we reify. But mind does not ponder reality: minds ponder ideas *about* reality. We also learn that whether or not something *feels* true may no longer be a matter of how closely something corresponds to an absolute truth, law, or principle but be a matter of how *consistent something is with the depths of personal experience.*

To hold the ambiguity of experience in this way is to experience mystery, and this is an understanding of a specific order: vis-à-vis *personal* life, it implies a contemplative stance. The subjective experience of wonder is a message to my rational mind that an object of wonder is being perceived and understood in ways other than rational. Of course, both ways of human understanding remain necessary and reciprocal. In Iain McGilchrist's *The Master and His Emissary*, he traces this reciprocity through history, underscoring contemporary imbalances between right and left hemispheric modes of perception that affect our culture today. Earlier, Erich Neumann expressed his understanding of an absolute necessity for an experience of this duality in terms of 'cortical human' re-linking with 'medullary human' or the archaic human within; and Jung expressed *his* understanding by personifying the evolutionary history of our species as a 'two-million-year-old human being in us all,' an imaginal personage still active in our dreams, myths, psychiatric symptoms, and all those traditional healing practices that re-link us with our instincts. I've imagined this same duality of experience as 're-linking' with the shaman.

Lost souls and dissociated affect

As we have seen, shamanism employed a kind of intuitive knowledge that taught that reality consisted in the relatedness not of a person with things but of human beings with human beings and of all people with spirit. Apparently, traditional cultures found interactions between person and person to be the locus par excellence of order, predictability, and regularity, and they based almost all their explanations of reality on observations of human relations or relations with spirits, including animal spirits. Traditions of peaceful living with neighbors, abstention from breaking taboo, and obedience to the laws of gods and human beings became essential for the protection of oneself and one's family.

But a shaman defied the norms of relatedness and behavior. Forced out of the roles and expectations that bind most people into outwardly traditional relationships, a shaman plummeted into an inner world where souls had been lost and hearts had been broken. Because of this, individual shamans were flooded with archetypal affects ranging well beyond those usually called forth in ordinary human relationships. Through agonies of their own suffering, a shaman was forced to see people differently: they saw them *sub species aeternitas*, so to speak – as ensouled human beings who were suffering various forms of sickness and despair.

Although a shaman underwent initial experience unconsciously, flooding by such intense affect left traces in mind, memory, body, and soul, and similar traces of similarly unbearable affects led Jung to decide that there were two kinds of complexes: soul loss on the one hand and possession by a spirit on the other.[5] However, Jung seemed to think that possessing spirits were mostly demonic and negative, whereas in an archaic shaman's experience, spirit was informative, opening another world and revealing a source of soul. This is to imply that the same spirit that invaded the shaman also *informed the shaman: it possessed their inner world while it presented them with another – or an Other*. In my view, it is possible that Jung's two kinds of complexes happen – or express themselves *in and of psyche* – at the same time, in a kind of third- door-of-both-at-once experience that is relative to Jung's stance of *either* a complex of soul loss *or* a complex of spirit possession. (For my own speculations on spirit encountered behind a 'third door,' see the brief entry on an Inuit shaman's experience of *Sila*, in Chapter 2.) Hence, for me, the whole realm of split-off affect falls under the shaman's purview, because in the time of the archaic shaman, rituals of initiation worked with embodied *albeit unfelt and barely registered experience of such affects*. Semi-conscious and unfelt though archaic shamanic experience may have been, it led to an inevitable enlargement of *a feeling capacity* in an archaic shaman: subsequently, a shaman turned their seemingly inherent ability to receive and integrate such an enlargement into trance-inducing shamanic techniques. When this feeling capacity is consciously registered *as such* today, the same human experience leads to an enlarged capacity of heart in a contemporary shamanic personality. Sometimes we see this happening in psychoanalytic training.

That we can't love another person without first loving ourselves – at least to some degree – is a psychological truism, and it follows naturally that we can't relate to other people when we are not self-related or related *within* ourselves, *including* relating to formerly split-off affect, as well as 'parts' of ourselves. This process of in-gathering into inner self-acceptance is what the old alchemists meant by undergoing a continuing process of *coniunctio* and what Jungian therapists mean by someone becoming 'psychologically married' or finding one's sense of self-integrity.

To be able to fulfill ourselves in relationship to others and the world, we must not only be outward turning, toward others, but also in touch with our innermost selves, and the bridging instinct that I am calling the shaman is what makes this possible. All real relatedness is both inward to oneself and outward toward another. When we are infants, a nascent symbolic process emerges to link and mediate both between us (infant) as an emerging individual and the self within *and* between us (infant) and a mothering person without. Discovering and realizing oneself always coincides with an ability to recognize and relate to other 'selves.'

So, in a therapeutic situation, the shaman constellates a vessel of transformation and determines its symbolic dominants – whether the mother-child matrix or the father-child matrix is constellated, for example. As the projection-making factor in the psyche, the shaman also determines when other archetypal relational configurations are activated: at certain times, levels of the personal unconscious are paramount, accompanied by shadow projections offering themselves for integration; at other times, levels of the collective unconscious emerge, accompanied by projections or personifications of the multileveled creative and generative energy of the contra-sexual functions of animus or anima. Gradually, over time, the difference between the archetypal and the personal realm clarifies.

A shamanic personality with a differentiated shaman instinct can aid or constellate Erich Neumann's centroversion in another person, activating a tendency toward healing and individual wholeness. As a 'differentiated' (conscious) shaman, a therapist can also guide a patient to truly question, or even fear, an unmediated encounter with the self rather than romanticize it. In fact, when the shaman instinct is raised to consciousness and differentiated, it is the most convincing mediator of the disillusioning idea that the self is not necessarily in business for the ego. Therefore, blindly following a sense of destiny, or heeding the call of an unconscious and compelling sense of fate (as often happens when the self is projected) is often to court sorrow and pain, if not grief and annihilation, not only for oneself but for those who are near and dear as well.

Within the temenos of self-projection a shamanic therapist may help negotiate between our familiar ego and our whole self by intentionally relating to the aspect of personality to which we seem least related. Consciously companioning us where we are weak or where consciousness is practically nonexistent – where we are terrified of our own anger, for example, or where we are unrelated to our bodily reality – such a therapist helps us know more fully what it is that we are experiencing, what it is that we live. A shamanic therapist does this not so that we become more self-centered but so that we become more self-connected – more inwardly related, more humanly related to our own potential wholeness, which includes our fellow human beings and the wholeness of the world. This is what a 'shaman' sees in us from the beginning.

Reflections on soul, psyche, and the symbolic life

In archaic societies, a shaman was the soul's only companion, enacting what psyche later became. Later cultures (e.g., Greco-Roman) depicted psyche as a winged person not-yet-fully human or as an ephemeral butterfly. In our culture, psyche has become a reality in itself, the matrix of meaning between two worlds.

Poet Robert Hass (2017, 6) comments that mind, soul and self all create themselves as they come into being. What Hass leaves out of his picture is that mind, soul, and self, come into being only *as we relate to each other and to the world.* A mind in the mode of individuation can have thoughts that separate us from others and help us differentiate a sense of self, but the soul in the mode of individuation *feels connective urgencies* and depths of affect that expands it toward reconnection with the soul of another and merger with the soul of the world. To avoid the structural limitations of our language, I seldom imagine the soul as an object; instead, I try to imagine soul as a mode of relating.

On the other hand, we can think of the psyche as the linking factor that weaves the tapestry of mind and soul together. Poet Louis Simpson describes psyche as 'flitting' from one plant to another in the garden or 'lifting her little sail'; I imagine psyche flitting about between elements of Being over time, weaving heart and mind, matter and spirit, and inside and outside into each singular personality. Each and every one of us seems woven on an invisible loom into an inextricable pattern of matter, flesh, and spirit. When I glimpse this pattern, I call the pattern 'meaning,' and we ourselves 'mean' something: we feel 'meaning-*full*,' both to ourselves and to another person.

Therefore, rather than following certain conventions in analytical psychology that equate psyche with soul (e.g., James Hillman), I've been picturing psyche as soul's companion. Soul's embodied resonance and affective depth feel quite other in kind from psyche's airy meanderings from one place to another, from one person to another, from this object or image and that idea or dream – even from synchronicities.

I also think of the soul as someone's 'essence' – as the essential particularity or the 'this-ness' of a specific person. In the face of demons and darkness, or even the ecstatic allure of enlightenment, on a quest of their soul's return, an archaic shaman went in search of their lost, individual essence, including their particular, specifically embodied ability to love their life and cherish it. In every story I've read (and in my own experience) – even when Death is tempting and near – a real shaman returns from the spirit world to *this* world because they care deeply about this world and the well-being of their fellow human beings; they also care deeply about they own limited, particular, quite earthly life. Shamans turn toward what Neville Symington (1993) calls the life-giver, not away.

In Chapter 4, Journey and helping spirits, I listed soul as one of shamanism's four core notions. I elaborated on the notion that in archaic times, the soul was thought to give each living thing the particular appearance it had: the soul of a reindeer is given a tiny deer, or the soul of a human being is given a tiny human being, like the *homunculus*. Medieval Western theologians like Thomas Aquinas believed that the created order could best be understood as a transparent medium through which a divine light (from without) shines; on the other hand, Duns Scotus taught that everything is itself endowed with an inner light that shines forth from within. Theologian Mary Beth Ingham (2003) comments that the difference between these two points of view is like the difference between a window (Aquinas) and a lamp (Duns Scotus): both window and lamp give light, but for Scotus, the source of light has already been given to the being by the creator. Vis-à-vis an analogy of 'ensouling' and where soul comes from, I propose that our shamanic legacy insists on a *both/and* rather than an *either/or* position, because wrestling one's way through the shaman complex teaches us that it takes light to recognize light, darkness to recognize darkness, and soul to recognize soul. We need to imagine both window and lamp, just as we need to inhabit both inner and outer worlds: in our time, the soul often appears as a dream symbol – the child.

As I've said, soul has very much to do with specificity: the is-ness of a life, its particularity, its essence, its this-ness. We human beings don't feel love in general; we love one particular person rather than another, one particular place and not another, one particular someone or something that holds *significance*. And when we love someone or something, we don't somehow endow that person with soul, as if it were simply a matter of psychological projection. Loving another person grants that other person soul, sees soul in the 'other,' and lets the soul of the other person touch one's own. In loving another person, *we ourselves become able to recognize soul*. We must love deeply in order to recognize soul, and until I am able to appreciate and even delight in the soul of another – even the soul of a tree or an animal – I doubt if I have fully discovered my own. All this is simply to reiterate that soul seeks soul, sees soul, and recognizes soul and that soul is not discovered, uncovered, or recovered, otherwise.

Certainly, the archaic shaman had the instinct to relate, and so the image of the shaman now symbolizes the human person who is compelled to seek and find the human soul. That the archaic shaman had *more of that instinct* than anyone else in their tribe is what made them a shaman in the first place, and it is still what makes shamanic being and activity collectively effective. When a modern person works through the shaman complex (in or out of therapy), *the ensuing depth of experience and resulting self-integrity* is what makes true individuality possible. Only then can an inner voice of soul reveal itself in personhood. Naming the precious, hard-won reality of this 'inner voice,' (Neumann, 1990) believed that there was no better name for it than individual conscience.

And so, as we come to know our own interiority, we appreciate interiority in others: we recognize complexes within the psyche, and we acknowledge profound differences between our ego and those complexes *and* between our ego complex, psyche and soul themselves. In turn, these differentiations clear expressive channels within our personality for true human relatedness with others in the world. Not until we've experienced the full extent of our own depths can we realize how deeply our 'little' self interrelates with the depths of other selves. We gain not just an idea of depth but also a real, panoramic perspective.

Throughout this chapter, I have proposed that the conscious appreciation of and respect for the 'otherness' of other people – ensouled, just as we are ensouled – is a gift of self-integration by way of the shaman complex. When we become conscious of the shaman complex and sacrifice its seductive identifications, we have a right to 'call our soul our own.' No longer unconsciously meeting unconscious needs of others (because others carry unconscious aspects of ourselves in projection), in the deepest sense imaginable, we 'come home.' We have fought for a soul and won it; from then on – from soul's home base, so to speak – life's 'otherness,' inwardly and outwardly engaged, can be fully experienced, recognized, deeply respected, and enjoyed.

The next paragraph details my personal experience of how psyche weaves tapestries of inner and outer worlds on behalf of the soul, and how I felt companioned by psyche through a shamanic journey toward what I've come to understand as ensouled personhood. It is also a story that describes my first glimpse of a 'meaningful' pattern to my own life. This experience includes uncanny events that Jung called synchronicity, by which he meant experiences of meaningful connections between inner and outer worlds that seemed to defy rational explanation or material causation. My story starts with a vision.

Setting: I'm in my first analyst's office in Manhattan (Dr. P.), where for the first time in several years I've began to talk to someone about my despair, pouring out and giving voice to unconscious pain that I've been holding for a very long time. This is my third session, and undoubtedly, I have been talking nonstop, but nearing the end of this hour, I leaned back in my chair and suddenly felt as if every bone in my body gave way: a 'bottom' fell out of my world. The atmosphere itself became thick, as if I were breathing and speaking underwater. I said goodbye to Dr. P., walked home to my small Chelsea apartment, and lay down on the bed. Suddenly, I had a vision – an inner event that felt absolutely real. The vision was of a single image – a big piece of white, rutilated quartz lit up within as if the stone had been struck by lightning. Shadowy rutilations within the stone glowed.

I Immediately felt that the shining fractures in this luminous stone outlined the history of my life, as if the stone pictured my sense of 'having' a personal history. The white stone gave me a map of my inner world, a map including light and dark, broken and whole, personal history and impersonal circumstance. Psyche's visionary presentation of this image to me felt like a gift. I 'knew' I had a soul in pain, but I couldn't really *feel* what I knew until the psyche let me 'see' it, imaged in this shining vision of a piece of rutilated stone. I tried to describe the vision to my analyst, and she received me with interest and concern. And while the vision faded quickly, my 'inner and outer atmosphere' stayed thick, as if it were charged with powerful energies both physical and emotional. I did not sleep deeply (at least this is how I remember it) for close to fifty days.

This may sound odd, even now. I knew about dreams, and by that time, I knew about psychology; I had a master's degree in psychology, for goodness sake. I had studied archetypal patterns in poetry and written poems and published them. From the outside, it *seemed* as if I knew about 'the inner world.' But this was different. What had been missing for me all along was something like a *sense* of myself – a sense of personhood, I would say now – a sense of having a personal center, a 'place' inside where inner and outer worlds could come together. The process of feeling my way into relationship with that center was the gift of psyche's companioning.

One year later, I was in Zurich, Switzerland, about to begin auditing a semester of courses at the C. G. Jung Institute in Kusnacht. I was auditing classes for a year, preparing for later analytic training at the C. G. Jung Institute in New York. Years earlier, I believed that the only psychological theory that could encompass my life and experience was what I knew of Jung's, and although I hadn't known then that this interest would take me into training, I believed that I had to follow this path. The present Zurich sojourn was part of that effort. Very much alone, with limited resources, I rented a tiny third floor room in a lovely Kusnacht home from a woman named Frau Bodmer, and one day soon after classes began, someone knocked on Frau Bodmer's door. Because Frau Bodmer wasn't home, I answered the bell: there stood a small, wizened, bent, white-haired Swiss person wearing a Swiss hat and what looked like Swiss mountaineering clothes. He looked like a mountain elf of human size, and he held out to me a cigar box full of shiny white quartz stones. He talked and talked, and I couldn't understand a word – I knew no Swiss-German; as I tried to thank him and close the door, he picked out a piece of deeply rutilated white quartz from the middle of his box, handed it to me, turned away, and left.

The memory of my earlier vision flooded my mind, and I felt breathless. Here, with an actual stone from the outer world, delivered into my hand by a wizened little Swiss man, my inner and outer worlds came together in a shocking *coniunctio*, a pattern linking an uncanny matrix of connectedness. I told myself this could all be explained as a strange coincidence, but I did not believe that then, nor can I now. My previous life had led me to severe dissociation between my inner and outer worlds – a condition known to older cultures (and to the shaman) as a loss of soul. This *coniunctio* was another of psyche's gifts – a moment of healing integration between inner and outer worlds that let me feel that I was in the right place, at the right time. A synchronous incident brings news of the soul's return.

Soul simply can't fully come to presence until it is integrated within *a person*. If parts of a soul are missing, or lost in another world, we tip over into the shaman complex, and that's what happened to me. Witnessing a pattern between inner and outer worlds, between spirit and matter and between the unconscious and consciousness, is perhaps exactly what we mean by 'meaning,' and this was a second, incredibly meaningful coincidence, which is precisely Jung's definition of 'synchronicity.' But meaning means nothing without a person who finds something meaningful, and the shaman, mediating between the worlds on behalf of the soul, was the first individual in whom two worlds came together. (I had yet to stumble across the fact that white quartz was considered to be a stone for shamanic divination.) If I had further doubt about a shamanic pattern, it was erased eight years later, when – heralding another coming together of inner and outer worlds – the 'robin' taxi arrived to take me to my final examinations.

As in Theodore Roethke observes, 'things without hands take hands; eternity's not easily come by.'[6] When synchronicity is in the air, things without hands take hands in this life too: these two experiences – the first, of the white stone, one inner and one outer, the second my experience of the 'robin' taxi arriving at my door off the streets of New York City – formed a major inner signpost for me on my often confusing journey. Synchronicity is like that: it gives us hope. About such experiences, Jung writes,

> Reason evaporates and another power spontaneously takes control – *a most singular feeling which one willy-nilly hoards up as a secret treasure* no matter how much one's reason may protest [. . .] [Synchronous events] break through the monotony of daily life with salutary effects, [sometimes!] shaking our certitudes and lending wings to the imagination.
>
> (1963b, CW18: 787–789, italics mine)

Once in the early years of my training, as I marched around Joseph's music studio singing and humming to his accompaniment, I heard myself say 'well, in some profound way, everything is synchronous.' Since then, I have wondered what I meant. Now I would say that I was intuiting that matrix of uncanny connections between the worlds that surrounds us all the time. 'Psyche' can be a word for this *matrix of meaning* in which we live (mostly unknowingly), as if we were fish in water. This is a matrix that carries the meaning we find and feel as soul. But without a conscious personality that registers the psyche as such and 'tunes in,' the question of meaning is meaningless. Despite how frequently Jung talked about the necessity for consciousness and wholeness (the Anthropos) as a prerequisite of consciousness, he seldom mentioned that consciousness can take up residence only in a person, and the uncanny connectivity and archaic depths of psyche finds its affective ground only in personal love.

Perhaps the almost religious significance with which we regard 'the personal' today was best captured for us in the work of Dante, who – in the thirteenth century, nearing the end of his journey – glimpsed the 'love that moves the Sun and the other stars.' Staring transfixed into the eternal light, Dante saw *the human form* at its center, and in this moment, Dante's capacity to bear witness to his singular (personal) love for his singular Beatrice became a cultural beacon for the psyche's whole inner world. Perhaps the divine light and the human form *together* constituted Dante's experience of the Anthropos or the whole of human-being-ness; perhaps Dante even glimpsed the 'soul' of the human form he saw. But *Dante did not see himself seeing* the splendor of his wonderful vision, and that personal capacity, to see oneself seeing, is psyche's legacy to us.

To me, the image of Dante glimpsing the human form in the heart of the Godhead is as compelling as Dante's vision of the Godhead was to him. In our time, we understand that *psyche* allows us to see ourselves seeing, feel ourselves feeling, and sense ourselves sensing, and we believe that the pattern that emerges from this meta-vision is profoundly meaningful. Understanding the psyche as the matrix of meaning, we also understand that affect grounds the psyche in personhood. Because Dante channeled his personal passion into creativity, we – reading his book a hundred and fifty years after psyche's discovery – see Dante seeing his vision, and we become self-aware, recognizing ourselves with a symbolic apprehension that is psyche's gift to us in the twenty-first century.

Becoming a person is not the same thing as being an individual, although this is another distinction that Jung seldom made. Being an individual implies differentiation from the tribe, from the social collective, and embracing one's true 'orphan-hood,' but it doesn't mean developing our own personalities or becoming inwardly and outwardly ensouled people. As the shaman complex is brought to consciousness, wrestling one's way through it gives a modern person mutative openings toward new adaptive possibilities and new connections between inner and outer worlds. Perhaps alchemy pointed toward the distinction between individual and person in alluding to the 'small work' of individual development, on the one hand, and the 'great work' (*rubedo*) of living a passionate life with no holds barred as a person in the world in human community, on the other: becoming inwardly ensouled and outwardly related is indeed a 'great work,' and among other things, it means living a symbolic life. A symbolic life is not necessarily a good life, nor is it necessarily complete. More likely, a symbolic life has been broken and repaired, hopefully within a community of others whose lives have been similarly broken and repaired. But living a symbolic life *can* be experienced as living a healing life, and – perhaps – living a life that others value as being somewhat healed as well.

So it's back to tending kitchen pots – randomly broken but mending again with gold.

Notes

1 Eliot Weinberger's back-cover review of Clayton Eschelman's *Juniper Fuse*.
2 *The American Heritage Dictionary*. New York: Houghton-Mifflin. 1973; also *Webster's New World Dictionary*. New York: The World Publishing Company. 1953.
3 See Quinan, Clarence: 'The American Medicine Man and the Asiatic Shaman: A Comparison,' in *The Annals of Medical History*, New Series. Volume 10. New York: Harper and Brothers. 1938. 509.
4 See Vasilevich, G. M.: 'Early Concepts About the Universe Among the Evenks,' in *Studies in Siberian Shamanism*. Edited by Henry M. Michael. Toronto: University of Toronto Press. 1963. 46–83.
5 For a discussion of Jung's description of these two kinds of complexes, see Donald Kalsched, *The Inner World of Trauma*. London and New York: Routledge. 1996. 90–91.
6 'Infirmity,' by Theodore Roethke.

Part 2

Seven expressive attributes used by the shaman

Mask, rhythm, silence, respiration, movement, sound, and gesture

Chapter 7

Introduction to the attributes

The archaic shaman

Imagine the following scene: thirty-five thousand years ago, a *masked* figure emerges from dark shadows – perhaps from a cave – to dance around a fire burning in the center of a ceremonial space. Flickering light sculpts the faces of those who watch, *silently* attentive to their every move. The shaman's *posture*, *gesture*, and *movements* mimic the birds and beasts of the great desert surround. The *rhythmic* pounding of their feet rises and falls like the heartbeat of the animal they portray. Their own *breath* comes quick and fast, muttering the *sounds* of conversation with a spirit world. Tribespeople drum around the fire and around the dancer, echoing the heartbeat of a second world – their own.

This shaman has had a journey, unasked for though it was. They come now to tell their fellow tribespeople about the spirits the shaman encountered: what the spirits revealed, where healing plants can be found, where the great bison herd will next appear. Their journey would not have been undertaken had they not been a figure of exquisite sensitivity, able to register unconscious distress or suffering in the people around them. They are enacting a sacrament long before psyche, as we know it, came into being. We might say that because of shared unconscious pain, the human attributes that are italicized in the previous paragraph become, through the shaman, shamanically sacramentalized and thus imbued with unconscious intent.

Let's say that the archaic shaman's postures and gestures make visible an answer to their tribe's need to see a yet-to-be-articulated image of life after death that lies beneath the hungers or fears that make up the people's daily anxieties. *As an image carrier and an image maker, a shaman could enact qualities of human character that gave their tribe a collective, inner vision or fantasy that gave the tribespeople's lives meaning in the moment.* This happened as a shaman's gestures and postures elaborated the kind of rites and sacramental acts in which all our arts have their origins, in which social coherence might be founded, and in which would reside fossil imagery of nearly every religious conception that later civilizations would come to develop over time.

Such archaic communication was preverbal, nonverbal, and 'extra-verbal,' mediated through the attributes that are the subject of this chapter. From a later objective vantage point, we can say that the archaic shaman seemed to mediate immersion in the collective psyche directly into the senses and perceptions of their fellow tribespeople, thereby activating their deepest imaginings. We can also say that today, when someone behaves in ways that activate the deepest imaginings (including unconscious suffering) in another person and consciousness is lacking, that individual is behaving in a shamanic fashion, or – in the language of this work – that the shaman complex has been activated.

The modern psychotherapist must be aware of these shamanic ways of communication and how they become activated in the psyche. Otherwise, the therapist may become unconsciously fascinated with projected evil, suffering, or pain in another, and such fascination suggests mutual unconsciousness and lack of vision: hence, my efforts to differentiate various images of the archaic shaman from the shaman complex. When modern therapists sacrifice unconscious identification with the shaman's image, for example, the legacy of the archaic shaman becomes a symbol of the natural roots and channels of personality, offering deeper connections to primitive levels of the personal psyche. I propose that our acquaintance with the following attributes enables us to make these differentiations.

I have also proposed that an unconscious image of the archaic shaman 'dances' on the threshold of an individual's emerging consciousness. Earlier, I suggested that the figure of the shaman led the evolution of collective consciousness as well. In both cases, communicating preverbal, unconscious experience requires vehicles like the shamanic attributes that are the subject of the seven brief meditations that follow. Rooted in the human body, these attributes allow primitive affects, instincts, and images to express themselves relatively unhindered. It is almost as if such primitive energies 'want' to become conscious, but only individual consciousness can link personal history with emergent meaning and memory, and only when individual consciousness arises in the between space of a holding relationship is there safety enough to promote and contain the resulting emergent awareness.

Personal example

Fast-forward thirty-five thousand years to a here and now that happened fifty or so years ago, as I began to do vocal work with my voice coach Joseph (see Introduction). While I had few illusions about becoming a singer, I had been concerned about how little 'voice' I had in my personal life. So, in this initial session, I told Joseph that I thought my voice lacked authority.

'Can you simply strengthen it,' I asked?

'We'll see,' Joseph replied, and we got to work.

For several weeks, I easily sang the melodies that Joseph played on the piano, following with words from sheet music. Despite acute discomfort at making such funny faces and awkward sounds, the singing exercises mostly made me laugh.

Joseph always sang along with me. The studio was spacious, lit through big windows facing Lexington Avenue, and as I moved around, I began to hear my own voice more deeply, and I opened to the feelings that were stirred by uttering the words. Slowly, I became accustomed to taking deep breaths (and I immediately stopped smoking), as new muscles strengthened and a more flexible diaphragm began to develop. Then, abruptly, I entered a phase where I couldn't bear to hear myself give voice to the words that I heard myself sing.

'Hum, then!' Joseph said, 'Keep your voice going!'

So, I hummed, and Joseph kept playing and humming with me. I marched around the room to the pounding rhythm, eyes lowered and mouth closed, my body and breath moving in time with the music's beat, all the while experiencing the sound of my voice extending from the soles of my feet out the top of my head, forming a kind of vibratory backbone of energy that I could *feel*. It was as if I were feeling myself energetically reassembled as a 'whole being' for the first time, mind and body together. In retrospect, I believe that this was the experience that activated the archetype of the Anthropos in my psyche: the pattern of becoming a whole person was a sensate experience of *feeling* whole that flooded ego awareness. It also resulted in an eruption of affects, dreams images, visions, other sensations, and synchronicities. An experience of myself from within and without, and top to bottom all at once, was powerful indeed. And consciously holding all of this suddenly became a task of heroic proportions.

Looking back, those days were telescoped into one intensive year in which I was in both a highly charged verbal analysis and an equally highly charged preverbal 'practice,' as different from one another as chalk from cheese or silence from sound. I realized that these two 'practices' were mutually igniting, creating space for the copresence of parts of myself that had been separated for years. One time, my analyst worried aloud about split transference, but for me, this dual experience was anything *but* a split. In fact, the two situations created an opening that allowed space and place into which a new 'me' could – and did – emerge. This space provided a necessary gap into which all that previously had been dissociated from my personality development poured into my rapidly expanding personal consciousness, filling body *and* mind, making me feel like one embodied, personally sensate 'vessel' of sound.

Because I could no longer bear what I was feeling, or give voice to the impersonal phrases that sheet music presented, I could only move, marching around like a dancing shaman, inwardly personalized feeling emerging out of a highly activated bodily self, as into that self, impacted memories bloomed – emotional memories of which I held no conscious recognition. At home, I spent hours walking round and round my tiny apartment, practicing voice and thinking to myself, 'I'm not making mandalas, I'm *walking* mandalas, pushed into being through me!' Other mandala-like material (see the eye vision in Illustration 1) had been part of earlier experience, but now, Being-like mandalas came and went through my ego's sense of physical aliveness, and I was pacing them out. During this time, I also painted a few dreams, and I began work on a round, table-like piece of plywood, layering acrylic into a mold that covered randomly collected shells that I had arranged so that they flared out from the center, like rays in a sun disc. I meant this round table to convey what I imagined it might be like to gaze into the depths of an inner sea.

Foregoing experiences such as these allowed me to track shamanic attributes as they became activated in my own psyche and as they slowly changed. For example, my voice, originally experienced as weak and disconnected from my body, became more supple and more expressive, a stronger instrument for the expression of deeper sound; my gestures loosened, becoming smoother and more expressive of 'me.' My breathing became regular and deep. It was as if, in my case, the attributes became vehicles through which a consciously apprehended (and ultimately sacrificed) shaman complex led me through a deconstruction of a falsely adapted (and defended) self. The attributes underwent transformation too, and I slowly emerged with a more authentic, personal, and embodied sense of self.

It is fair to say that before working with Joseph, I had 'forgotten' my body; my conscious abilities to adapt and accommodate to my environment had served me all too well. And yet, over time, as the attributes underwent their various transformations, I also came to realize that everything that had ever happened to me was registered somewhere in the container of my body, carried in nerve and cell, impulse and memory, muscle and bone. I was the 'vessel' or container of myself.

The animal body

To repeat, these various attributes have their roots in a mute animal body that has not yet learned to 'speak' a language that we associate with conscious self-reflection. Our European fairytales suggest that we human beings once lived at peace with the animals and understood animal speech. In the archaic shaman's world, an animal was not only a creature or beast but also a vital potential for renewal and transformation. The unquestionable, instinctive integrity of an important animal – friend or foe, food or deity – was considered to be a fundamental resource. And participation in the splendor of such a creature was of the nature of religious experience from which new human energy emerged and new human beginnings were made.

After a primordial catastrophe comparable to a biblical 'fall,' we became as we are today, limited and defined, obliged to work to feed ourselves, and often at enmity with animals and our instinctive selves. Somewhere within we can imagine – or do we remember? – how it was when instincts were at peace with one another and 'the lion lay down with the lamb.' But we are far from the Peaceable Kingdom today. When we objectify ourselves, we separate from our innate capacity for instinctive understanding and rapport with earlier, more primitive levels of life and memory, as well as the psyche on which these depend. But even in states of alienation, the attributes serve as portals for channeling animal memory.

Psyche and soma

Psyche brings to the ego an introverted experience of body and an extroverted experience of the world in language that is generated by the shaman complex. Individually, we experience bodily life and functioning moment by moment over time as if over a wide river of shared reality, whether we name that river the objective psyche, the collective unconscious, the primary thinking process, or simply life itself. 'Knowing' bodily life, we name it as our 'earth,' in which autonomic and parasympathetic nervous systems function, and we know *of* bodily life when our capacities of intuition and sensation bring us a sense of bodily facticity. However, we forget this bodily awareness. Consciousness reigns. Yet only by way of an individual body ego can we personally experience ourselves as 'vessels' or containers of ourselves. And only by way of individual body egos can we realize that everything that ever happened to us is registered somewhere in our unique container, carried in nerve and cell, impulse and memory, muscle and bone. Our senses finger the world around us, and our bodies deliver the world to our minds by way of these attributes that I am calling shamanic.

Only an infant body can encode our earliest preverbal experience, to say nothing of the archaic antinomies of the archetypal psyche. The more deeply we explore layers of the collective unconscious, the more unified we find psyche and body to be. For example, unconscious conflict in the psyche can affect the body, just as bodily illness can affect the psyche, because a body is not a thing we have but rather an experience that we are. Psyche and soma are not separate: both express one and the same life, and this is especially so at the earliest stages of human existence. Contemplation of one's 'original nature,' therefore, means to consult one's implicit memory of primitive bodily being.

None of this is new knowledge – this knowledge of origins – including the origins of the psyche embedded in the body's reality. But it seems as if each of us has to forget what many human cultures take for granted. Many of our religions, particularly those with a mystical tradition, hold traces of the kind of wisdom we need and psyche we must recover: 'This body is the field,' states the *Bhagavad Gita* (XIII, i), and a verse from the Pali Canon reads, 'My friend, in this very body, six feet of it, with its senses, thoughts and feelings, is the world, the origin of the world, the ceasing of the world and the way of its cessation.' Ancient Egyptians referred to the body as the net, understanding the body as a device for catching what can be caught and as something in which we are inevitably enmeshed. Even today, Christian ritual tells us, 'Take, eat, this is my body,' and what the figures of Buddha and Jesus hold most in common is the idea of becoming an individually embodied carrier of human consciousness. More currently (1854), Chief Sealth, a Coastal Salish person, wrote in a letter to President Pierce,

> One thing we know which the white man may one day discover . . . our God is the same God. You may think now that you own him as you wish to own our

> land. But you cannot. He is the Body of Man. And his compassion is equal for the red man and the white. This earth is precious to him. And to harm the earth is to heap contempt upon its creator.[1]

With a wisdom that puts to shame our current treatment of the planet we call home, Chief Sealth equates God and the body of humankind with the earth itself, mother of us all.

For early human beings, bodies were sacred, whether as ornamental vessels or dwelling places of power. Therefore, images or color painted on the body portrayed graphic, dynamic, inward transformation. The bodily attributes listed earlier were the shaman's most potent implements of ritual power – sounds, gestures, facial expressions, movements, and other forms of sacramental action employed by a shaman in a ritual calling. Foremost among an archaic shaman's collection of sacramental paraphernalia (e.g., rattles and drums, batons, magical items) were costume, headdress, and animal mask. When covered or masked, a shaman's head was understood to be a seat of transformative power, the site of transformation itself: to put on another head was to admit another spirit, and the loss of a shaman's everyday shape and physiognomy made this transformation evident.

Thus, I suggest, the more consciously we are able to relate to psychosomatic levels of our own experience, the more consciously we will relate to an activated shaman, because an activated complex emerges at primitive levels of preverbal, embodied expression, and it will be pictured or symbolized by various unconscious behaviors that are expressed by way of the attributes to be described in the following seven chapters or meditations.

What exactly *is* an attribute?

By definition, an attribute is an embodied quality or characteristic of a person. Attributes are situational, individually expressed, and, in that we all partake of attributes, they are collective in nature. Detached from a person, agent, or enactor vis-à-vis another person or world, an attribute has no substantial reality. I've thought of the attributes as pools of participatory being that we experience *with* each other and *in* each other, often as personal characteristics or personality traits. They are participatory pools of human experience of self and other, inner and outer, by which we are able to access deep levels of the unconscious and mythic dimensions of life. There may be as many ways of perceiving attributes as there are people or as many ways as there are leaves on the artichoke of my earlier dream (see Chapter 5).

That we cannot conceptualize or intellectually formulate an attribute's ultimate nature means that, ipso facto, we will experience it as ineffable. We can only sketch an attribute's essence, surrounding it with images, associations, and symbolic amplifications. While I treat the attributes separately in the following pages, and while one may stand out or be more apparent in a situation than the others, in reality, attributes overlap and occur together all the time. A good image of a human being experiencing themselves through several overlapping attributes at once can be seen in Messina's famous little painting of the *Annunciation* from the Palermo Museum in Sicily. In this particular portrait of the Virgin, Mary is shown at the moment she is inspired by the Holy Spirit. Unlike other painters of his time, Messina does not separately depict a spiritual power (e.g., the angel Gabriel) inspiring the event. Instead, Messina depicts a very human Mary, inwardly 'seized' by psyche's world. In Messina's luminous depiction, several attributes overlap, as they do in life. Clearly inspired (respiration), the Virgin looks within, her mask depicting her inner experience with an instinctively silent (silence) gesture (gesture/posture, movement). The rhythm of Mary's (and Messina's) inner experience resonates with the painter's inspiring use of color, composition, and brush.

Attributes in the shaman's domain

Each attribute that we will explore was a principle of existence or a dominant expressive factor in the great unconscious domain of the archaic shaman. When it was used as an unconscious instrument, each attribute became a sacrament, depicting an aspect of the shaman's implicit professional task of realigning and balancing the collective psyche of the group. When they become imbued with unconscious intent in a contemporary person, these common human attributes may still be understood as shamanic sacramentals, which means that their dynamics act directly and autonomously from and on whatever unconsciousness is present.

Under certain circumstances, and particularly with trauma, a specific form of expression may become fixed and rigid precisely *because* it has become valuable to the *psyche's* survival, which means that the attribute has not developed into something valuable to an individual *person's* aliveness and individuation. Things like habitual facial expressions, habitual gestures and postures, and habitual sounds still serve the psyche's intention. It also means that such unconsciously fixed 'forms' have become repeatable – and often obsessional – instruments that serve the unconscious intent of a personality's survival rather than a person's conscious ego intent. Ego choice is not yet possible, and they do not serve a developing, conscious personality. In this sense, when a shamanic attribute is fixed and rigid, it has become a repository of *unconscious defenses* that lead to an unconsciously primitive quality of personality, and its activation indicates the shaman un-sacrificed and on the rampage. 'Shamanic primitivity' implies both merger with and alienation from the unconscious, since we cannot relate to something if we are identified with it. Paradoxically, a primitive mode of experience may be total, but if it is unrelated to a conscious ego, it cannot become personal experience that can be remembered. Unconscious primitivity is barbaric because it depicts a dangerous and lonely condition of rootlessness. The philosopher Santayana tells us that to have no memory of the past is to be at the mercy of the past, and in a psychological paraphrase, to have no conscious experience of the depths is to be at the mercy of the depths: similarly, to have no conscious experience of the shaman complex is to be at the mercy of shamanic energy.

As we slowly bring the shaman complex into consciousness, the process of wrestling one's way through it provides modern people with mutative openings toward new adaptive possibilities, and by becoming aware of the attributes within themselves, psychotherapists are given the opportunity to cultivate psychological and emotional literacy. How, when, and whether an attribute 'ignites with significance' will point us to unconscious, personally shared backgrounds of unconscious suffering and possible shamanic sacramentalization, and it will warn us against fascination with the unconscious needs of another and of shamanic, enacted behavior. For all of us, working through the shaman complex is equivalent to giving up one's innocence (i.e., unconsciousness) in a slow, deepening process of gaining psychological wisdom (i.e., emotional maturity). Reading about the attributes, pondering them, remembering them, and meditating on them, whether in or out of therapeutic hours is the equivalent to undertaking a kind of 'yoga of consciousness.' After using the attributes as lenses through which to look at personal memory and experience, therapists may assume an attribute as an imaginative *asana*, a psychological position that therapeutic consciousness can fruitfully assume.

Note

1 Quoted in "Myth and the Quest for Meaning: Earth and Spirit," in *Parabola*. Volume VI. Number l. Winter. 1967. 7.

Chapter 8

Mask

The cultural history of the mask and its dramatic representations ranges throughout the world, from Egyptian zoomorphs, and the Hindu elephant-headed, human-bodied Ganesha, through the Minoans with their legendary minotaur, to our modern theatrical masks, comedy and tragedy, implying the cleansing release of laughter and tears. Earlier images in the form of animal powers hearken back to our archaic beginnings, as if to remind us that the mask carries the numinous power of nature itself. Later images of the gods remind us of the great dramatic plays of the Greeks – where the powers of nature were brought 'down' into human cultural forms – manifestations that began to inform the archetypal stories of people the world over. Because it occupies this threshold between the natural and the human, the mask is one of the most powerful of the shamanic attributes, and it can be dramatically illustrated in many facets of the psychotherapeutic dialogue, as we will discuss.

The mask as intermediate reality

The experience of seeing a masked human being is probably as old as the first shaman and as recent as last Halloween. But the different ways we've thought about this experience – in history and in clinical situations – have evolved over time. We find perhaps our earliest portrayal of a masked human being in the sketch of the beast-human figure of the Sorcerer of the Trois Freres Cave in Ariege, France. There, peering out from behind an erect reindeer form, stands a startled-looking human being who stands on human feet. The question is, do we see this masked human as we suppose our earliest ancestors did – as a living mask whose covering proclaims an identity of its own – that is, as a 'god' appearing in the flesh? Or do we see a person whose identity is hidden by wearing a mask? In the latter case, we are obliged to hold two views at once – and this is the beginning of a symbolic attitude.

Joseph Campbell (1969, 33) writes,

> In the primitive world, where the clues to the origin of mythology must be sought, gods and demons are not conceived of in the way of hard and fast,

> positive realities. The phenomenon of the primitive mask . . . is a case in point. [On the one hand] it is revered as an apparition of the mythical being that it represents, yet everyone knows that a man made the mask and that a man is wearing it. . . . In other words there has been a shift of view [from a literal identification] to a theatrical or play sphere . . . and the logic is that of 'make-believe' – 'as if.'

In terms of the psyche's evolution, the movement over time of the first way of 'seeing' to the second parallels how the personal psyche began to emerge from the collective psyche over time: in turn, psychotherapy echoes this emergence in how our patients develop a sense of personal awareness of the difference between their transference projections onto the 'mask' of the therapist's face and the personal reality lying behind it. This personal awareness accumulates and leads to a deepening sense of personhood within the patient, making them feel more real in a world becoming more real as well.

Idealizing energies that elevate the image of one's therapist to a godlike 'mana personality' are likely to be disillusioned over the course of psychotherapeutic treatment, but hopefully not all at once. One experiences oneself moving from enthrallment with the power of the mask as a projected image to seeing through to the hidden human being wearing a *persona*. I remember my shock when I realized that I was taller than one of my idealized analysts, someone who had loomed over my interior and exterior landscapes for several years. My unconscious 'magnification' of him masked my ability to see him clearly. This experience was an important increase in my sense of my own personhood and myself. In other words, we cannot progressively see through what we project into an outer object or person without simultaneously accruing progressive insight into an inner world and ourselves.

Frank Baum gives us a wonderful example of this in his stories of *Dorothy and the Wizard of Oz*. Through volume after volume, Baum depicts a child's (Dorothy's) experience of magnified voice and power rendered by a 'wizard's' oracular mask. When Dorothy finally recognizes the little man who actually lives behind her 'great expectation' of a wizard, she sees through 'two worlds' twice over: a mist of projection clears, shards of archetypal reality fall about Dorothy's feet, and the psyche's creative 'act' unites 'two worlds.' Dorothy suddenly feels like herself again, aware that she is facing a simple, worried man behind a mask. Becoming conscious places Dorothy back in Kansas into the midst of a personal life.

Mask as power: where between space is reified

In ancient ceremonies of the mask, the wearer of a mask functioned as a psychic conduit, personifying the contents of the collective unconscious to others and sometimes becoming virtually identical with them. In other words, the mask itself had power. In some societies, a mask might have its own house; food might be left for it, and it could be approached and handled only by special guardians. If a mask appeared in your dreams, you had been approached by the numen itself, because the mask was a repository of sacred power.

One contemporary myth from an Indigenous people in what is now called Delaware, the Lenape, presents a situation in which the mask as such is experienced as a god. For the Lenape, Misinghalikun (Living Solid Face) is a fur-clad figure with a wooden face – a living mask, rather than representing a deity with a human face or an animal disguise. Following disaster, Misinghalikun teaches his people how to make a mask like him, promising that when they wear his mask, his spirit will enter in. It is as if among the Lenape that the mask itself had become something of a daimon, a powerful intermediate being with its own peculiar ontology (*Mystical Rites and Rituals*, 1975, 98). For this tribe, Living Solid Face is a teacher and a moralist, a healer of children and a beneficent guardian over tribe and hunt.

The Greeks had a different point of view. Among the Greeks, the mask was no longer a one-dimensional power but had begun to evolve into human self-reflection. In the Greek theater, for example, actors wore masks only while depicting dramatic roles in a play. When 'speaking aside,' the chorus embodied a change of view, dropping their masks as if to imply that while the mask itself belongs to unreflecting, transpersonal, nonhuman beings (a character in a role, in a play), beneath a mask is a human self, who comments on what happens. In the Greek imagination, under the aegis of a mask, action and behavior remained autonomous and transpersonal, but conversation, consideration, and reflection began to become human privileges.

Mask and '*original time*'

Psychologically, a masking image always faces in two directions, and although the image flirts both with inner and outer reality, divine and human, the image itself stays 'in-between.' This intermediate, in-between-ness conjures up what Patrick Harpur (1994) calls daimonic reality, which we might think of as the paradoxical space of the human imagination. D.W. Winnicott (1971) called this space transitional space.

The mask's blurring or co-inherence of boundaries is the essence of magic, and it embodies the double function of all imagery, whether in art or in dream. In one form or another, magic always explores the mysterious bond 'between' an image (spirit/psyche) and its material or human object. Thus, on the one hand, when a shaman put on a mask, they occupied the threshold between 'two worlds.' One world embraced a paradisiac age, *in illo tempore*, a sacred mythic time when the gods mingled freely with men – a time before 'the fall,' or a mythic event that caused a rupture between heaven and earth – a time when humans and animals spoke the same language. We might call this a world of *original time*.[1] In the second world, a shaman was a person behind a mask, 'ordinary,' separated from animals and gods like the rest of their people, consigned – like others – to sickness and death.

Mircea Eliade (1964) makes clear how important the shaman and their mask were in mediating *original time*:

> we know that, *in illo tempore* ('in *those* days,' parentheses mine), in the mythic time of Paradise, a Mountain, a Tree or Pillar . . . connected Earth with Heaven, so that primordial man could easily go up into Heaven by climbing it. Communication with Heaven *in illo tempore* was simple, and meetings with the gods took place *in concreto*. The remembrance of this paradisiac period is still vividly present to these primitives. The Koryaks remember the mythical era of their hero Great Raven, when men could go up to Heaven without any difficulty: in our days, they add, it is only the shamans who are still capable of this. . . . The shaman, during his journey, returns to the paradisiac condition. He reestablishes the communications that used to exist *in illo tempore* between Heaven and Earth. . . . Lastly, the shaman renews the friendship with the animals. . . . In this respect, the mystical experience of primitives is equivalent to a journey back to the origins, a regression into the mythical time of the Paradise lost.
>
> (65–66)

When a shaman wore a bison mask, for example, they danced a story about where the bison god would grace his people's hunger with lifegiving food, thereby bringing the power of the gods into human presence, connecting this world with the next. Poet W. H. Auden (1944) says, 'We who must die demand a miracle,' and by linking the finite and the infinite through the medium of the mask, an archaic shaman 'storied' just that miracle; that is, they narrated an intermediate 'between' space that recovered *original time* for their people – thus, a shaman's extraordinary mana, or charisma.

Ritually worn, an animal headdress and mask conjoined human and nonhuman worlds, bridging the gap between the natural (transpersonal) and human order of things. So strong was the belief that wearing a mask actually transformed the identity of its wearer that the use of a mask was strictly confined to rituals that marked crucial events of tribal life, where the space between worlds was thin. Tribal customs and strong taboos ensured that when put to ritual use, any adornment with animal parts had magically powerful significance. For example, wearing antlers could bestow powers of swift running or sexual potency. Both wearing and seeing a horned head drew on powers in the natural world that were thought to be both demonic and benign.

A mask magnified the shaman's voice, lowered their accessibility to oxygen and severely restricted their field of vision, so the very act of wearing a mask enabled them to focus on an inner world to a point where they represented particular animals so concretely as to make them reappear. Mask's ceremonies allowed shamans and those participating through shamanic mediation to evoke an experiential zone of *original time*, wherein the usual radical differences between human and animal, Earth and Heaven, no longer held. The idea was never to *return* to that time – that would have been a literal regression – but rather to revisit it, so that the people might recall *original time* and benefit from it, absorbing its healing power and meaning.

Mask and psychotherapy

The psychotherapeutic structure presents a similarly charged situation. For example, as therapists, we know that we can never 'be' a patient's mother or father, but we also know that simply by being who we are, we are apt to 're-present' a parental mask, inviting our patients to revisit an earlier, often unremembered version of *original time* – that is, the deep unconscious. We invite them to revisit *original time symbolically*. We also imagine that repeated experiences of *original time* will enable a patient to recover preverbal (dissociated) material and that a slow, patient, and repeated recovery of dissociated 'pieces of self' promotes a sense of psychological wholeness, including the implicit possibility of what Michael Balint (1968) called a new beginning. Balint points out that a new beginning means both (1) going back to something 'primitive,' to a point before a child's faulty development started – that is, regressing, but not in the usual pathological sense – and (2) discovering at the same time a new, better-suited way, which amounts to a progression. Balint's famous example (132) is a patient who, in an act of spontaneity and aliveness, suddenly got up from his couch and did a somersault in Balint's consulting room.

Personal experience of mask (a new beginning)

When I entered training, perhaps my biggest discovery was that psyche's natural defenses had been masking my whole life all along. When I really began to experience what Dr. E. called the reality of the psyche, my outer life adaptation was unmasked, or so it felt: I knew that my tendency was to take situations and people at face value, but my 'innocence' masked gullibility and blunted instinct, not trust, just as my 'shyness' masked radical disorientation and fear. At the beginning of our work together, Dr. E. asked me to write my anamnesis, so I dutifully wrote pages that took me to the age of twelve, and then I had to stop, because I found no words to describe the confusion I remembered from that point on. It seemed as if somewhere along the way, I had so misplaced my sense of 'I' that a collective, impersonal self-definition that Jung called *the persona* masked 'me' from that time on. At the same time, I wondered – I had been reading in the Jung Library – could someone have a persona of *not* having a persona? This simply meant that I became acutely aware of how inadequately defined I felt – now and for so long – and how defended I must have been against living the ordinary, undefended life for which I longed. As Maud Oakes (1987, 75) declares in her story of personal transformation, the first mask that I took off was what I believed the world wanted me to be: a mask that seemingly came about with a sense of 'ego' itself.

I've had little experience with actual masks but a lot of experience with 'masked' human faces. Early memories include myself as a small child, standing by my mother at the kitchen sink and reading her anger from her tightening jaw. No one ever raised a voice in my family, except to call the dog. When my father returned from WWII with a classic case of posttraumatic stress disorder (PTSD), his face also seemed oddly masked. It was hard to tell just what he thought or felt. Of course, in our house, feelings – personal or general – were never talked about, either.

So psychoanalysis with my earliest New York training analyst was challenging. Dr. E. was an introverted man, a quiet person by nature who was not very expressive. His dark eyes were warm, but his mostly impassive and expressionless face made it easy to imagine that he had all kinds of wisdom as well as all kinds of unspoken judgments about all kinds of things – including me. Still, an impassive face, though hard to read, is better than nothing at all: I'd had an early fear of working with anyone 'on the couch'; imagining myself in unrelated space outside a face-to-face encounter troubled me still. Seeing Dr. E.'s face, expressionless or not, anchored me in time and place when I had little knowledge of, let alone trust *in*, an 'inner world' of any kind.

Anyone who has been unconsciously identified with the role of the shaman/healer is troubled to begin with, since wounding and being wounded are the dark premises of healing, and this is practically a standing definition of someone with a shamanic personality. Perhaps this unconscious equation also defined the link between my analyst and me, both of us sharing a shamanic vocation. That these archaic channels activate in therapy as a matter of course is the open secret of the archetype of wounded healer, who has assumed the forms of gods and heroes and their destinies as far back as the early physicians of Greece (Majno, 1975, 39).

Perhaps I was drawn to Dr. E. because his face reminded me of my father's face – similarly formed and similarly expressionless – particularly after my father returned with a Purple Heart for being wounded in battle on the Island of Leyte during WWII. He 'came back' from overseas when I was seven years old, and I remember asking to see his 'scar' as I proudly showed him one of mine, a scar from a bout of acute appendicitis that had neatly divided my seven-year old abdomen in two. And probably that's why I began my work with Dr. E. by telling him all about my father, who had unexpectedly died of a brain aneurysm in his early fifties, long before I was ready to let him go. Dr. E. encouraged me to write letters to my deceased father, and the writing helped me 'tell' my father things that I hadn't had a chance to say, particularly how much I loved him, just because he was my dad. And at some time during that first year of training analysis, I pondered a line in a poem I was fashioning idly, something about looking at myself in a mirror and seeing my father's face begin to be.

A year later, simultaneous voice lessons with Joseph began, and there couldn't have been a greater contrast between facial expressiveness than there was between Dr. E. and Joseph R. Joseph's face was somewhat mask-like in repose (an orphan, Joseph suspected that his father might have been Japanese), but Joseph's intentional use of facial muscles and expressively magnified voice poured such rich affect into his teachings that I felt freed up, face and body both, simply by being in his presence. This led to my earlier comment on a striking, *feeling* difference between these two 'practices,' like chalk and cheese.

Recently, a patient of mine (a busy psychotherapist herself) described her experience under ayahuasca as seeing that she was a holograph of herself, beside a true self that she didn't know how to find. Given her early experience of a predatory, sadistically inclined father, she and I mused together about early trauma and dissociation, but I also offered Thomas Merton's words (Merton, 1966, 11–12): 'Many of us live lives of self-impersonation,' and these descriptive words struck a chord with her as well. It is possible to wear a mask of yourself that masks your real self.

Describing what his writing means to him, another 'wounded healer,' Parker Palmer (2018, 99), tells us that 'writing allows my mask to fall away so my true face can appear and get a clearer look at things I need to be facing into.' Palmer is right, of course, but almost any other creative discipline also allows the mask to fall away, and the practice of psychotherapy, no matter which chair one occupies, is a case in point. Good therapists let themselves be used as mirrors by their patients, and hopefully what patients see back is *themselves*. Therapists whose true inner reactions to another are unreadable are likely to be unconsciously shamaning. Those of us who have seen Ed Tronick's stunning still-face experiment (Tronik, 2007) have been exposed to the devastating effect on an infant or toddler of the mother's sudden, unexpected 'still face.' The mother's sudden 'mask' of unresponsiveness causes an attack of disorganizing anxiety in the children that grows only worse until taking off the 'mask,' the mother's truly responsive, mirroring face returns. Other psychologists place great emphasis on the gaze.

Jung wrote extensively about the phenomenology of the mask under the general category of the persona, which for him was the social face an individual presented to the world. One's persona was designed, on the one hand, to impress others in favorable ways according to the collective role one identified with and, on the other, to conceal the 'true self.' Jung also felt that having a flexible persona was a sign of psychological development, whereas identification with the persona was the sign of a person who has no awareness of a distinction between the 'face' they show the world and their inner self. Thus, 'saving face' and 'losing face' are concepts that refer to an unconscious identification with the persona.

How often have we (unconsciously) peered into our own faces? How often do we glance in a mirror, over a lifetime? A friend of mine, having ingested a dose of LSD, terrified herself by looking in a mirror, where she saw no reflection of herself at all. D. W. Winnicott would say that most likely, her experience was a 'memory' from the kind of *original time* the shamans knew, a memory that now, for the first time, entered consciousness. Winnicott reminds us that often the things we imagine and fear happening in the future are things that we have experienced already in an *original time* of an infancy that we do not remember. We may dread a psychosis, for example, because we've already experienced moments of nonbeing. The psyche's endless creativity brings us news of life already lived, so when we dream, psyche simply masks itself, lending us images to which we can cling and that we seldom forget. Terror itself masked my friend's pre-memory of self-erasure.

I suspect that many analytic experiences over many years of training, and years of conducting psychotherapy myself with hundreds and thousands of face-to-mask encounters and face-to-face encounters, have helped me discern the 'true face' of my soul – the inner companion that represents my true life, since the process that Jung called individuation continues for me – as it does for all of us – outside therapy of any kind. Understanding how I, and others, 'live' and enact the shaman complex, including the powerful attribute of the mask, has been crucial to this discernment. Ultimately, when masks of unconscious defensive identifications and collective ideals fall away, we search no longer for ourselves in other faces but instead glimpse ourselves in the reflections of a very different 'mirror,' the mysterious mirror of what Jung called the self within.[2]

Inner mirroring

This mask-less 'seeing' of one's own face mirrored from the self-side of things – a kind of mystical, inner mirroring by an ostensibly 'objective' observer – found room in early Christianity in one of two images that have been important to me. For example, the Russian painter Andre Rublev's original painting, *Trinity*, had a small mirror positioned on the canvas at the bottom of the round table around which the three figures of the Trinity gather. A viewer of this painting could glimpse their own reflection, *implying the presence of a 'fourth person'* at the Feast of Love, the *perichoresis* (circle dance), the ongoing exchange of love between the people of the Trinity (Rohr, 2016).

The second image comes from the Hindu world. The statue of the Cosmic Creator, Aditi, Mother of All the Gods (*Devamata*), hides a similar, small mirror at the very back of her veil. Aditi rewards the supplicant who braves the darkness of her rock-cut chamber in Kerala to pull her veil aside with a glimpse of the supplicant's own face, as if to say to the viewer, 'My real face is yours.' In both these cases, Christian and Hindu, the self-reflective viewer is pulled out of individuality *into a relational field*, be it a field of the divine exchange of love in the Trinity, or a field of becoming – with Aditi – a source of life in the River of Life. Dante also believed that 'on the farthest wall of the cave' that centers our interiority, what we see is our own face.

I want to end this chapter with two personal examples of this kind of mystical experience – coming face to face with oneself with no mask in between – through an inner process of self-reflection.

As a first example, twenty years ago, I flew to Boston for a week of training in eye movement desensitization and reprocessing (EMDR) therapeutic techniques. To me, the techniques seemed effective but remarkably impersonal. Attached as I was to my own predilection for working interpersonally, I never used EMDR in my practice. However, near the end of training, I had an experience that made me appreciate what EMDR techniques might bring about.

Submitting myself to the ministrations of two fellow students practicing their newly honed techniques, I focused inwardly on the target issue I wanted to explore, the loss of my father. This loss was something that happened to me twice. The first loss was in *original time*, when I was three, when with no warning to wife or family my father was shipped out with his battalion to fight in WWII. Inconsolable the following morning, I reportedly cried myself into a fever. The second, later, loss was in my early thirties, when my father suddenly died of a brain hemorrhage.

As I watched the moving finger of one of my colleagues-in-training, suddenly – without sobbing – I began to weep. Copiously, endlessly, silently, tears simply poured from my eyes, and the line from that long-ago poem about glimpsing my face in a mirror and seeing my father's face swam into mind, these new tears of summer-melt falling on old icy grief. Though long-stored in 'implicit mind,' these tears held the memory of loss, and a mask of denial slowly slipped away. What a relief it was now – simply to weep, below words, beyond reason.

The second example of a mask-less encounter with myself requires more background. Early in my analysis with Dr. E., I had a dream of C. G. Jung, a little white dog, and me. In that long-ago dream, Jung and I are in a room, and Jung watches me as I settle cross-legged into a yoga position to meditate. Then he rises, shaking his head and as he says, 'That's all well and good, but who will take care of the little white dog in the kitchen?' and he leaves the room. (End of dream.)

Fast-forward fifty years: one spring, not long ago, I went on a three-day Zen meditation retreat in nearby Tesuque with a small group of people and a visiting Roshi. On the first night of the retreat, I went to bed and dreamed that I was a little girl again, maybe four years old, pulling my red wagon. I often gave my baby brother a ride, and he was in the wagon now. Nearby lay a little white dog. Someone had performed a cruel experiment on it, removed its liver, and left it for dead. I knew that if I could find my mother, the little white dog could be healed, so I gathered the dog into my arms, placed it gently in the wagon with my baby brother, and set out to find her. (End of dream.)

The next morning, first thing after breakfast, Roshi John T. asked for dreams. Along with several other people, I told my dream of the little white dog and her terrible plight. (I did not remember my earlier 'white dog' dream then, but I was embarrassed by the violent imagery this 'little white dog' dream contained.) I had no idea what this specific dream was about, but I knew it pointed to wounds of my own, so after I spoke and the day's activities began, I held it in the back of my mind. We spent hours together that first day – meditating, talking – not to each other but 'into the group': eating together, walking outdoors to observe a 'pour' at Tesuque's nearby Bronze Foundry, meditating again, eating our evening meal together, meditating again, and then to bed. The second night I had another dream, and I woke in the morning with tears streaming from my eyes – again without sobs and again without images, except for my dream. But these tears clearly felt as if they surged from some 'great happiness,' a spilled-over gratitude simply for being alive. Tears streamed down my cheeks and dripped from my chin all morning long, and I mopped them with a fistful of tissues until it was my turn to speak. Still weeping, I told the group my last night's simple dream, of a small brown spider, sitting on the right-hand shoulder of a tall straw broom. (End of dream.) This little spider was innocuous enough, except that her two tiny eyes were clearly made of turquoise stone, echoed by, on her belly, two tiny, also-turquoise, spinning ducts, for spinning webs. Surely, Spider Woman visited me in last night's dream – a local version of the Great Mother, for whose arms I longed. She wore the guise of a wisdom goddess beloved by nearby the Navajo people. But I simply told the group that the dream 'felt' wondrous to me because my spider's tiny turquoise eyes and spinning ducts were made of 'living, seeing stone.'

'Kensho,' murmured one participant ('seeing one's Buddha nature'); 'ordinary mind,' murmured Roshi John T., from a koan we'd spoken of before. A moment later, the Roshi rose from his chair and wandered to a nearby window. With his back to the group, the Roshi spoke to a clearing Santa Fe rain shower beyond the glass: 'We *did* it!' he said, and Jung's story of the Taoist rainmaker flooded my mind. Had I used this group, I wondered, as my 'mother,' so my little white dog could find healing? Was my temporary community serving as gold to mend my broken pot? At the workshop's close, a friend drove me home by way of Keshi, Santa Fe's Zuni fetish store, where I just 'knew' that my little brown spider waited: and there she was, small and green-brown, with glowing turquoise eyes. To this day, she sits on a bookshelf in my office, as if to remind me always – always of what?

What do I make of all this, here and now? In a dream fifty years earlier, an image of Jung had said to himself, almost as an aside, 'Who will look after the little white dog in the kitchen?' A 'little white dog' wasn't even *in* that dream! At that time, I had no idea how to work with that dream or how to take care of a little white dog in the kitchen, even if I had found one. But something remembered: something in the psyche knew what it was doing – then *and* now – to 'image' a 'little white dog' needing care that my four-year-old dream self provided as best she could, as she searched for a mother to heal a wound at the center of life (the liver).

I now understand the little white dog as an image of my pretraumatic innocence. On the first night of the Zen retreat (the dream of a wounded little white dog), the psyche depicts my innocent early attachments, my instinctive love of life and those around me – a self of *original time*, 'forgotten' through everyday traumas of growing up. But somewhere along the way, this little white dog had been badly wounded, its trauma as deep as a cruel experiment. In the accidental context of this retreat, my little white dog returned in (my) flesh, informed by a dream of how it could heal. I mulled this dream in my mind's eye for a day, and then came my Spider Dream, bringing her healing into my life.

No consciousness can summon implicit wounding at will, since psyche alone plumbs the depths of a healing dream. Can a dream be a well, or a cauldron, that channels an uprush of love? My dream of a little brown spider somehow embraced me like a mother, and my tears overflowed in a river of gratitude. In Tibetan culture, turquoise – being both a 'living' stone' and susceptible to destruction (like human beings) – has profound symbolic value; it represents vitality and death and is a support to human life itself (Jest, 19). Had I been healed in that mothering space that only a group provides? Or was I shamaning for others of my kind – wide awake, this time? Or maybe both? Wisely guiding her people, Spider Woman taught them the arts of the loom and the planting of seasonal fields. In Jungian lore, the unconscious mothers us all, and she had sent a dream to remind me/us that she is alive and well. Upwelling tears proclaimed the psyche's spontaneous joy, and I, with unabashed openness, felt fully alive. Perhaps there had been times I had 'known' feelings like these, at home in my young mother's arms.

In illo tempore – in *original time* – such early encounters with intimate love are veiled in darkness. For example, in the Eros and Psyche myth, Psyche was not to look upon Cupid's face nor see his form until much later (Hooper, 1956). In C. S. Lewis's remarkable novel *Till We Have Faces*, Oural asks 'How can (the gods) meet us face to face till *we* have faces' (italics mine). I think what Lewis means is that until we know our own true feelings, we can't meet each other face to face, unmasked. Lewis himself explained the meaning of Oural's words by saying that we must speak 'with our own voice, not one of our borrowed voices; we must express what we actually desire, not what we imagine we desire . . . we must "be for good or ill itself, not any mask."' Lewis's meaning echoes Apostle Paul writing to the Corinthians (C13:v12): 'For now we see through a glass, darkly, but then face to face: now I know in part; but then shall I know, even as also I am known.' Wholeness can always be found beneath the broken surface of people and things.

But this experience wasn't primarily *about* my meeting the people of this group, face to face – symbolic mother though they may have been. Somehow this whole process felt like *me*, like finding the truth of my feeling life so that my own 'true face' looked back unmasked at *me* – unmasked. At age eighty-five, analyst Florida Scott-Maxwell wrote (1973, 42), 'You need only claim all the events of your life to make yourself yours. When you truly possess all you have been and done. . . *you are fierce with reality*' (italics mine). *Joyfully* 'fierce with reality' comes closest to what I experienced in that moment – as if the *feeling* of pure joy was what I'd missed my whole life. The best I can do, given Jungian schemas and concepts, is to suggest that as I offered my joy to the self, the self blessed me back.

A Buddhist teaching from *The Record of Linji* (Discourses, III) comforts my mind as well and gives me hope: Linji muses, 'There is a true person with no rank who is constantly coming in and out through the gates of your face.'

May my 'true person' hold hands with my *fierce reality*, and may all of this be so.

Notes

1 Eliade refers to this as 'paradisal time,' a mythic time of paradise lost as contrasted to time in our present 'fallen' world, ruled by laws of chronological time and history.

2 Jung often defines the self as a virtual center of a mysterious constitution. He writes, 'I have called this center the self . . . a psychological concept that serves to express an unknowable essence which we cannot grasp as such. . . . It might equally well be called the God within us.' (CW7:398–399)

Chapter 9

Rhythm

Inherent rhythm

From the moment we are conceived until the moment we die, an inherent tendency toward repetition in muscle and nerve is as innate to our bodily structure as flesh and bone. Thus, I perceive rhythm to be a basic feature of human nature, a pool of participatory being, and one of the shamanic attributes. From a rhythmic point of view, every movement we make is an experience of measured energy, a rhythmic release that happens according to laws of structural functioning that have been set up within a natural timing: work and rest, control and release, begin and end. Other internal rhythms manifest themselves in muscular tensions that we become aware of by noticing built-in kinesthetic sensitivity or as we express a simple sense of 'how it feels.'

When I was in first grade, I was an awkward, knobby-kneed, skinny little girl whose ankles turned in, so my mother enrolled me in dancing lessons in El Monte's one and only tap dance studio, run by Mrs. Haughton, the wife of a town judge. My early associations with rhythm are colored by memories of Teach, as we called her, seated at an old upright piano pounding out measures of something like 'Tea for Two and Two for Tea,' and calling out at the top of her voice above the music a sequence of steps that fifteen young tap dancers had spent the last thirty minutes trying to memorize: *step* (left foot), brush right, step, brush back (*right* foot, this time). From my usual place, third row center (at least not the *last* row), of struggling little girls collectively known as The Haughton-Tots, I tried hard to learn to tap dance. Being dyslexic didn't help, but the rhythm and music did, and soon movement rang through my bones. So, for me – and my best friend, Alice – music carried rhythm early on, and rhythm carried music, and these two and the presence of Alice carried me through class after class since I never managed to keep a dance routine in mind.

Words came later, along with an innate sensitivity to the rhythmic sounds inherent in language. I also reached for metaphor – images of likeness from the realm of bodily sensations. One or more of my senses had allowed me to perceive rhythm in the first place. Such 'felt' senses are what constellate the subjective unconscious, summoning sensations and emotions into awareness. Ivan Pavlov, reaching for words to describe the primitive exuberance that he perceived in rhythmic movement, came up with the graceful phrase, 'muscular gladness,' while somewhere the philosopher Immanuel Kant referred to music itself as a 'quickening art.' We also 'quicken' when we experience rhythm in action. Something 'feels right,' we say, as if we were listening with our muscles. In the *Timaeus*, along with number, Plato proposed that rhythm organized the cosmos, and several old Western myths present rhythm as having come into being at the same time as the first and oldest of the gods, because surely rhythm was present as Eros ordered Chaos, and the round dance of the stars began.

More recently, neurologist Oliver Sacks (1984, 219), contrasting his 'neurology of soul' with 'Sherrington-ian' neurology (the study of 'trigger puppets') and 'Lurian' neurology (the study of 'self-activating robots'), relates how, as he clambered down a mountain with a badly broken leg, rhythm and music came to his aid:

> Before crossing the stream, I had *muscled* myself along – moving by main force, with my very strong arms. Now, so to speak, I was *musiked* along. I did not contrive this. It happened to me . . . I got into the music, got into the swing, and this ensured that my tempo was right. I found myself perfectly coordinated by the rhythm – or perhaps subordinated would be a better term: the musical beat was generated within me, and all my muscles responded obediently. . . . And even when it was not literally (audibly) music, there was the music of my muscle-orchestra playing – 'the silent music of the body,' in Harvey's lovely phrase. With this playing, the musicality of my motion, I myself became the music – 'You are the music, while the music lasts' . . . a creature of muscle, motion and music, all inseparable and in union with each other – except for that unstrung part of me, that poor broken instrument (his leg) which could not join in and lay motionless and mute without tone or tune.
>
> (Sacks, 1984, 30–32)

Galen of Pergamum, a prominent Greek physician, noted that the human heart is rhythmically organized with a similarity between systolic and diastolic beats of the pulse and the *arsis* and *thesis* of a metrical foot. Whatever Galen's exact meaning may have been, he deemed that the pulse that threads through each human wrist is a built-in measure of rhythm. Centuries later in another country, counting his own pulse as he idly observed a chandelier swaying to and fro, the Italian Galileo discovered that each oscillation – small or great – had the same duration. In this discovery, Galileo used his sense of blood rhythm as a first-ever clock, demonstrating stress and time to his observing mind (Rovelli, 2017, 180).

Rhythms of heartbeat and breath guide the root grammar of our parasympathetic and sympathetic nervous systems: our passions and depressions rise and fall as if with inner planets, waxing and waning to an inner moon. Intimately tied to and integrated within these systems, the remarkable muscle of the human heart consists of a heart's mysterious power (inherent in each fiber and independent of impulse arising elsewhere) to contract and relax in a self-generated rhythm. Surely the unknown source from which this power rises lies close to the origins of life itself.

Indwelling circadian rhythm is widespread, shared by all organic life. Related to alternations of day and night, circadian (meaning 'about a day') rhythm articulates a dim awareness of a cyclical time that runs through almost every species of plant and animal. Molecular rhythms control a body's circadian rhythm, adjusting our biological rhythms to synchronize with planetary gravity. With exquisite precision, inner clocks adapt our physiology to the dramatically different phases of the day, regulating critical functions such as behavior, hormone levels, sleep, body temperature, and metabolism.[1] Curiously, the life patterns of bacteria and viruses possess neither rhythm nor a sense of time. These formless, blind life patterns are as unrhythmical as cancer cells, the growth of which affects so many of our lives (Mukherjee, 2010).

Organic characteristics of rhythm are also present in other natural activities. Thoughts and feelings proceed by rhythmic pulsations: animals 'mate in season,' women menstruate in lunar time, and plants appear and disappear with seasonal change. Lest we underestimate the effects of rhythm on a cosmic scale, the Large Hadron Collider was unable to function until its engineers remembered to factor in the pull of our moon on the earth's *bedrock* (forget about the moon's pull on ocean tides!) Until minute fluctuations in solid rock had been accounted for, rhythmic gravity phases between our planet and its moon repeatedly jostled the LHC'S carefully structured apparatus and delayed its initial operation.

Rhythm and the psyche

On a more human scale, potent sources of inspiration like poetry, song, and the cadence of human speech manifest themselves organically, as do breathing, walking, and any other whole body, muscular activity. Oliver Sacks comments that

> The fundamental object of rhythm seems to be to minister both to the stimulation and to the expression of feeling. . . . Thus rhythmic form is the channel for reflecting mental experience. To a certain extent *the rhythm of emotion determines the rhythm of motion*. . . . It is unlikely that the internal rhythms of any two individuals are the same. . . . Individual variation of the basic rhythmic patterns are what give unique value and interest to every individual's expression. If inner and outer rhythm are one, communication is rich and complete; if not, something like the dance is likely to be too physical, too much body, not enough mind through the body. . . . The source of this union between feeling and movement is a sensitive comprehension of idea, mood, rhythm and movement.
>
> (1984, 30–32, italics mine)

So, let us imagine that rhythm organizes the psyche too. Each day, every one of us fluctuates in energy, mood, well-being, and performance. Every one of us undergoes prolonged, subtle psychological alterations, every day, week, month, season, and year. Longer undulations in emotion and cycles of more subtle psychological change also occur, unnoticed. Our internal rhythms have been synchronized within a rhythmic environment from very early on. For months before birth and breath, we rocked to the heartbeat of a mothering body, sharing its pulsing blood. Echoing the mythic arrival of winged Eros, each of us proceeded out of a containing body into the chaos of a newborn world, inseparable from a world of a newborn. Once on our own, our every response to being cradled and rocked reorients us in the same way we were oriented by a mothering womb, heart centered in chemicals that swaddle and seep through us from conception onward, influencing our later health, moods, and the span of life.

An innate sense of rhythm seems to appear long before language. Babies drum on their cribs or respond to music. The sounds and cries of babies have rhythms of their own, consonant with tiny heartbeats and steady breath. A musician once told me that his father had played the saxophone to him while he was in his mother's womb. Later, as a growing infant, nothing stirred or comforted this man as quickly as the sound of the saxophone. Some infants rock themselves rhythmically, cradling themselves in and out of sleep. I remember rocking my own bed gently, gently, one six-year-old foot out of the blanket against a nearby wall, until I fell asleep.

Sometimes, moving body, spirit, and the gods, rhythm spills itself into dance. Watch how children dance, chant, march, and sing with rhythmic repetition. Not only *children* love to swing. In once-open fields, reapers sang to the rhythm of their scythes. Rowers keep the rhythm with their oars. Within such movements, instinctive energy is concentrated and released, the energy rhythmically transferred to an activity or another person. Scenes of our contemporary world may differ in goal, but discotheques present us with a similar spectacle – imagine all the energy released and channeled by repetitive rock music. Rhythm literally sweeps us along, transferring itself to everything and everyone under its influence.

Through a Jungian lens, rhythm dwells in the magical levels of psyche, relating us to what European alchemists called the vegetable soul. Rhythmed even below what we know as our most basic instincts, like sex and hunger, this realm displays itself in our relatedness to the world, to significant others, and to ourselves, overlapping in a kind of eternal present of infinite dimensions. Imagine the layers of a large red onion or a set of carved Russian dolls, one inside the other. Unfolding like plants unfold – out of air, earth, water, light, and warmth – the vegetable soul has dominion over organic growth and reproduction, deep levels of being beneath and before a separation of outer and inner worlds. This does not imply that eating or sexual activity is necessarily unconscious or involuntary but rather that all our unconscious, involuntary processes belong to the rhythms of the vegetable soul. The vegetative levels of the psyche operate within us as silently as a plant feeds directly on the soil and chemicals of the earth, out of awareness, perhaps, but formative of archaic reality, as if psyche itself rests on a bedrock of stone.

Unconscious bodies remember what we cannot. Therapists try to tune themselves, as inner and outer seasons of past experience rhythmically unfold into present awareness, in themselves as well as their patients. As if engraved into unconscious mind, anniversaries of love and loss may erupt to surprise us, flooding a distracted or dissociated ego with memories. One woman told me a dream on the anniversary of her long-ago miscarriage, an event for which at the time she was simply relieved and grateful – no big deal. Now tears overwhelmed her. Aspects of her past unknown to her present felt loss deeply and needed to grieve. Who knew? Deeply personal loss began to live in memory instead of haunting an absent broken heart. When deep grief can assume the shape of personal history rather than impersonal fate, all of us are less burdened by our collective past. And the rhythm of moving implicit experience into explicit memory differs, somehow, from that of seeing through projections.

Rhythm's shamanic legacy

Examining rhythm as a subjective experience, Jung's words suggest that few of us actually feel all we are 'given to feel' from moment to moment:

> Libido forced into regression by an obstacle always reverts to the possibilities lying dormant in the individual. A dog, finding the door shut, scratches at it until it is opened, and a man, unable to find the answer to a problem, rubs his nose, pulls his lower lip, scratches his ear, and so on. If he gets impatient, all sorts of rhythms appear: he starts drumming with his fingers, shuffles his feet about . . . when libido is forced back by an obstacle, it does not necessarily regress to earlier sexual modes of application but rather to the rhythmic activities of infancy which serve as a model both for the act of nutrition and for the sexual act itself. . . . Strictly speaking, since the rhythmic activity can no longer find an outlet in the act of feeding after the nutritional phase of development is over, it transfers itself not only to the sphere of sexuality in the strict sense, but also to 'decoy mechanisms' such as music, and dancing, and finally to the sphere of work . . . the rhythmic tendency does not come from the nutritional phase at all, as if it had migrated from there to the sexual; *it is a peculiarity of emotional processes in general.*
>
> (Jung, CW5:218–219, italics mine)

Archaic shamans felt the instinctive push of burgeoning affect in themselves instinctively and they 'knew' how to arouse it in others, often expressing this 'intuitive' knowledge in relation to a drum. Imagining their drums as 'steeds,' they rode the rhythm of drumbeat into trance – lords of magical flight soaring up and down the World Tree. Thought to be a repository of divine power, a shaman's drum poured out its rhythms over love and war in ritual behavior like dancing and sacrifice. When a shaman of the Ostyak Samoyed people sought to acquire such a magical drum, he was to stumble into a forest with closed eyes, drawn blindly on until he bumped headlong into *the* tree from which *his* drum was to be fashioned. Chance could play no part: supernatural guidance drew him on. Having transformed his destined tree into his destined drum, '*the drum's rhythm then transformed the shaman*,' opening the shaman's being to a second world (Eliot, 1976, 56, italics mine).

Sensitive therapists work between these two worlds, and they know the role of shamanic trance in this intermediate space. They sense how changes in consciousness correlate with changes in heartbeats; they know that the texture of consciousness that accompanies the rapid heartbeat of fear or excitement differs radically from the kind of consciousness that companions a slowing heartbeat into deep concentration or meditative trance. HeartMath[2] is a contemporary science devoted to developing simple techniques to help us slow down our minds, attune to our inner feelings, and refine our intuition. These techniques suggest that experiences we commonly refer to as 'hunches,' 'heart feelings,' 'gut feelings,' or a sense of inner knowing or intuition can be developed intentionally.

Simple efforts to become attentive to the deep, internal rhythms of heartbeat and breath help us perceive the subjective imagery of an inner world, and meditative disciplines have made use of this knowledge for centuries. Jnana Yoga offers techniques purposely designed to manipulate the rhythms of heartbeat and breath in order to bring about a direct experience of magical levels of the psyche. This procedure may go well for a creatively stabilized ego or for someone who is adequately prepared, but if we are *not* well prepared, immersion in the magical dimensions of the psyche can be dangerous. Analytical psychology refers to what the Hindus call cosmic consciousness as the collective unconscious, and therapists who are sensitized to rhythm know that suggestions to turn inward and relax *may* be appropriate (perhaps to accompany active imagination) but sometimes are not. Discerning therapists discriminate between times when activating unconscious contents (by definition uncontrollable) might weaken an inadequately developed ego or – on the other hand – when a flow of unconscious material might help a hide-bound ego relax. Dancing Shiva's drum symbolizes creation and destruction both: beneath *the terror* of nonbeing lurks Nonbeing itself.

Rhythm and awakening

Animate life quickens to, by, and with rhythm, and the return of rhythm to a frozen life is memorable. Years ago, I dreamed that a large gray stone burst into pulsating flame along one side: something not living lived, and something immovable moved. The paradox this dream presented me with was heart-stopping: even the inorganic undergoes transformation.[3] In this dream, psyche's use of metaphor and image to describe the undoing (or transformation) of something that had been petrified, frozen, or stuck heightened my awareness that while dreams may call forth consciousness, consciousness alone can never be 'king': consciousness alone is never 'all there is to it.' Powerful dream images *move* us. The sheer presence of change and transformation in the psyche proceeds from – and is accompanied by – a deepening sensibility of kinship with the surrounding world. A deepening sensitivity to nature's organic rhythms widens the field of self-reference.[4] Later iterations of my dream-stone's ongoing transformation appeared in dreams of a naked woman walking rhythmically along a beach, the skin of one shoulder and one hip flushed with flame. The transformative procession of such images fed my ego, thawing my frozen personhood with rhythms of aliveness.

As a defense, psychological petrifaction manifests itself as frozenness, numbness, or lack of feeling, and it symbolizing a congealing flow of rhythmic affect. Theologically speaking, petrifaction indicates sin and stagnation – a detention of moral progress or a devolution of soul – that can force spiritual evolution from its proper course. In biblical stories, sin petrifies and stagnates, or it sours one's heart into a rebellious longing: imagine Lot's wife, becoming a statue of bitter salt. For the Greeks, the stony glare of an agonized Medusa petrified all who beheld her. More hopefully, a Zen koan states, 'The Stone Woman Gives Birth,' and cycles of legends from Indigenous Peoples in what is now called the United States place special emphasis on the motif of a stone body, or animated stone. Alchemically speaking, animation of the stone symbolizes a process of coming back to life, wherein a deeper rhythm reanimates all that has been petrified, hardened, or dead.[5] Depths such as these form the rhythmic texture of life itself.

In some situations, rhythm communicates more deeply than words. A withdrawn nine-year-old autistic boy obsessively tapped his hands on his body, the furniture, and every instrument handed to him by his befuddled music therapist. Trying to reach the boy by taking drumming as a language, the therapist tells us he *tuned himself* to resonate with the boy's world, slowly leading him through trickier syncopations and volumes of sound. Because rhythm is such a basic component of speech and vocal sound, as his sense of rhythm loosened, the child also became more daring and expressive in other areas of his life (Bloom, 1987, 62). For this particular child, this therapist functioned as a conscious shaman.

As long as magical behavior is effective, we seldom challenge it, so repetitive behavior tends to continue its until magical intent has been consciously assimilated. This attribute is intimately involved in the psyche's complex-building processes of identification and introjection, and a therapist's sensitivity to rhythm tends to heighten as the collective unconscious unfolds.

Describing a man's passive-aggressive attitude (gesture, posture, and sound – all imbued with sacramental intent), analyst Geza Roheim wrote of his patient, 'If he were a sorcerer in a primitive culture, he would at this phase be wearing his clothes like a child and performing an incantation, saying "I am a good boy," and the aim (intent) of the performance would be to make his stepmother love him (result)' (Roheim, 1970, 64). In this passage, Roheim intuitively perceives that the shamanic, symbol-making aspect of his patient's unconscious mind is *engaged in trying to affect Roheim's unconscious mind*: this is shamaning, pure and simple. When repetitive behavior fails, as it does here because of Roheim's symbolic sensitivity, unconscious anxiety becomes accessible to the now-stressed patient, compelling the patient into ego awareness of meaning hidden behind instinctively enacted behavior. As Roheim's patient comes to understand his symbolic behavior, our expectation is that *he will simultaneously experience the difference between 'relating' to the symbolic process and 'being' the symbolic process*, because this quantum leap from unconscious 'enactment' into conscious 'relating' assumes the form of unconscious sacrifice of influence that underlies everything we call becoming conscious.

In the example from Roheim, as one aspect of his former magical (made 'sacred' or shamanic) personality dies, Roheim's patient is being called upon to become conscious of a previously shamanic or magical, unconscious mode of behavior. And as the magic fades, an earlier identification with an unconscious image of symbolic enacting disappears, freeing energy to become consciousness itself. Roheim's description also gives us a graphic example of how what I've been pointing to as unconscious shamaning substitutes for real relatedness between one person and another.

Of course, verbal communication manifests rhythm. As guardians of tribal lore and the early narrator of tribal tales and stories, the historical shaman was the ancestor of all our orators, storytellers, bards, and singers. The effectiveness of a shaman's tales lay (as it continues to do in all oral transmission) in the hypnotic effect of repetition. We know what this is like, instinctively. We've all been children, insisting that a story be told exactly as it was before: 'tell me again how I was born, Mommy,' or '*seven* dwarfs found Snow White, not *six*!' as I had to admit to my small son. Even accidentally expressed words have an effect. The rhythms of organized speech are compelling, and metrically organized words develop concentrated power. Prayers solemnly formulated over centuries retain as much effective power as fairytales from the past, and both these forms of 'oral tradition' resonate today with magical levels of the psyche (Huizinga, 1924, 116). Curses and blessings work deep in the psyche, and the 'old ones' may affect us still. Both the giving and the receiving of words has tremendous emotional impact. If prayers and fairytales are the stories we inherit through culture, we can imagine that the stories that we weave ourselves – those stories that slowly emerge in therapy, hour by hour – as if personal stories are 'woven by hand.' Such hand-woven personal stories told during therapeutic hours help us weave our lives together again, making us feel *coherent*.

Rhythm's power strengthens through repetition and parallelism, alliteration and rhyme. Writers consciously employ such literary forms to achieve aesthetic purposes, but Gerardus van der Leeuw reminds us that in the past, these forms were magico-religious means of retaining and controlling power (van der Leeuw, 117ff). Ancient Egyptian sacrificial texts and Indian ritual-healing formulas exhibit parallelism, and in both, the obligatory repetition of spoken words had to be rhythmically exact. We also repeat incantations, as we have done since ancient times. As a remnant of the magical level of consciousness today, repetition manifests itself in compulsive behavior.

As Jung discovered in his early association experiment (Jung, 5:219), in no matter what phase of life energy and excitement appear, repetition, assonance, and the alliteration of complex-toned reaction words display a tendency to rhythmic expression and perseveration. We too, when strongly moved, repeat 'I love you, I love you,' 'I'm so, so sorry,' or (usually in crowds) 'Hurrah! Hurrah!' Common wisdom formulated in meter and rhyme repeats itself unceasingly in the refrains of our popular music, not to mention our TV ads and limericks, and these make up the collective everyday *mantras* that we hum silently to ourselves or sing aloud. Such odd little self-songs repeat again and again, containing the words of a popular song, jingles meant to sell cars or dog food, and so on, and they inform our unconscious minds. How often do such collective furnishings of our inner worlds reach individual consciousness?

Another therapeutic rhythm to keep in mind can be found in the natural alternation of introversion and extroversion. In its own peculiar time, it is almost as if the psyche 'breathes' – in to a center, out to an external world – a natural alteration of personality orientation with a rhythm of its own. Those of us who have a passionate predilection for outward movement tend to grossly undervalue an introvert's equally valid, vital flow of subjective feeling, while those of us who are more at home with introverted ways of being may be overly dismissive of undue attention to the outer world. Yet everyone's psychotherapeutic task is to understand and learn to value (somehow) whatever is dark or unknown. In an extroverted personality, introversion often begins with an outer world slowly losing the overwhelming fascination it has always held, while external things begin to appear inwardly as 'images.' For introverts, on the other hand, images from dreams and waking life have moved naturally through an inner world like servants of the invisible, full of secret meanings that flow toward a center, flooding and regenerating soul, so an extroverted turnabout may appear to be a desert of despair. Yet as strange and unnerving as alternation between the two can be, neither can be overvalued, because each alternation – whether introverted or messaged from an outer world – is part of psyche's whole.

The rhythms of therapy

The catching and netting of divergent psychic elements into an organic order that takes place in therapy happens because psychotherapy is the rhythmic setup par excellence. That the constancy of presence and behavior of one person affects the rhythms of another person is practically a psychotherapeutic axiom since therapy is a virtual paradigm of reciprocal, rhythmic dialogue between two people, including the conscious and unconscious aspects of each. Slowly, the rhythm of weekly or bi-weekly sessions, and the repetitive, peculiar quality of the time spent in session assumes importance and relevance to one's life as a whole – hence, our distress when a therapy hour suddenly changes, or vacation happens, or illness interrupts the flow. Constant, consistent therapeutic companioning in a dependable rhythm anchors us in effective interactions with other people and relates us to an inner world.

But each person has an idiosyncratic tempo too. A therapist has to be able to differentiate themselves from a patient's rhythm of being in order to relate to it, sensing the other's personal tempo through their therapeutically informed awareness of psychological complex building and consolidation. They sense the *quality* of compensatory companioning that might be needed for each person they work with – a quickening or slowing, a speeding up or a holding back, an upbeat or a downbeat – whatever tempo might best accompany the other's usual, even if irregular, pace. Personal tempo differs depending on the patient too: one may need an enthusiastic drumming up, while another needs quickening interest and attention; still another tends to relax into a receptive quietude in which anxiety simply runs out of steam.

Developing their own sensitivity to this attribute is one way that a therapist's training helps them relate to the rhythms of a session rather than shamanically enacting it. We struggle to become more conscious of how we express our personal rhythms: how and when do we present ourselves to each other? If I'm a patient, do I present yesterday's experience first, and then my dreams? If I'm a therapist, do I tend to greet a session with words or with silence, and why one and not another? Within an hour, two people can rhythmically alternate intensive work and receptive relaxation; two people also experience the nuances and subtleties of sound and silence, and laughter and tears. These rhythmic alternations weave the ongoing dialogue of individual rhythms of speech and rhythms of procedure that happen between conscious and unconscious material. If patient and therapist are badly mismatched, unconsciously misdirected energy in one person is apt to overwhelm the innate rhythm of another, and a sufficiently catalytic counterpoint may depart. The therapy stutters to a stop.

Rhythms of inspiration and quietude embrace the ebbing and flowing of archetypal energy, and they define the limits and the capacities of our personal disciplines too. Deeply creative energies are engaged in psychological work and active imagination. Psyche unfolds beneath all this, rhythmically becoming itself, dream after dream, fantasy after fantasy, and hour by hour, in session and out. If we don't learn to deal with the psyche in consciousness-making dialogues such as these, we tend to remain at psyche's mercy.

Rhythm and trance

By mastering dancing, chanting, beating the drum and sharing rhythm between themselves and others, archaic shamans brought about the equivalent of collective trance. As a trance master, an experienced shaman could invite an initiate into trance, and in psychotherapy we do much the same. In therapeutic hypnosis, we too are lulled, carried unresisting along regular waves of sight (motion) and sound. This is not unlike the hypnotic effect that poetry, music, the soothing sound of a waterfall, or the sound of waves on the shore has on us. The whole therapeutic setup is exquisitely designed to lower the threshold of everyday ego consciousness, inviting a patient into a rhythmic field of potential wholeness, a field we think of as the field of the Anthropos, the whole human being, or Jung's self.

As a modern practitioner I do this consciously, not as the archaic shaman did, but (and here is my main point) I do it with familiarity with how the shamanic attributes operate through the objective psyche *in both myself and my patients* as well. I know that compensatory information about our work together lies in the objective psyche: perhaps I will be guided by a dream (my patient's or my own). The quantity and sequential patterning of a series of dreams may indicate that my tempo of companioning is too much, too little, too personal, or not personal enough. Or perhaps the psyche is going about its business relatively undisturbed. I won't always be able to tell what is happening 'objectively' – after all, consciousness is never king. But above all, the conscious apprehension of this attribute requires me to maintain a dramatic sense of the emotional ups and downs within each hour, which is to say that I know that I will be called upon to try to identify with the emotional substance of whatever I apprehend. I imagine that this capacity for dramatic apprehension is simply a noble form of the great human art of placing oneself inside another (consciously *identifying* with another), a capacity that is as basic to a personalized experience of relating to the field of the Anthropos by way of the shaman complex as it is to any religious discipline I know.

Like the other attributes, rhythm attends to our own developing, personal lives as we attend to conscious restoration. A rhythmic interchange of subjectivity and objectivity underly dialogue of every kind, freeing up self-created worlds of mirroring, while a rhythmic alternation of self and other actualizes aliveness in both. Last but not least, an awareness of sharing this attribute with others and the world at large can save us from becoming self-serving models of ourselves, cut off from a larger, open-ended quest for personal meaning. I want to end this chapter with a poem I wrote years ago. The poem, 'Shaman Song' sings my personal experience of rhythm when I had little sense of wholeness of any kind, inner or outer, and rhythm brought a vision of the world:

Shaman Song

Rhythm brings a vision of the World.
Snow. Poem. Bird. Tree. Journey. Night.

I'm the time I measure, I myself
Road. Bridge. Fire. Beast. Water. Light.

Original Time begins with every breath.
Sun. Moon. Dark. Rain. Voyage. Heat.

Breath unfolds time's rhythm to itself.
Cold. Wind. Stars. Cave. River. Beat.

Rhythm told my heart how Light begins,
Cloud. Song. Drum. Dust. Music. Stone.

Locked within the cells of my own skin.
North. South. East. West. Flower. Bone.

Cold. The snow, and northern light, and
vast plains shadowed by a fluid run of caribou,
their steaming bodies shuddering a silver steam
into the air long after they have gone.

Out on the steppes the great Siberian Tiger moves,
muttering her love of cold, the muscle in her
measured flank articulating, like the sound of
linked chain in a sack.

And south: the flat, clear heat, and spare shadow,
the endless Altiplano, level and blunt for undulating
miles, equivocates to sky.
Rough coated as the sere gold grass and
yellow-eyed, a puma stalks
the high plateau.

Unrolling silver sheets of Pampas grass
the land continues, resonate and lean.
Yet in the hollows, brown deer hesitate,
the small and larger, pale and darker,
moving without fear,
hushed to cadence like a stream.

Road becomes river, step becomes flow,
I am myself the hungry animal.
Hunter and hunted, arrow and bow,
seeker and sought, wounded and caught,
a wide mind's delta ends the drought.
Tears allow the trees to grow.

Love and hate, light and dark,
swerving through a weaving heart
cast long shadows, eddying whirls
of river-wrack and image flow.
Above, below, without, within,
hung by a rope
that flows through my wrist
I spin.

Breaking apart and coming together again,
Words wheel and flock, like birds in flight.

Here star is stone, and stone is star,
and living is the metaphor:
I travel light.

Shattering sunlight, quartz becomes cascade,
arcades of laughter, spilling into sight.
Deliquescence of the Stone
creates a world's archaic ecstasy,
coercing heartbeats,
sounding depth and height,
the pounding blood-bell
beaten like a gong
to arabesque'd imagination's flight

till I am bodied home
to my original cell of skin and bone.

Lord of the Narrow Gate
and Needle's Eye,

may I pass by.[6]

Notes

1 Kolata, Gina: 'Nobel Prize in Medicine Awarded for Discoveries About Circadian Rhythm,' *New York Times*. 2017, October 2.
2 HeartMath Institute offers products, tools and techniques dealing with the psychophysiology (heart rhythm patterns and emotions) of stress, emotions, and the interactions of these between the heart and the brain.
3 In addition to alchemical imagery, several Indigenous wisdoms think of stone as being alive. For example, the Ojibwe word for stone, *asin*, is animate. Stones are addressed as grandmothers and grandfathers, and the universe begins with a conversation between stones. See Louise Erdrich's poem 'Asiniig' in *Original Fire: Selected and New Poems*. New York: Harper Perennial. 2003. 153.
4 I refer to this dream elsewhere among other self-directed dreams (van Löben Sels, Robin: *A Dream in the World: Poetics of Soul in Two Women, Modern and Medieval*. London and New York: Brunner-Routledge. (2003) 2012). Here I want to convey the ego-self axis as a process that is analogous to repeated shamanic journeying up and down the World Tree.
5 See Erich Neumann's 'Mystical Man' for articulate aspects of mystical experience in Western, ego-bearing people in *The Mystic Vision*, Bollingen Series XXX, Volume 6. Princeton: Princeton University Press. 1968. 375–415.
6 Published in van Löben Sels, Robin: *Wanting A Country for This Weather and Other Poems*. Lampeter, Ceredigion, Wales: The Edwin Mellen Press, Ltd. (1993) 2003. 43.

Chapter 10

Silence

When I began to write about silence, a specific dream came to mind – one in which even a flaming angel made no sound (see Chapter 2). Like night and day, dark and light, or cold and warm, this dream formed two parts of a silent whole. In the first part, I stood alone on a hill under a dark night sky. I have been waiting – for what, for whom, I didn't know – for a long time. In the second part, from far away, I saw a fiery light coming toward me: the light grew gradually until it flared into a flaming angel, who wrapped me in an all-consuming embrace: *I felt myself warmed and held and able to speak*, telling the angel everything.

I painted this dream and called the painting *The Skin of the Angel* (Illustration 2). And I imagined the dream – as I described it to my first analyst – as 'me coming to life again, or life coming to me again.' In the embrace of a flaming angel, I reencountered a world that held 'myself.' Looking at this painting a year later, my second analyst exclaimed, 'But there's nothing there to see!' And, indeed, in my rice paper, watercolor depiction of an angel's flaming skin, there *was* very little to be objectively conscious *of*, yet the feeling quality of that dream held me fast for years. In that dream, I discovered myself again, and that discovery enabled me to speak, but where psyche may have brought the dream, silence returned my soul.

D. W. Winnicott might have suggested that in a dream like this, the dreamer glimpses (tastes? feels?) their true self.

Silence and feeling

Feeling itself is usually silent, as is caring. So too is appreciation, and so is reverence. Our various gut reactions are silent, and so are intuitions, as is much of the information we take in through our senses from and about the surrounding world. In all of us, male or female, old or young, the desire as well as the capacity to maintain ties between oneself and others, between inside and outside, between a personal world and a collective world is something that we live silently and seldom voice – something that we *feel,* but seldom think about. Feeling tends to stand for a secret side of life.

Venturing home from outer space, the Russian cosmonaut Aleksei Leonov tells us that what struck him most was a silence so vast and deep that he began to hear his own body – his heart beating, his blood pulsing, the rustle of his muscles moving over each other – unlike any silence on earth. Feeling 'struck' is a sensate, *feeling* term, as if Leonov's description is suggesting that the silence of space enabled him – hearing and feeling himself *alive* – to rediscover his 'original' embodiment.

Robert Sardello (2006) thinks of silence as the ground of the world, a 'palpable surround.' What we tap into in dreams, and what astronauts seem to tap into as they return to their home planet from outer space – is a *felt* access to the inner world of silence that rests below all sound, as if it takes an inner earth to remind us not only of the palpable body with which we each began but also of the palpable surround of the outer earth we live in and have come to know.

But feeling can be difficult to assess. A quality of feeling cannot be proven, only recognized by feeling of equal quality. All of us are faced with a profound need of this something that we cannot measure – indeed, that we can barely describe – but whose presence or absence changes everything. This difficulty of recognizing and honoring feeling also forms an intangible aspect of what Jungian therapists refer to as the feminine principle. While all hope of communication and security rest on our ability to relate consciously to one another, we nevertheless value each other differently. Culturally speaking, we have come to regard the feeling bonds between people and between individuals and the world as precious, if silent, bridges across which reason and trust occur, take place, and pass. That reason and trust are dear enough to value indicates that feelings have been 'lived' over time, in that feeling 'lived' indicates a slow distillation of emotional experience.

Feeling has always been associated with fire in all its incarnations, perhaps because it is hard to tell where a just sense of feeling ends and the heat of emotion begins, and emotion is fed from irrational sources. Archetypal emotion flares, for example. Boiling up from unfathomable depths, archetypal emotion is usually uncontrolled and often uncontrollable. Powerful emotions can render us helpless as well as violent. Clear feeling, on the other hand, can truly assess value and thereby maintain a living relationship to experience. Above all, feeling lets life flow healthily, always allowing for movement and the entry of the unexpected.

Tending the silent flame of feeling in oneself, as well as in others, seems to be central to healing of any kind. Yet feelings may always represent the hidden side of life, and rapport with feeling may not be easily recognized or can be easily lost. When a feeling rapport is paralyzed by discord, feelings that once seemed alive and stimulating flee. When we cannot fully feel what happens to us, we cannot fully live our lives.

Silence and the sacred

For centuries, the kind of silence that feeds feeling hid in our religions. Max Picard describes human voices moving along a 'wall' of silence, a silence that signifies a kind of 'primary speech' in which God and humanity speak to each other:[1]

> God became man for the sake of man . . . a layer of silence lies between this event and man, and in this silence man approaches the silence that surrounds

> God himself. . . . It is a sign of the love of God that a mystery is always separated from man by a layer of silence. And that is a reminder that man should also keep a silence in which to approach the mystery.

Simone Weil, a contemporary mystic, writes, 'There is a silence in the beauty of the universe which is like a noise, when compared with the silence of God.'[2] Perhaps Weil's 'silence in the beauty of the universe' now inhabits our psyche, permeating us in a silken sheet of dreams. During therapy, these silent dreams unite us with ourselves and relate us to each other while psyche flows between. Images of animals and trees entwine us more deeply with our own nature and with the nature of a world that embraces all the life we've ever known and more.

Earlier in history, sacred groves embodied silence. Perhaps silence made the groves sacred to begin with. Then came temples, churches, and shrines. Even today, amid sprawling cities, churches and temples stand like empty secrets – tranquil places that are strangely still. Upon entering them, silence invites us to be silent, to listen attentively and rest, simultaneously inviting us to enter our own presence in the presence of another. Not only does a soul seek silence in which to hide; it incubates there too, in that any possibility of imagination lies on the other side. When I flew to California to attend my father's funeral, I left my beloved St. Bernard dog, Katrina, in a veterinarian hospital to undergo minor surgery. When I got home several days later, I went to the hospital to pick her up only to be told that Katrina had unexpectedly died under anesthesia. I fled the hospital halls onto busy Manhattan streets and spied a nearby empty church where I could weep in peace. In all our cities, it seems, extraordinary churches still stand, framing an emptiness of space that seems to bear witness to a still center of being, and the soul – all souls – need the silence of such space. Perhaps poet Paul Elouard's 'another world, in this one!' points to the world of silence.

Dividing our human selves into unconscious bodies and conscious and unconscious minds, Freud and Jung discovered psyche as their guide. Psyche silently unrolled Royal Roads before them, and dreams led them to underworlds that silently held sway. In an earlier underworld, silence reigned because in the Greek Hades, shades did not speak. The Psalms (115:17 and 94:17) tell us that She'ol, the Hebrew Underworld, was silent too. Centuries later, James Hillman suggested that images of the Underworld refer us not to another world after death, or simply to an afterlife, but to the silent presence of another world that lies *beside* everyday life – a life that lies alongside the life we know, an underneath, or an undertone that echoes in each earthly step we take.

Even our scriptures picture creation as an ongoing process of coming-to-be out of silence: 'In the Beginning was the Word.' But mystical thought depicts a second world of interior awakening. Fourteenth-century mystic Meister Eckhart, for whom God was 'the simple ground, the still desert, the simple silence,' – insisted that the Word is born and reborn in our hearts.[3] A 'second birth' initiates us into a silent heart of Being. Any mysticism that goes beyond, behind or beneath the Word directs us toward a world of silence that lies before and beyond language, a world that we feel within, for much of the psyche's 'inner world' consists of our dawning capacity to open ourselves to our own beginnings and the mystery of a silence that is neither known, nor seen, but only felt.

Silence and presence

Silence and presence bring us close to paradox. On one hand, we can experience silence as presence – a renewing companion that restores, and deepens our bodily response to internal and external worlds: meditators of various disciplines know what that is like. On the other hand, silence that is presence can also draw us into it until words fall away: 'The Lord is in his holy temple; let all the earth keep silent before him:' or, 'Silent night. Holy night.' Silence implied by familiar phrases like these is a silence that is somehow contained by time. This kind of silence has a beginning and an end, as if it enclosed itself in the form of a pause, or a rest. Nor is this the silence of someone who has never spoken; rather, it is the silence of someone who *falls silent in the presence of that which silences* – the silence of someone who holds her breath, or has been silenced.

In the outer world, sudden silence like this can indicate the presence of danger. Bedouin travelers used to 'bell' their camels so that their loping progress across the dunes continually 'sounded' a melodious tinkle. At night, the camels' rhythmic breathing kept the bells sounding ever so faintly 'til morning – a constant background reminder that all was well. A sudden silence meant the camels held their breath – intruders or other creatures on the prowl? So sleeping travelers woke to silence as to a warning. And here is philosopher Kathleen Dean Moore, sleeping outside as she often does: 'But it was a sudden silence that woke me up. The night was very dark. What had quieted the frogs? A raccoon? A coyote? A human intruder? I lay still, listening the way prey listen. There was a rumble from the west. . . . The storm blew in.[4]

Silence and danger also join hands when the presence that stills us feels negative or diabolical – the dark *numinosum*. In our Western culture, when Yahweh finally revealed himself to Job, Job was stricken with silence. Job's experience of sickness unto death included the loss and death of all that he held dear – not only all that he thought his life ought to be, but all that he had thought about God – all the ways he expected God to be, in terms of images given him by Yahweh himself – Yahweh as just, Yahweh as compassionate, Yahweh showing kindness to someone who had respected the law and followed his ways. Job's experience of Yahweh was not dissimilar to the challenge faced by archaic shaman, called upon by otherworldly spirits only to be dis-membered and re-membered in an initiatory ordeal.

Whenever we fall silent before mystery, negative or positive, silence *becomes sacramental*. Many cults hold this kind of sacramental or 'holy' silence to be the highest form of worship and the deepest form of communication with God. In Antonello da Messina's beautiful *Annunciation*, the figure of Mary slightly turns and raises her hand in a gesture of recognition as an unseen messenger imparts a world-shaking message – in silence. Then again – in a religion that posits no god – Buddha once felt he could indicate the essence of his teachings to his disciples with a gesture (holding up a flower), a smile – and silence.

The very nature of ritual and oral disciplines that were used in several mystery religions – Orphic, for example – imposed on participants of initiation a silent, conditional knowledge in which comprehension entailed an *actual change of being*. The root of our English word 'mystery' is *muein*, a Greek verb that means 'to close the mouth.' Dictionaries usually explain this connection by telling us that initiates to ancient mysteries were sworn to silence, but at root, *muein* may also indicate that what is learned at a mystery initiation *cannot* be talked about. In other words, we remain ignorant of such mysteries not only because secrets have been kept but also because neither dogma nor description could possibly impart all that was accomplished by these ancient ceremonies, any more than an eyewitness or written account of an archaic shaman's animal dance could give us a shaman's personal experience of daimonic participation today.

Among humans, keeping silence can have a powerful effect on others, intentionally or not. A shaman's silent trance (unconscious prostration) told others (was read by others to indicate) that they were journeying – to another world, a sacred realm – where they either underwent initiation or communicated with spirits. Unconscious themselves, an entranced shaman constellated the unconscious in others, sharing a highly potentiated, imaginatively silent world. Once initiated, however, the shaman could bring about trance-like states again, in themselves and others intentionally, because they had mastered a 'technique' (Eliade) that – when skillfully honed – proclaimed the reason for their 'being' within the unconscious surround of their tribe. In the last century, our Western culture dubbed Marcel Marceau, the world-famous mime, a master of silence. Marceau's silent character, *Bip*, delighted audiences for decades, mostly making them laugh at themselves and each other. But deeply rooted in Marceau's personal experience of WWII, *Bip* also carried great pathos: as an ever-silent figure encountering our world without words, the 'masterly mime' was always a tragic comedian, never simply a clown.

Silence, secrecy, and waiting

Keeping silent can also be a way to hide. If we go back in history, we find implications of secrecy and 'secret knowledge' that unite the image of the archaic shaman more closely with silence per se. For example, Old Norse literature embodied silence in mantic images of Hoenir the Silent, friend of Odin and companion of Mimir the Wise, designating Hoenir as a sign of wisdom. Ancient Egypt depicted Horus, son of Osiris and Isis as a child with his finger across his lips in a gesture of silence. Later, Greeks and Romans designated the child Horus as God of Silence, Harpocrates. In his infant aspect, Harpocrates had his finger in his mouth or his finger to his lips, gestures childish by convention but also understood to indicate that the god demanded silence. In the Roman Sanctuary of Pleasure stood a statue of the Roman goddess Angerona, her mouth bound and sealed. Angerona's uplifted finger touching her lips pointed to silence and suffering, and Russell

Lockhart characterized Angerona not only as 'silent suffering' but as an image of 'the suffering of silence'[5] as well.

Secrecy can be symbolic, as it is in initiations where those who speak do not know, and those who *do* know do not (or cannot) speak. An Egyptian hymn to Thoth compares Thoth to a well that cannot be found by the talkative or noisy – a well that is a sweet spring for the thirsty in the desert, closed for those who speak there, and open for those who keep silence: when a silent person enters the scene, they find the spring. Some fairytales, like Frau Halle or Baba Yaga, bring us a third child – often a daughter – who quietly does whatever she must do, taking in all that she sees but asking no questions. Just so, when we are speechless and close our mouths, we may both embody and reveal a mystery that we are – simply by being human – to whoever can see.

Another aspect of silence – a silence of waiting – can denote inner concentration and detachment from manifold outward distractions. Rudolph Otto suggested that this kind of silence has value as a 'preparation of the soul to become the pencil of the unearthly writer, the bent bow of the heavenly archer, the tuned lyre of the divine musician. This kind of silence is not so much a dumbness in the presence of deity,' Otto writes, 'as an awaiting of His coming, in expectation of the Spirit and its message.'[6] Great accomplishments of the human spirit have been born from what mystics have called the silence of waiting.

Artistically, a silence of waiting may be experienced as a time of aridity, a desert, or a drought, since creative energy alternates with fallow fields that seemingly persist forever. 'Forty days and forty nights in the wilderness,' may signify a prolonged time of mourning or a long depression. In my own history, a dream 'foretold' a silent time of waiting by showing me a beautiful, solitary white horse standing in the exact center of an enormous, circularly plowed black earthen labyrinth. In order to reach the white animal in the center, I had to walk round and round, in an endless alchemical *perigrinatio* (circular perambulation) – in silence.

Culture itself is born out of silence. As shadow is to light, or darkness is to the visual arts, silence is to music and the verbal arts. Hamlet's soliloquies and Beethoven's symphonies did not suddenly appear as simply bigger and better noises in a noisy world; they took form out of a vast environmental space around them, a space of contemplative minds and the largeness of an intensely spiritual environment. Although we hear music *in time*, music itself seems to proceed from timeless silence, and from this point of view, the simple occurrence of sound marks resistance overcome. Take language too: as an implicit context out of which all language emerges, silence holds unsuspected depths. Every use of language about language produces more language, but the deepest purpose of all language produces a kind of soul understanding – a silent consent between speech and its object as between a speaker and a hearer – in order to bring about that sense of 'it is as it is' that seems to be the end of every great work and a spiritual statement of life rooted in soul. In literature, silence concerns itself with what is between the lines. Just as it is in conversation, silence may often be 'the art' of saying something by saying nothing, or very little.

Interpersonal silence

Interpersonal silence is multifaceted. For either partner in a relationship, silence may show absence or communion, vacancy or calm, awkwardness or restfulness, acceptance or bewilderment and condemnation. Silence can be experienced as full and vital or merciless and barren – as encompassing as water or as dry as bleached bone. All of us know when interpersonal silence feels safe and when it does not. We know what a receptive, space-giving silence *feels* like, just as we recognize deafening silences that thunder like the roar of an abyss into which we fear we are bound to fall. In the presence of some silences, memories rise up like air through water: ideas surface and images resonate, bearing emotions that may range from pre-birth, uterine bliss to feelings of dismemberment constellated by the agonies of unmediated contact with reality or dimly remembered terrors of infantile abandonment or pain. Memories of profound oblivion can be as death-like as nonbeing itself.

All of us know something about the silent suffering that occurs in mute places of dissociation that follow trauma. When an awareness of suffering *as such* is lacking, suffering is numbly endured. Perhaps a dream pictures us entering a dry desert or lost in the snow; a rainstorm approaches and we have no shelter; or we can't get out of a dark, still, room without windows or doors. Mute in themselves, dreams bring us news about places rendered silent by trauma – places of 'speechless horror,' as some describe. Perhaps dreams inform us that faraway grief and pain live elsewhere – out in the barrens or out in the cold; or unconscious feelings seem to be closing in around us, as if a depiction of torrential rain were an aspect of ominous weather rather than unshed tears. Dreams like these picture just-so landscapes through which we happen to move; because feeling is dead, we find them 'hard to understand.'

The most powerful scream I have ever experienced is void of sound: Edvard Munch's painting of *The Scream*. Talk about speechless horror. Many of us fall silent upon looking at this canvas, as if silence communicates between the painting and those who see. 'What we cannot speak about,' says the philosopher Ludwig Wittgenstein in the famous ending to his *Tractatus*, 'we must consign to silence.'[7] But in the body of his work, Wittgenstein emphasizes that we can (and must) *show* that for which we cannot find words: what can be shown, in other words, often cannot be said. 'My whole tendency, and, I believe, the tendency of all who ever tried to write or talk Ethics or Religion was to run against the boundaries of language' (4.1212). Things like the meaning of life, 'the good,' or what is truly valuable can *show*, Wittgenstein realized, meaning they may be thought, be felt, be experienced, but not articulated, in silence.

When after a time of silent suffering feeling is quickened again and we learn how to recognize and express feeling in the body and in relationship, the silence that follows has become a psychological accomplishment. This kind of silence punctuates our experience and renders it deep, like the pauses that create the melody in a score of music. 'Silence is not native to my world,' writes Wayne Oates

(1979, 3); 'silence, more than likely, is a stranger to your world too. If you and I ever have silence in our noisy hearts, we are going to have to grow it . . . we will do so on silence's terms for growth – terms which are not yet our own.'[8] The Norwegian writer and explorer Erling Kagge, who walked in silence fifty days solo across Antarctica to the South Pole, discovered something about this slow growth in the slow growth of his own capacity for developing this attribute: 'I no longer try to create absolute silence around me,' he writes; 'the silence I am after is the silence within' (25). Kagge ends his remarkable memoir with 'You have to find your own South Pole' (175).

In psychological development, therapeutic situations, and natural, everyday relationships, silence and speech mark rhythms of natural growth. Blindness to the natural place of silence in personal interactions can close potential space of the imagination – an elusive 'third' space that must be potentiated if healing is to occur and play is to be actualized. In sand-play therapy, the therapist holds a space for psyche to emerge by silently witnessing a client's creative constructions; the same is true of the silent witness in authentic movement therapy. Talk therapists hold a therapeutic silent space, in which psyche may be sheltered and nurtured in darkness and allowed to mature. In therapeutic space, desire can open, deepening into feelings kept at bay; as this happens, *we* deepen too – for example, as sadness from the past wells up into here and now, becoming more authentic, more three-dimensional, and more present to experience.

In alchemy, an alchemical process itself protects the secret treasure, and to approach this secret is to approach the soul's silent solitude. Members of a high order of contemplative activity, medieval alchemists worked in secret and always held the alchemical secret in silence, hidden away in ancient places of the psyche still alive to the resonant silence of truth. Silence was one of an alchemist's closest companions, without which the Philosopher's Stone could not be found. When we connect with this kind of silence and solitude, we connect with psyche and its secrets: hence, the poet John Keats refers to psyche as a 'bride of quietness.' Companioned by quietness, the alchemists connected with the earth and its transformations; not by accident did ancient Western alchemists create chemistry, the science of earth's mysterious, silent, inner properties.

Clinical silence

Freud famously employed therapeutic silence and anonymity as a powerful tool in the evocation of transference neurosis, and analysts practicing in this tradition have remained mostly silent ever since. With the shaman complex in mind, however, this classical position may also be interpreted as a countertransference phenomenon that springs from the analyst's unwitting participation in the sacramental nature of unconscious shamaning. Despite a rationalization of necessary 'neutrality,' such an approach may simply betray the therapist's fear of using their personality in a more open and transparent way.

Unnecessary silence can be self-indulgent on the part of a therapist and wounding to a patient's soul, particularly when someone has been badly shaken or inadequately formed to begin with. The legend of the Grail offers us a mythic paradigm. When Parsifal met the injured King Amfortas, he simply did not think to open his mouth and ask what ailed the king or whom the Grail served. At one end of the egoless corridor yawning between the two, Parsifal's silence failed the king; at the other end, Amfortas would remain speechless (wounded) until he was addressed (Majno, 1975, 39.). When silence is shamanically sacramentalized, each participant undergoes unconscious weakening or feels abandoned; that's what shamanic silence *does*. Through a therapeutic lens, Parsifal has to go away and develop an individual ego. The second time around, Parsifal speaks, the silent impasse between him and Amfortas is addressed, and the paralyzing archetypal stalemate is dissolved.

Freud interpreted silence in keeping with his hermeneutic of suspicion – that is, no mystery was allowed. Sometimes silence meant death; sometimes it meant an inability to speak. Sometimes Freud understood silence as an image of the feminine – the 'bride' a stand-in for his own ability to accept death and the reality principle, thereby turning the threat of blank extinction into his ego's mature relation to reality.[9] Famously, Freud referred to his healing method as a talking cure, but I've often thought it might better be called a listening cure, because in my experience, the silence of my listening therapists was as healing as all the talking either of us did. C. G. Jung hardly mentions silence, except to speculate that a patient who kept silent for years simply had no desire to share or explain their 'strange experience' (CW3:356). But in my experience, I've found silence powerfully therapeutic, and possibly harmful. A therapist who unwittingly remains so silent that another person meets no reciprocity is probably behaving shamanically, exploiting the power of silence. If therapists hide behind theory or esoteric procedures or seek to generate mystery through concealment or innuendo, the shaman heaves into 'unconscious view' through identification with the shaman as a guardian of secrets of the sanctuary, and this will be registered by the unconscious, for better or for worse.

Another way of saying this is that when therapists use silence to compensate for their own lack of relatedness, they flirt with sacramental influence and unconscious power. Without this awareness – be the situation therapeutic or personal – a therapist risks shamaning in potentially destructive ways. Under the auspices of the unconscious, silence may loom, sacred and mysterious, feeling as if it will pull one into a vacuum. Like other attributes, if silence isn't personally mediated, the impersonal, transpersonal, archetypal nature of silence will predominate. The constellation of emotionally latent contents of the collective unconscious – meaning emotions we didn't know we had (or were capable of having) – can stir us to depths we haven't been able to imagine. Such contents strike us dumb: we're too overwhelmed to express them.

Clinical understandings of silence have come a long way since Freud and Jung. Writing about the silence of patients as important communications, psychoanalyst

Masud Kahn (1979, 168–72) differentiates between muteness, which he feels can have a destructive or aggressive and belligerent tone to it, and silence, that indicates a more benign or neutral state of being - one that can serve the function of recollecting, integrating, and working through very early relationships. Perhaps the silent patient (usually interpreted as resistant) is not 'running away,' but running toward – which implies a silent state that eventually produces something of a 'creation' – not necessarily a creation that is profound or artistic but a creation nevertheless, something that is a product of the psyche's creativity. Analyst Michael Balint (1968, 39) also relates silence to primary psychic creativity. Balint knew that silence always opens onto psyche and the world of the imagination.

Silence in the consulting room can indicate a therapist's sensitive personal restraint, an ability to hold a quiet, uninterrupted 'space' into which stories can flow. The shaman (symbolic process) of the two people meeting negotiates a *kairos* moment, wherein whatever it is, dancing between the subjectivities of two psyches, is joined by an invisible third – an intersubjective 'third' that Thomas Ogden called the analytic third.[10] Jung used the maxim of Maria Prophetissima, the first Western alchemist, as a similar metaphor for wholeness and individuation: 'Out of the One comes Two, out of Two comes Three, and from the Third Comes the One as the Fourth.'[11] Imagine sparks of affection; imagine shared marveling; imagine silence present, and then parting, as if on a silent rush of wings.

When silence proceeds from a patient, there are marked differences in how an analyst listens. A real listening cure allows for empty moments. It allows for pauses – breaths held and released between utterances – each phrase weighted with individual pace and rhythm. Other therapies differ in what they label 'inter-psychological communication and exchange.' Kahn suggests using a sentient, concentrated, alert attention, listening with both mind and body to the paradoxical wisdom that silence speaks. That means that as therapists, we must remember that when we keep silent, we are speaking a language that humans did not invent. Plutarch's words come silently from a Greek world now centuries removed from ours but remain relevant: 'From human beings we learn to speak; from the gods, to keep silent.'[12]

Creative silence

Creative silence implies inner riches and a savoring of impressions, yet inner forms of personal creativity may make no sounds at all. We can track inspiration in the shush of a brush across a canvas and imagine ideas in the scribbly sounds of a pencil or pen, but the energies flowing through brushes or pen are as silent as owls in flight and as elusive as still trout finning in the shadow of a stream. Silence is 'like space,' says Florida Scott-Maxwell, 'an intensely alive something that contains all . . . from the first pause of understanding to the quiet of comprehension' (1968, 143). This is a kind of silence that we can't do without. Suddenly, we find the energy to *create something* rather than pathologically accommodating what is expected of us or unconsciously serving a psyche with a purpose of its own. In Winnicott's words, our energies begin to make use of transitional space; we imagine turning our newfound freedom of spirit into cultural terms. When we've solved (at least for the moment) the vexing problem of being isolated without being insulated, creativity ensues, creativity that begins to build bridges between imaginative life and everyday existence. We write. We paint. We dance. We Sing. We play. We pray. We build. We think. We dream. We live more fully than we ever lived before. Creative energies flow between our inner objects and the worlds we share out there – inner and outer, personal and collective – while silence embraces us all.

Notes

1 Picard, Max: *The World of Silence*. Translated by Stanley Godman. Chicago: Regnery. 1952. 219, 227, 229–230.
2 Weil, Simone: *Waiting for God*. New York: Capricorn Books, G. P. Putnam Sons. 1951. 213.
3 Meister Eckhart, as quoted in Cassirer, Ernst, *Language and Myth*. Translated by Susanne K. Langer. New York: Dover Publications, Inc. 1946. 74.
4 Moore, Kathleen Dean: *Wild Comfort: The Solace of Nature*. Boston: Trumpeter. 2010. 132.
5 Lockhart, Russell A.: 'Eros in Language, Myth and Dream,' in *Quadrant*. Volume 2. Number 1. Summer 1978. 41.
6 Otto, Rudolf: *The Idea of the Holy: An Inquiry into the Non-Rational Factor in the Idea of the Divine and its Relation to the Rational*. Translated by John W. Harvey. New York: Oxford University Press. 1970. 211.
7 Wittgenstein, Ludwig: *The Tractatus Logico-Philosophicus*. New York: Dover. 1922. 4.1212.
8 Oates, Wayne: *Nurturing Silence in a Noisy Heart*. Garden City: Doubleday. 1979. 3.
9 See Freud's interpretation of 'The Theme of the Three Caskets' (Freud, Sigmund: *Collected Works*. Standard Edition. 12. London. 1053. 291–301), referred to in Ricoeur, Paul: *Freud and Philosophy: An Essay on Interpretation*. Translated by Denis Savage. New Haven: Yale University Press. 1970. 330.
10 Ogden, T. H.: *Subjects of Analysis*. London: Karnac Books Ltd. 1994. 61–95.
11 Von Franz, Marie-Louise: *Number and Time: Reflections Leading Towards a Unification of Psychology and Physics*. London: Rider & Company. 1974.
12 Plutarch. *De garrulitate*. Cap. 8.

Chapter 11

Respiration

Definitions and history

Defined most simply, respiration is the process of breathing air into and exhaling air from our lungs (inhalation/inspiration and expiration). Our first act after birth is to draw breath, and our last act is to breathe forth our last at the moment of death. Life's very possibility depends on the grace of breath's rhythmic recurrence. Like the presence of a pulse, the fact and rhythm of breathing is one of our vital signs, signifying life's vitality, and the mysteries of respiration have been a stimulus to the human imagination for centuries. Of course, ancient philosophers assumed what modern scientists are beginning to prove: breathing affects our mental and psychological well-being. The oldest Chinese medical book, the *Nei Ching*,[1] written around 2600 BCE, calls lungs 'ministers who regulate one's actions'; in another place, the lungs are called the seat of sorrow. Later Chinese texts suggest that deep breathing clears the intellect and perhaps prolongs life.

People have speculated that our word 'is' originally came from the Indo-European root word *as-*, meaning 'to breathe.' From the French *aspirer* and the Latin *aspirare* – both meaning 'to breathe upon' – we derive our word 'aspire,' which means to long for or seek, and 'aspiration,' which means a strong desire or ambition. We all aspire to ideals, ideas, and images of self-realization (e.g., intelligence, imagination, and sensibility) that we hope will complete and deepen the totality of our nature. Jung's ideas about the self as the totality of the psyche were anchored here and found expression as such in the last century.

A general interest in respiration on the part of ancient peoples probably derives from it never having been easy to decide whether our breath comes from within or without. Understandings of our earliest conceptions of soul, spirit, *anima*, *animus*, and even consciousness itself rely on the phenomenology of this attribute.[2] Many ancient Greek theories of breathing stemmed from Aristotle's observations that 'the soul is air' or 'air moves and is cognizant,' and for the ancient Greeks, lungs themselves were organs of consciousness. We still use the phrase 'I need to get something off my chest.'

When both feeling and thought were understood to be the work of the lungs, breathing in literally brought inspiration. To take a deep breath could make courage palpable, while to be breathless was to be faint and powerless. Inspired by Aristotle's notions, the Pneumatists concluded that air was pneuma (spirit, a vital force), and pneuma was the source of all health and disease. The Latin *spiritus* means both spirit and breath, as does the Greek pneuma and the Hebrew *ruah*. When we say that someone is spirited, or high spirited, we mean that they are full of vitality. In Christian theology, the third person of the Trinity is thought to be spirit – literally, the Breath of God. One is baptized with the Holy Spirit. And in Pentecost, the Breath of God can become visible as holy fire.

In *Genesis* 1, we learn that the human being, the *nephesh*, is dust of the earth that is elevated to human form only when it is inspired by *ruah*, the divine breath.[3] God breathes the breath of life into the nostrils of the *nephesh*, and *nephesh* thus becomes a living soul. *Ruah* thus signifies that spark of divinity in the creature that ties creature to Creator, a primary connection between God's inspiring force and a creature's vital being. Commonly, the *ruah* – a procreative life soul with a wisdom of its own – worked in the belly: the spirit of Yahweh entered in the belly to possess someone to prophecy, to fill them with wisdom or strength, to trouble a person, or to lead someone astray (Onians, 485). In the Hebrew tradition, then, to breathe is to assimilate spiritual power.

Pantanjali, the Indian sage who first codified the rules of yoga in the second century CE, linked control of thoughts and emotions to breath control that is gained in mastering various *pranayamas*, or methods of regulating prana, the life force. Master yogis have always particularly emphasized breathing, believing that breathing enables one to absorb not only air but also the light of the sun. In yogic thought, the two movements of breathing – inspiration and expiration, positive and negative – connect with the circulation of the blood and other important symbolic paths of involution and evolution. Difficulty in breathing may therefore indicate difficulty in assimilating basic principles of spirit and cosmos. We can associate the 'proper rhythm' of yogic breathing to the 'proper voice' demanded by ancient Egyptians for the ritual reading of sacred texts, or the 'proper' pronunciation and articulation that was demanded by one of our earliest languages, *Sanskrit*, a language that is specifically based on breath control.

Spirit and wind

In Indian mythology, the breathing cosmos is seen as alternating periods of activity and rest: The Days and Nights of Brahma. In the intervals between successive creations, Vishnu reclines, withdrawing the universe into himself. A little Gouache from the Guler School, c. 1760[4] illustrates Vishnu sitting within a golden egg in a threefold aspect: as himself, as the serpent Ananta-Shesha, who forms his bed, and as the Cosmic Ocean on which both he and the Ananta-Shesha float. All of creation is pictured as if it were a dream within Vishnu, ready, as he breathes out, to manifest from the potentiality of Primordial Waters as the Spiraling of the Cosmic Serpent. This symbolism amplified my recent dream, wherein I am moving in and out of what appears to be a holograph of a ghostly great white snake: perhaps during all my years of psychotherapeutic practice, I've really been practicing how to dance with spirit and inspiration, and (perhaps) with life itself.

In its active or violent aspects, and by virtue of its connection with the creative breath, or exhalation, wind was once believed to be a primary element. Qualities of bodily wind that have been attributed to breath are age-old indicators of sickness or health. Dry breath implied alertness and sobriety, for example, while a wet breath implied intoxication or the damp heaviness of sleep. Odor on the breath can indicate health or sickness. An entire Hippocratic treatise (translated both as *On Breaths* and *On Winds*) closes with the statement that 'winds are, in all diseases, the principle agents' (Majno, 310). Many ancient peoples thought that disease, like courage, was something that could be inhaled into the lungs from without. A similar theory appears in Plato's *Timaeus* (85), where tetanus was believed to be because of air that entered from without and caused the sinews to swell and strain. We moderns, contagiously coughing and sneezing ourselves through winter months, apparently continue this theory, believing that many diseases 'enter from without.'

Ancient Egyptians as well as the Chinese also considered spirit as 'wind' to be a possible cause of disease. For early Egyptians, our ears were part of our pulmonary system. In a rather skewed anticipation of right-brain/left-brain theory, one ancient manuscript states that the breath of life enters by the right ear and the breath of death enters by the left (Majno, 310). According to the text of the *Smith Papyrus* (possibly the world's oldest discussion of causes), when a disease or injury enters from the outside, it is the breath of an outside god, or death itself, rather than the intrusion of something engendered by flesh. Here the commentator, obviously distinguishing between internal and external causes, suggested that if even an open wound can imply the 'breath of an outside god or death,' treatment by magic was clearly indicated. The Egyptian goddess Isis was the patroness of such therapy (Majno, 125).

As in Hindu thought, in Chinese thought the internal *ch'i* was breath that was not all that different from meteorological wind. 'In estimating people,' muses the unknown writer of *The Seventeenth Century Mustard Seed Garden Manual of Painting*,

> the quality of spirit [*ch'i*] is as basic as the way they [people] are formed, and so it is with rocks, which are the framework of the heavens and of earth and also have *ch'i*. That is the reason rocks are sometimes spoken of as 'roots of the clouds.' Rocks without *ch'i* are dead rocks, as bones without the same vivifying spirit are dry are bones.[5]

And in the *Nei Ching*, it is reported that 'winds contribute to the development of a hundred diseases' (Majno, 310).

Breath as spirit and soul, including aspiration, inspiration, and expiration, have always been experienced culturally as *both/and*: as positive *and* negative, as creative *and* destructive, and as possible agents of death and disease as well as sources of procreative energy. Here are some examples: an old superstition I am unable to trace tells us that the breath of the panther is so sweetly fragrant that it allures (to their extreme danger) humans, beasts, and cattle to inhale it, yet the sweet breath of life or the Holy Spirit itself also figures in the panther's breath. From the word *Hurakan*, meaning 'the Mighty Wind' worshipped by Indigenous Peoples in what is now called South America, we get our word for dreaded 'hurricanes.' The Buddha alludes to a double aspect of the breath in *The Secret of the Golden Flower*: instructing his disciples on the necessity for 'fixing the heart,' he mentions the necessity of *refining* the power of breath with the heart:

> When you fix your heart on one point, then nothing is impossible for you. The heart easily runs away, so it is necessary to gather it together by means of breathing power. Breathing power easily becomes coarse, therefore it has to be refined by the heart. When that is done, can it then happen that it (the heart) is not fixed?[6]

In a psychological community, we instruct ourselves similarly. In a kind of psychological take-off on an Ignatian 'discernment of the spirits,' we value the making of consciousness and acknowledge the necessity of becoming conscious in order to live a personal life. The implication is that 'fixed' personal feeling and the ability to make conscious choices reflects a refinement of impersonal spirit.

In more recent cultures, like Bali, the ceremony to consecrate a Brahmana priest is a matter of breath control, postural immobility, and vacant concentration on the depths of being, a ritual that is thought to display a reach toward numinous transcendence.[7] And D. T. Suzuki, in his comments on the image of the 'fat belly' in pictures of Zen masters in connection with concentration on the *hara* as the center of being, suggests that a 'fat belly' indicates the significance of diaphragmatic breathing – the sort of breathing that is done with the whole body or the whole person; but diaphragmatic breathing also signifies breath that enters the body as fully as possible, as if to sound the depths of the inner world.[8]

Breath and the inner world

Historically and linguistically, there are explicit connections between the attribute of respiration and the inner world, meaning the world of unconscious spirit and soul. If I stop to reflect on my own breathing, I discover that its rhythm remains smooth and regular only as long as I don't pay attention to it. Implicit in this discovery is the indissoluble connection of my breath with my inner world. Our everyday language is filled with allusions to the union of breath and expressing instinctive or unconscious emotion: when angry, we 'bellow,' we 'breath fire,' or we 'fume with anger'; more mythically, we 'breathe forth vengeance.' We 'breathe a secret,' or if – in confidence – we pledge 'not to breathe a word.' We describe ourselves as 'panting' with eagerness, 'gasping' with astonishment, 'whistling' with amazement, 'snorting' with indignation, 'sobbing' with grief, 'yawning' with weariness or boredom, 'laughing' with mirth, and 'sighing' with sadness and think nothing of it. If we are suddenly tired, we're 'winded.' We 'catch our breath' at a sudden sound. We 'hold our breath' in suspense, and we 'become breathless' with anticipation or anxiety and then 'breathe freely' again. Every sudden emotion can quicken the action of a heart and, with it, our respiration.

As we know the inner world today, it has deep origins in our instinctive experience. In its collective nature it is rooted in bodily functioning, and in its personal nature it is rooted in somatic memories of embodied experience. In part, the quality of instinctual experience accounts for our attitude toward whatever exists inside. Acute instinctual or archetypal experience gathers the personality together from within: thus do we gasp in pain, sigh with relief, hold our breath in anticipation, feel breathless with excitement, or feel inspired by ideas. In each case, the way that we feel – *not just physically but emotionally* – is directly linked to how we breathe. Whether a breathing pattern is rapid or slow or deep or shallow or whether it predominates through the left or the right nostril determines our susceptibility to illness, the strength of our beating heart, and the depths of our depression.

Breath and imagination

I propose that metaphorically and symbolically, all our imaginative activity rises and falls in concert with respiration. Under the rhythm of breath's turn and return, creative inspiration moves in and out of our consciousness. This means that while creative inspiration remains deeply connected to respiration, it also relates us to revelations of the inner world – revelation as a second breath and a second sight. Just as the Buddha thought of breath as coarse or refined, we can regard our imaginative inspirations (or aspirations) as coarse or refined as well, depending on whether we use them for good or ill. The function of imaginative expression is to reveal images of an inner order that is shared by all of us, that opens to each of us those ways *in*; but always the creative imagination is a child of unconscious forces rather than conscious will, so imaginative inspiration is impersonal, too. This means that the creative spirit can be as primeval as the inspiration of a bodily breath, and its use may describe and enrich reality, distort and deny reality, or a little of each. Creativity can terrorize as well as inspire.

Truly expressive images are released from within. When an inspired act or expression is successful, it is as if it produces a second showing of the external world – a showing from another world that contains, holds, and reveals an inner world. Dame Julian of Norwich, in her rapturous *Revelations of Divine Love*,[9] called her showings, *Shewings*. Whether we call the inspiring force the Holy Spirit, the psyche, the Muse of Apollo, or the unconscious matters little; whatever we call it, it *acts on* those who receive its impact, arriving as an invigorating and informing force that provides new energy and knowledge, or it erupts with ruthlessly destructive energy that clears away what stood before and scours the remains. Once I dreamed that a white wind made of light spiraled down from the sky to move in and out of every last crevice and cranny of a dark earth that was also somehow myself, scouring it clean of all that did not belong: that's the kind of 'ruthless scouring' I mean.

Always moving in more or less the same way, inspirations of the inner world visit us at unexpected moments – awake, asleep – so that they startle us into action, surprise us into utterance, or (as in dreams) unfold a new awareness. And Jung tells us, from a psychological point of view, inspiration seems to act most deeply from and on whatever aspect of our personality is least differentiated along the lines of Jung's four functional personality types. The fourth function, he suggests, is not only the least developed (consciously) but also the most primitive and often the most creative.

Personal experience

I was an unwitting child of the respiratory domain. Having undergone three tonsillectomies and repeated bouts of strep throat – not to mention several episodes of childhood pneumonia – before I entered my teens, I grew up to think of my lungs and throat as my weak spots. To add to repeated experiences of being operated on under ether and feeling unable to breathe, I had an emergency appendectomy before I was seven, and upon returning to school, I promptly fell off a merry-go-round in the school yard, broke open my stitches, and had to go back under (anesthesia) to have the scar and stitches repaired. So many bouts of unconsciousness and feeling radically 'acted on' took their respiratory toll, leaving memories of fear of suffocating and not 'waking up' again.

So childhood breathing felt precarious, and breath was precious. Once doctors told my young mother that my lungs might 'have a spot.' (Tuberculosis? Back then, it was a possibility; my mother's father had died from tuberculosis when she was three!). And I repeatedly 'got' colds and sore throats until my late twenties. My adenoids were taken out too – I forget just when. In early adolescent yoga classes, I came to think of my 'throat chakra' as my weak link, elaborating on an idea of myself as a girl who could move (e.g., dance, ballet, and acrobatics) but seldom speak, someone who could sing in a choir with others (and – later – write well enough) but essentially rather die than get up in public and sing (or speak). This accruing self-image came to inhabit my inner world. In addition, I came from a family wherein many things were to remain unaddressed and unspoken, even if one *could* have found words enough to tell them. True to form, I seldom 'breathed a word.'

In general, a child who discovers that she can affect caretakers by withholding emotional expression – by *not* crying, laughing, breathing, or sighing – is not that different from the child who discovers that she can get what she wants by loud, prolonged crying or tantrums. Both 'children' (of whatever age) have begun a shadowy functionalization of native, emotional expressiveness that skews a developing personality toward fixed, persistently unconscious modes of respiratory behavior – for example, a characteristic laugh, a tremor in the voice, or a marked tendency to withdraw into silence. Until such a child can become aware of the ideas and attitudes that underlie their behavior, it remains sacramental, used 'magically,' and ritually connected to archetypal energy. A child may write a poem, for example, unaware that what they are really doing is asking for love and attention. Poem in hand, their attitude may convey something like 'now, are you proud of me?' (meaning, 'now, will you love me?') My mother's reception of my first poem was mixed. As I remember, 'My Little Sister as Ten Pink Toes' was the scribbled outcome of my buckling down to feel 'as I ought' to feel about the arrival of a second sibling, God having failed to 'at least let it be another boy!' as my seven-year-old self so fervently prayed, walking round and round the swing set in the back yard. In similar fashion, a musician may perfect his ability to play an instrument because, as a person, he can hardly speak, and when he is asked to speak, he experiences anxiety and helplessness. Some actors play an endless number of roles searching for the one that will give them a sense of singular identity since they are much more at ease in a role than when they appear people; and a therapist may speak to many, many patients for a long time rather than address their own psychological situation.

As I mentioned in the Introduction, the first thing in my respiratory repertoire that happened when I began voice lessons with Joseph was that I stopped smoking, and I've not smoked since. Beginning in college, I smoked: everyone else smoked too, and in my early world, smoking was 'adult.' In several WWII neighborhood blackouts, my brother and I were sent to play in a closed-in, well-lit hallway closet for the duration. When we emerged, I could tell where the grown-ups were sitting in the dark by the glowing ends of their 'ciggies,' as they called them. Our family purchased cigarettes, C- rations, and chocolate at the local army canteen. Today the mere thought of inhaling smoke pains my lungs; thus, I avoid visiting Beijing, and the smoke of wildfires on a horizon makes me drive in the opposite direction. On September 11, 2001, my husband and I were in Manhattan, New York, during the World Trade Center catastrophe. That day, the air became so laden with smoke that we could hardly breathe. Weeks later, walking the streets of Toronto, Canada, and breathing clear northern air, I said to Don, 'Something is wrong with my lungs; I suddenly can't breathe!' At home, my doctor called it 'adult-onset asthma' – not all that uncommon – but I could hardly bear the thought, let alone own my condition. I feel as if a ghostly 'breath' of ghastly smoke of the 9/11 destruction haunts me still.

Respiration and the shaman

Shamanic personalities seem to have an instinctive apprehension of the symbolic effects of spirit and breath. Among early peoples, the archaic shaman – the 'chosen one' – was the person who influenced others through inspired power over the spirits (archetypes), and they often expressed the degree of their connection with the spirit world in respiratory language and respiratory ways. By way of excited breathing (the effects of hyperventilation); more shallow, trance-like breaths;

using ritualized sobbing and sighing; or hypnotic singing and chanting, shamans communicated to others their experience of an inner world. Because such unconscious, expressive respiratory manifestations were also how a shaman could fulfill their task of realigning the collective psyche of the group, they easily became fixed as sacramental modes of respiratory behavior. Familiar with (and using) all of breath's meanings and manifestations, shamans became respiratory technicians, specializing in the respiratory domain.

As a lord of magical flight, a shaman was also completely identified with inspirations and aspirations – with their own creativity, bright ideas, and intuitions – and prone to unconscious identification with collective images. In this domain, a modern person's unconscious identification with the shaman likely takes the form of unconscious identification with *the psyche's creativity*, and all kinds of erratic behavior is 'acted out' and acted on: trips are taken on whim, therapy is ended without notice, emotional responsibilities are left unanswered, and relationships are turned inside out. Sudden changes of all kinds happen 'out of the blue.' In other words, when shamanic personalities today evince little value to a personal life, they follow suit. Like an archaic shaman, the porous nature of a shamanic person finds it all too easy to identify with the psyche itself – with its rivers and currents, its products and dreams, its inspirations and revelations, its instincts, its unconscious patterns, and its gods.

In archaic times, a shaman's song represented a profound relationship between spirit and matter. Emerging from within as a song or a chant, we can liken the spirit of a shaman's breath to an illumined soul, shining through the eyes of a human face. Orpingalik, a shaman-poet, told Rasmussen,

> Songs are thoughts, sung with the breath when people are moved by great forces and ordinary speech no longer suffices. . . . How many songs I have I cannot tell you. I keep no count of such things. There are so many occasions in one's life when a joy or sorrow is felt in such a way that the desire comes to sing, and so I only know that I have many songs. All my being is song. I sing as I draw my breath.[10]

Often a shaman's mask had a distinctive mouth; some have animal teeth, while from others a tongue protrudes. Sometimes a shaman's face peered out from within an animal's open jaws or the beak of a giant bird. Presumably, empty or O-shaped mouths were *not* empty, since this configuration was associated with a shaman's breath and breath's inherent power. From our earliest beginnings, then, having breath or not has meant the difference between life and death: hence breath's direct association with soul or spirit. Someone's soul might be the same as that person's breath, so that in trance – while the soul left the body – a shaman was considered dead. Ancient Finns called the shamanic state *olia halitosa*, meaning that the ecstatic state itself could be understood as the act of 'being named by a spirit':[11] and being named was comparable to having one's soul formed (or – as we might say – having one's psyche complexed),[12] in that 'soul' comes from a Gothic word root that denotes 'wind' and the word for 'name' derives from another word that means 'to blow.' As both name and soul consist of breath, writes Briffault (4–11), one's name must be comparable to one's soul.

Even before the advent of shamanism, breath had special power. Certain mythic figures cured the sick by blowing on them or farting ('break wind.')[13]

'With visible breath I am walking,' sings Pte Ska Win (White Buffalo Maiden) as she appears, walking from sky to earth, bringing the prayer pipe to Indigenous Peoples in what is now called the United States – the first of seven gifts: 'I walk and my voice is heard. I am walking with visible breath. I am bringing this sacred pipe; with it, I walk to you. For you I am walking with this pipe . . . so that the breath may become visible.'[14]

Some shamans cured by blowing, for the power of a shaman's breath could blast forth like a fire. In practice, the shaman's mouth was the most frequently utilized opening of their body: a spirit helper might live in a shaman's mouth, or a helper had been swallowed, or was kept in the mouth for 'storage.' From a shaman's mouth, power was emitted as visible or invisible breath, as flame, or as an animal soul.

Among our fellow mammals on this planet, only dolphins are distinguished by purely voluntary breathing (my dream of the ghostly great white snake contained a dolphin, but I was dancing with the snake). Dolphins do not sleep as we do, lest they drown. Our breathing, while not voluntary, forms an odd link between the voluntary and involuntary functions of our brains. Although our breathing is regulated by the nervous system in the same way that our heartbeat, blood flow, and other autonomic functions are, breathing seems to be the only one of these that we can consciously alter. By consciously controlling our breathing, we have some control over other functions of importance, like brain waves, hormonal secretions, and metabolism. Breathing is the key to the amazing feats of bodily control that yogis perform, and it is directly related in strategic ways to the functioning of our internal organs, emotions, and minds.[15] Through using proper exercises to relax our muscles and allow for proper breathing, we release pent-up emotions and deal with them.

Psychotherapy and respiration

Strictly speaking, respiration and its extended meanings enter the scene the moment a psychotherapeutic relationship begins. Both analyst and patient participate in respiratory behavior every time they breathe, cough, sneeze, sniffle, speak, laugh, or cry. A psychotherapist of my acquaintance was working with a highly anxious, obsessional patient who had recently been destabilized by an interaction at work and now obsessed feared that she would be fired. In her session she could barely sit still, cycling through her anxious thoughts so fast that no self-reflection was possible. The therapist asked her patient to close her eyes, focus on her breathing, and then – as she had done before – did a slow 'body scan,' asking her patient to follow her breath into various parts of her body and notice where tension was, directing her breath to those places and letting her breath 'refresh' and relax them. The patient calmed noticeably, and as her breath entered her lower abdomen, suddenly she 'saw' her younger, little girl self and burst into tears. The rest of the session was spent exploring her sad feelings and remembering a traumatic history that left her lonely and sad, threatened by abandonment.

This scenario gives us an example of how the shaman as symbolic process can link a patient's distressed ego with feelings in the body, then with an image, and then with unconscious personal history, dissociated until made explicit, riding up into the patient's imagination on the little surfboard of her breath. This also gives us an example of how a therapist's explicit attention to respiration as a vehicle for entering the inner world can open the unconscious in therapy. We can imagine that breath and respiration were so effective here because both of them are under voluntary control and are simultaneously involuntary. Both implicitly unite conscious and unconscious worlds, and *both* describe the respiratory domain through which the shaman dances.

Explicit attention to the breath and the non-ordinary realities of unconscious life that breath can open within psychotherapy is also found in the work of Christina Grof and Stanislav Grof. The Grofs' breath work confirms Wilhelm Reich's observation that psychological defenses (character armoring among them) use mechanisms of restricting breathing so that 'opening up the breath' seems to loosen psychological defenses at their roots and open the unconscious. The Grofs' call their method holonomic integration, or holotropic breathwork therapy (Grof, 1988, 169). In holotropic work, after having been prepared by therapists who serve as guides, a client is asked to relax in a safe setting and simply accelerate their breathing while they surrender to music and focus on their inner world, accepting whatever emerges. Significant healing results have been reported, including mysteries such as the remarkable story of Gladys, reported by the Grofs from an experiential seminar held at Esalen Institute, in California.

For many years, Gladys suffered from serious attacks of depression, accompanied by intense anxiety. In the session that Grof describe, as Gladys descended into holotropic breathing, she responded with an extraordinary activation of physical energy, including violent tremors, screams, and fighting motions. Slowly her screams became more articulate and began to resemble words in an unknown language. The group encouraged Gladys to let the sounds emerge (which seemed to her nonsensical), and she began to chant them in powerful, repetitive sequences that sounded like prayer. Inexplicably, the chant moved the group so profoundly that many members were in tears.

Later, Gladys reported that she felt an irresistible urge to 'speak' this apparent language and that she had no understanding of what she uttered. An Argentinian psychoanalyst who was participating in the group realized that Gladys chanted in a perfect Sephardic language, which he happened to know. This language, also called Ladino, is a Judeo-Spaniolic hybrid consisting of medieval Spanish and Hebrew. Gladys had never heard about Ladino, nor was she Jewish, nor did she know or speak modern Spanish. She did not know such a language existed or what it was. But here is a literal translation of the chant that so powerfully affected the group:

> 'I am suffering, and I will always suffer,
> I am crying, and I will always cry.
> I am praying, and I will always pray.'
> This episode and the profound influence it had on Gladys have remained a mystery for her as well as for us.
>
> (Grof, 1988, 169)

Grof's case gives us a perfect example of shamanic activation in a shamanic personality within a 'tribe' down to its archetypal bones: clearly Gladys channeled collective *and* personal material. Gladys could have made a perfect archaic shaman, dancing in the firelight, unconsciously activating the unconscious of her surrounding people as she articulated spirits of suffering and sorrow. All the members of her 'tribe' were deeply affected, even though only one member of her 'tribe' could read a narrative into the spirits, and Gladys could not. In this situation, it was as if respiration opened a worldwide net of connectivity. And moments like these – where we glimpse an expanding domain that interconnects us all – return us to the mystery that we are.

Other 'respiratory' professions

Relevant imagery of this attribute is frequently found in the psyches of those whose professions specifically depend on the expressive capacities of the respiratory domain. This includes singers, actors, musicians, teachers, writers, and speakers of all kinds, including therapists – creative personalities all, who depend on access to depths of unconscious creativity. Professions like these cluster around the field of the shaman as a channel of symbolic expression and communication, so it isn't remarkable that shamanic aspects mark off cryptic expressions of emotion like fixed habits of breathing around unexpressed indignation or anger, characteristic sighs that indicate boredom, despair, or helplessness. Others also employ creative faculties from the respiratory domain in life and work, whether in artistic terms or not. And we all have habits of nearly ceasing to breath around concentration or reverie.

On the other hand, we may find ourselves taking breaths so quickly that we seem on the verge of hysteria discover ourselves in the midst of periodic bouts of sniffles or throat clearings instead of assertive articulations, or be overcome by elaborately stifled yawning rather than voicing our outspoken opinions or irritations. As small and unimportant as they are when they are consciously related to, when such respiratory mannerisms are employed unconsciously, they function as fixed 'habits of expression' that communicate bundles of unconscious affect.

Breathing problems of all kinds, including allergic reactions, asthma, and other respiratory conditions that once resulted (and still do) in tuberculosis or consumption, or in pneumonia, bronchitis, or sinusitis, are exacerbated when they are hosted by a person whose unconscious use of the respiratory attribute borrows from attitudes and assumptions that underlie the symbol of the shaman. Involuntary muscular spasms have always been associated with emotional stress and nervous tension mediated through the autonomic or involuntary nervous system, and the bronchial spasms that are characteristic of asthma attacks are involved in other diseases of the respiratory system, including emphysema, bronchitis, and pneumonia. Breath is life, so it is small wonder that our patients (and ourselves) who suffer from serious respiratory disorders experience fear and panic. Our emotional states and breathing patterns are so deeply interrelated that our respiratory patterns become irregular with anger, slow and deepen with relaxation, and quicken with fear or stress.

We take it for granted these days that physiological symptoms function as somatizations that are symbolic of psychological issues: asthmatic personalities wrestle with dependency issues, for example, while singers who periodically lose their voice, or writers who lose inspiration, usually contend with complicated issues of personality development. In personalities like these, the shaman complex usually mediates subjective aspects of personality inaccessible to consciousness by channeling such implicit material into enacted respiratory behavior.

Plain and simply speaking, someone suffering from asthma simultaneously suffers a psychological and a physiological condition. Whatever the *facts* may be, their shamanic behavior will tend to compensate for it, employing respiratory phenomena sacramentally in a 'dependency' complex. Unconscious projections of 'the feminine' as nurturer – negative or positive – may fall onto their therapist, onto their personal mother or women in general, onto the animus, on their own body, or onto the unconscious itself, as in Briffault's realm of 'The Mothers.'

To accompany the psychogenetic predisposition of an asthmatic person 'within,' I know I will have to help them dig up memories, since our individual bodies are containers, vehicles, and memory banks combined: thus, shadow material will lie in the patient's unconscious use of bodily symptoms. When all the emotions and affects that may surround such a condition in terms of the past and whatever it all means now have entered consciousness – including awareness of how the shaman complex affects others – an experience of 'self-relatedness' lies within this person's reach. The psychological meaning of their asthmatic condition in relation to the totality (wholeness) of their asthmatic personality has been approached by therapist and patient together.

Writer's block (or other blocks that deny access to a spontaneously emotionally expressive life) may seem less extreme, but writer's block is no less pertinent to the respiratory domain. Usually, such a creative block indicates the presence of an unconscious demand that one's own emotional expressiveness be *functional* – that is, one's creativity work to achieve some end, like making an impression on others, maintaining a mask, being worth one's time, earning a good deal of money, or producing fame or public notice. To place such an expectation on oneself ends up being an example of what Bernard Brandschaft calls 'pathological accommodation' on one's inner world (Brandchaft, 2007). Such a demand places an excruciating burden on one's native capacity: not only will creative inspiration have little chance to inflame one's imagination, but under such pressure, something in our instinctive nature also rebels.

Here it helps me to remember that the functionalization of cryptic emotional expression was one of the primary strongholds of the archaic shaman. As a physically individual container for revelations from the collective unconscious, archaic shamans had inspired experiences that they expressed through images, words, songs, movements, rhythms, gestures, and sensations of all kinds. Shaman repeatedly experience a return to the origins, and given significant depth and import, their 'realizations' have the force and value of living myth for those who receive them through the shaman's embodied person – see, for example, Grof's patient, Gladys, mentioned earlier. The archaic shaman's image may symbolize the creative presence of a mediating personality within any group or society, but we have choice today in how – or whether – we step into such a role.

Notes

1 Shampo, Marc A., and Robert A. Kyle: *Nei Ching – Oldest Known Medical Book*. Mayo Clinic Proceedings, Google; also, Ingher, Dina: 'Brain Breathing,' in *Science Digest*. June 1981. 75.

2 Onians traces an evolution of psychological understanding: the ancient Greeks understood the breath of the living as well as the soul (breath-soul) of the dead as the *anima*, while the *animus* was the vital life principle of a living person. For Romans, the vital life principle was also in the *anima*, which resided in the head with the *genius*. Romans, however, called the *animus* the principle of consciousness that included all variations of emotion and thought: to contemplate an action was to have it 'in one's *animus*'; to turn attention toward something was an act of *animus*; courage, despair, pride, spirit, thoughts, words, and logos were matters of *animus*. The *animus* was concerned with consciousness, while the *anima*, the vital life principle, was not.

3 *Nephesh* is closely related to the Assyrian *napistu*, meaning the throat through which one breathes: the larynx. *Ruah* has the root sense of blowing – of wind, blast, merger, spirit – and only sometimes breath (Onians, Richard B.: *The Origins of European Thought*. New York: Arno Press. 1973. 481).

4 Purce, Jill: *The Mystic Spiral: Journey of the Soul (Art and Imagination)*. London: Thames & Hudson. Perfect Paperback. Illustration 1.

5 Mai-Mai, Sze: *The Way of Chinese Painting: Its Ideas and Techniques with Selections from the Seventeenth Century Mustard Seed Garden Manual of Painting*. New York: Random House. 1959. 191.

6 Buddha: *The Secret of the Golden Flower: A Chinese Book of Life*. Translated by Richard Wilhelm. New York: Harcourt, Brace and Company. 1932. 46.

7 Geertz, Clifford: 'Deep Play: Notes on the Balinese Cockfight,' in *Myth, Symbol and Culture*. Edited by Clifford Geertz. New York: W. W. Norton and Company. 1971. 29.

8 Suzuki, D. T.: 'The Awakening of a New Consciousness in Zen,' in *Man and Transformation: Papers from the Eranos Yearbooks*. Bollingen Series XXX. Volume 5. Edited by Joseph Campbell. New York: Pantheon Books. 1964. 201.

9 Julian of Norwich, also known as Dame Julian or Mother Julian, was the greatest of all the English anchorites of the Middle Ages.

10 Halifax, Joan: *Shamanic Voices: A Survey of Visionary Narratives*. New York: E. P. Dutton. 1979. 16, 321.

11 Briffault, Robert: *The Mothers: A Study of the Origins of Sentiment and Institutions*. Volume 1. New York: The MacMillan Company. 1927. 4–11.

12 In these amplifications, the action of spirit on the psyche is depicted as an act of having one's psyche 'complexed,' or formed. Later mythological manifestations similarly assert that spirit 'fathers' ego consciousness, not ego intent; e.g., Yahweh's visit to Sarai results in Isaac, son of the spirit, not son of Abram, and the Holy Spirit's visit to Mary results in Jesus, son of God, not son of Joseph.

13 Rasmussen, Knud: *Intellectual Culture of the Iglulik Eskimos*. Quoted in *The Coming and Going of the Shaman: Eskimo Shamanism and Art*. Winnipeg: The Winnipeg Art Gallery. 1979. 182.

14 Freesoul, John Redtail: 'The Native American Prayer Pipe: Ceremonial Object and Tool of Self-Realization,' in *Shamanism: An Expanded View of Reality*. Edited by Shirley Nicholson. Wheaton, IL: The Theosophical Publishing House. 1987. 204.

15 Ingher, Dina: 'Brain Breathing,' in *Science Digest*. June 1981. 75, 110–111.

Chapter 12

Movement

Movement and aliveness

We are born moving, and for us animate creatures, movement is almost synonymous with life itself. News that something or someone is *still*born brings a chill, and a body that is utterly without movement summons the specter of death – life's sister mystery – into a living, moving world. To see and feel movement, then, evokes the depths of our human existence; and because it can happen only across time and space, immediately apprehending movement evokes, and is accompanied by, conscious and unconscious memory in psyche and soma both.

Movement that we can apprehend also implies stillness – something that does not move. Yet even apparent stillness may be a fiction, because apparently everything moves, all the time. Alan Lightman (2018) writes out of this paradox, imagining that he is standing at the North Pole 'in the shoes' of Robert Edwin Peary, who lived near his home on an island in Maine. Musing on stillness and motion, Lightman reminds us that even when we imagine ourselves locally at rest relative to the center of our planet – 'at the precise point where that imaginary axis emerges from the interior and punctures the ice' – the center of the earth itself is still in motion, hurtling around its own center star at 65,000 miles per hour and that *that* star, in turn, revolves around the Milky Way, the center of our galaxy. 'Do I know too much, or too little?' Lightman wonders; 'I look up into space, as the cave dwellers did, and am transfixed by the infinite. Although I cannot touch it, I *feel* that I'm there. This resting yet unresting pole is quite a spot for viewing the universe' (31, italics mine). In his night sky reverie, Lightman feels 'moved' by forces larger than himself, and this fact lends emotional power to his experience and ours.

We don't usually think about movement; we just move. We can imagine the attribute of movement as a basic element of life in which children simply swim, for example, unconscious and un-self-reflecting. As children, we *are* movement: we just 'Be.' My early memories of movement include turning cartwheels every school day, rain or shine, from my house to Cherrylee Elementary School, two blocks away, and home again. I also remember swinging high and low on the swing set in the backyard every evening after dinner, pumping and pumping on the swing set that Grammy gave us (until I was old enough to help with the dishes). In the chapter on rhythm, I mentioned becoming a Haughton-Tot and learning to tap dance, but real self-awareness of my body in motion came only later as I grew up a little and began formal lessons in ballet and acrobatics. Not until then did I become aware (or capable) of self-discipline, and the difficult sensations that accompanied hard work accomplished, the stiff tendons and sore muscles that accompanied the physical activity in which I had formerly, mindlessly, moved. Reflecting on how hard it was to loosen up sore muscles grown stiff from regular lessons in acrobatics and modern dance in my early teens, I wrote a little article for *Seventeen Magazine* that I titled 'How to Move Like a Glass Giraffe' (a title that was oddly sensate and 'frozen' at the same time, it occurred to me later).

Movement in history

Perhaps the earliest historical evidence we have of the human capacity to apprehend movement appears in prehistoric rupestrian art. Strewn like starry constellations across sky-dark walls of unmoving stone, shamanic petroglyphs of people and animals are important not only because of their anthropological significance but also because they depict movement, indicating that some kind of psychological differentiation of time from non-time (or dream time) had already occurred. Somewhere in the remote past, a first, brief apprehension in human consciousness made possible both an impulse and an ability to dramatically represent the monotonous but heart-stirring rhythms of movement and countermovement, the eternal cycles of life and death pulsating in sheer nature and human life. In essence, movement and countermovement express the most ancient drama of all: a dialectic of the living and the nonliving, the mysterious and the known – even of god and human. Our Judeo-Christian heritage, for example, posits God as Mover and ourselves as moved: God begins, and we respond; it is as if when God came to earth, puppets on the earth began to move, and all the bones danced in Ezekiel's dry valley. This heritage also tells us that when we imagine that *we* are the ones who give impetus to this drama, all sense of the dramatic vanishes from our lives, and we ourselves can *become* as rattling, dry bones: without a 'moving' sense of the divine, life and movement make no sense.

Moving body, moving psyche

As bodily movement is to motion, so psychic movement is to emotion. Though this was not always so, today our notions of motion and movement are as native to the inner world as they are to the outer. Common parlance equates motion and emotion when we find something moving, or when we say, 'I was deeply moved.' However, psyche's movement – since the time of William James, thought of as a *stream of consciousness* – is not really something that streams (movement) but a streaming *in* consciousness. Herbert Rorschach discovered that many of the subjects who responded to his inkblots saw movement in them and described movement as activity of some kind in the world. Rorschach's subjects also responded to the colorful inkblots with feeling, so that both movement in the outer world and movement in the inner world (emotion and feelings) are involved in reading and scoring Rorschach's plates of projective technique. Feeling and movement, or emotion and motion, are like two balancing pans of the psyche, inner and outer aspects of this attribute. Every thought and every emotion we have finds expression in movement, whether the expression consists of the gross muscular transformations that are usually involved in expressing rage or fear, the inspired or repetitively disciplined movements of creative work, or an infinitesimal change that occurs in the pupil of an eye, caused by a fleeting thought.

With growing awareness, we find we can develop a capacity for self-witnessing and emotional literacy, slowly attaining a greater capacity for objectivity and detachment, and our sense of urgency to express all the 'moving' emotions we feel begins to diminish. I imagine that this acquisition is something of a cultural gain, but whether we become healthier or whether we are the better for it is another question. This question was dramatically highlighted for me in an experience of major cultural differences. When I was in Russia in 1988 before the collapse of the Soviet Union, my husband and I attended a rock concert in a local theater. In response to the music, we Americans, sitting together in the balcony, virtually danced in our seats – legs swinging, arms gesturing, hands clapping. Then I happened to lean over the edge of the balcony, where I looked down at a solid bloc of Soviet patriots below, sitting stock still in their seats, gazing straight ahead. There was not a movement to be seen among them until the polite, cautious applause that accompanied the conclusion of the show. I wonder if such collective displays of frozen movement are different today.

Movement and culture

In ancient Greece, many great thinkers pondered movement. Aristotle defined movement as the actualization of potential in things: more importantly, the movement of 'things' indicated the presence of an unmoved mover (Buckley, 1971). Epicureans reached their awareness of the 'god' through the movement of the archetypes in the mind – that is, though those things that human beings *thought of* as movement. Somewhat differently, the Stoics found the 'Ultimate' (Aristotle's Unmoved Mover) in change that was apparent in all things; academics found it through the coming about of traditions of state; and Cicero found it though the implicit movement of discourse and debate.[1]

Among Western thinkers, apparently it wasn't until Hegel that the motion of the human mind was identified with the movement of objects. For Hegel, the movement of objects *united* subject and object: therefore, movement lodged at the substructure of reality. For Hegel, *movement itself* was the life of every concept and the soul of every proof. Because contradiction was a law of life itself and dialectic was a necessary movement of mind, Hegel declared that motion had to be the soul of matter, putting forth branches and fruits organically.[2] In contrast, much of our current psychological thinking tends to speak of psychological movement more in terms of unconscious fantasies or living images that trouble the psyche. Writing about embodied cognition and the aesthetics of human understanding, philosopher Mark Johnson (2007) reminds us that,

> From the very beginning of our life, and evermore until we die, movement keeps us in touch with our world in the most intimate and profound way. In our experience of movement, there is no radical separation of self from world . . . we are in touch with our world at a visceral level.
>
> (2007, 20)

In other words, movement gives us knowledge about the world and reveals important insights about our own nature, culture, capacities, and limitations. Understanding that psychic feeling and bodily change (movement) are two sides of a unity requires us to understand the psyche as a dimension of reality in which both psyche and soma have cumulative and reciprocal effects on each other and have never been separate; nor are we ever separate from our world. 'There is no movement without the space we move in, the things we move, and the qualities of movement, which are at the same time both the qualities of the world we experience and the qualities of ourselves as doers and experiencers,' says Johnson (20). In the primacy of psychic experience, there exists no split of self and other or self and world.

Dance as sacred movement

Long ago, perhaps when early human beings first became actively concerned with the powers of life, ordered bodily movement occurred, and dance became a universal, all-inclusive form of human expression. The oldest of all the arts, dance has apparently accompanied and stimulated all processes of life, from hunting and farming to war, fertility, death, and love. As sacred movement, dance was originally part of seasonal celestial observances. The corn and rain dances that are still performed today by some Indigenous Peoples in what is now called the United States give us living examples of such symbolically enacted, participative rituals. To this day, in Pueblo, Hopi, or Zuni ceremonies, entire villages partake of ritual ceremonies. Either as dancers or as the audience, everyone – the young, the old – dances in rituals that continue from sunrise to sunset with unfaltering movement and rhythm. Within the houses that surround the square, pregnant women move, and babies rock within their bellies, sharing rhythm before they are born. Outside the door in the audience, caretakers bounce infants on their knees for twelve and fourteen hours at a time.

No wonder particular tribal movements are felt to be inherent to the heart's deep rhythm from birth; after all, the movement and rhythm of tribally significant dances has been experienced from the beginning of human life. When my husband and I began our lives in New Mexico, I visited several Pueblo dances.

Usually a dance began at the crack of dawn. If I were lucky (or brought a chair) I had a seat, but I often stood with other onlookers hour after cold hour at a ritual distance, watching everyone – parents holding the hands of tiny ones – whose moccasin-clad feet pounded the same earth that had been pounded in the same fashion at the same time of year, generation after generation, for eons upon eons. (I wished *my* children could have experienced that kind of collective cohesiveness!) Then as now, only the words 'deeply moved' come close to describing how watching those dances made me feel.

In one translation of the *Odyssey*, Homer tells us that Eos, goddess of dawn, had her 'residences and dancing places,' implying that dance is a basic parental movement of all life. For Homer, the Muses and the Graces danced, along with Apollo and Dionysus. In India, Krishna danced, and Shiva, a noble incarnation of ecstatic movement, was also called Nataraja – king of the dance. Shiva dances, 'full of yearning, like the hidden fire in firewood, pouring his power into spirit and material and setting each in turn to dancing. In Shiva, pictured as dancing within a circle of flame, the whole world, completely caught up, dances to the same compelling rhythm of life and death.'[3]

The intoxicating nature of one kind of movement was vividly brought to life in the Dionysian rites. According to Aristotle, souls who devoted themselves to the service of Dionysus became enthusiastic (*entheos* – filled with the god). Plato cautiously agreed that mania or madness might be a necessary precondition for any contact with the Muse, but ecstasy, as inspiring and overpowering as it was, could also empty and discard what it conquered. A 'person' could become lost, while it felt as if the narrow confines of body and environment were extended to infinity. The Bacchantes danced until every human feeling was lost.

But another kind of intoxication with ecstasy happened under the aegis of Apollo – not Apollo the sun god, but his darker, more shadowy aspect – Apollo as healer and lord of the lair – had to do with shamanic arts. Under Apollo as incubator and (along with Morpheus) a master of dreams, ecstasy took the form of extreme stillness, as in trance. Then ecstasy was deeply individual and inwardly directed. Under Apollo as healer, ecstasy had to do with stillness, with lying in a cave barely breathing, like an animal, as in hibernation, and sleep. These were states of incubation and waiting, states of stillness and trance, associated by later mystery religions with experiencing 'death before you die' (Kingsley, 182–183).

With Lightman's meditation on the first page of this chapter, I suggested that our idea of stillness might be a fiction, but I made that suggestion in light of our present culture and modern world. The world of ancient Greece was different. While Dionysus inspired groups of ecstatically intoxicated dancers, Apollo as healer guided individuals into ecstatic trance – the stillness of waiting until the entrance to the underworld appeared, the stillness of another state of consciousness. Scholars like Peter Kingsley[4] trace this kind of inner movement back to shamanic traditions of Central Asia and Siberia. Apollo's ecstasy related to entering a state of suspended animation like the shaman's trance, entering a different world – a world that was concerned with 'indivisible oneness' (Kingsley,

111–115). In India, says Kingsley, 'this state that could be called a dream but isn't an ordinary dream, that's like being awake but isn't being awake, that's like being asleep but isn't – had its own names.' In Iranian tribes, and in Siberia and Central Asia, this shamanic, trance-like state of being is traceable back to even older shamanic cultures and prehistoric times.

Other arts have sprung from early dance: music, song, verse, and drama. Some claim that medieval folk dances were survivals of pagan imitative and generative magic. Yet dance itself remains the simplest unity, and like all artforms, dance generates and regenerates the very subjectivity it portrays. All our emotions, from lowest to highest, can be expressed and evoked by dance, and dance has often been experienced as a form of prayer. To dance, we need nothing – neither paint nor instrument – other than our bodies. We stamp our feet and clap our hands to produce rhythms that induce our bodies to move, the movements echoing in essence our beating hearts. Before we learn to use any other instrument, we use our bodies as instruments, and much individual experience of movement is not only visual but also kinesthetic. My kinesthetic experience of aching muscles stimulated my article about the glass giraffe.

Because we are literally made to move, the attribute of movement is active in creating and maintaining the health of the psyche/soma. I taught dance for a short time and saw for myself how dance lessons could become a vocabulary of self-discipline for my small students. I saw them try hard and become proud of themselves. Lessons in movement increased their self-esteem. Most young children move to music instinctively, anyway, especially if they see adults respond.

Movement and the shaman

Probably the first to gain access to the spirit world through ecstatic movement, the shaman was also the first ecstatic dancer. One meaning of the Tungus word *saman*, from which 'shaman' is derived, is 'one who is excited, moved, or raised.'[5] Early dances of early human beings (including shamans) imitated the motions of animals, for animals – especially birds – also dance. The instinctive certainty in the dance movements of animals must have impressed the first human dancers. In China, there were crane and monkey dances, in North America, dances of the buffalo and bear. We have our fox trot and our Pavan, or peacock dance. By dancing the movement of animals, a shaman mastered instinctive, animal rhythm; and by subjecting themselves to the animal order, a shaman added the power of the animals to individual human power, freeing deeply instinctive energies. By imitating an animal in dance, a shaman 'became' that animal.

In the frenzied dance of a shamanic ceremony, movement deepened and sometimes assumed control. Then movement became a sort of madness, sweeping first the dancer, then the others, along. Intoxication by movement, bodily *or* emotional, is highly contagious. Ritual intoxication (as in Dionysian rites, mentioned earlier) is easily transmitted from one person to the next, until finally the whole world seems swept along. Thus employed, movement releases power, dissipating it and emptying the soul so that the soul may be filled with the sacred. At the same time, raw elements of life are grasped and ruled. Dance unchains natural energy, but it also enchains it, making it possible for the movement and countermovement of passion to explode while being – at the same time – deeply controlled. And when movement becomes a sacred ritual or an ordered manifestation of the power of life, a place or the space for the enclosure and containment of movement becomes important too.

The archaic shaman 'found' shrines and dancing places already 'given,' intuiting holy glades and holy mountains already present in nature: 'this' is a holy place; 'this' is where the gods live or where god (an animal?) will visit again. A sense of the sacred rested between a shaman and a place, as if resting as *participation mystique* between someone who apprehended their subjective reaction as relevant and an object or place that *captured* their unconscious sense of relevance *out there*.

Early human beings deemed their first shelters to be enclosures of moving power. When building shelters began in history, any enclosed space that marked off inner from outer could become such an enclosure, understood to articulate potential movement 'held.' Some of the oldest surviving enclosures are dance houses in which – in that the dance house was built specifically to contain it – the power of motion was 'fixed.' Older still are enclosed dancing grounds such as the Maga in ancient Iran, where ecstatic singers and dancers assembled to develop their powers within a closed circle.

Movement and psyche

The real miracle of this attribute is the fact that inner movement or emotion becomes ordered, becomeing psychological by being perceived, experienced, valued, and understood to manifest unfolding, differentiating psyche. This is a movement from chaos to order. Whether we experience the psyche as rolling, dying, laughing, sleeping, or crying, the experience of psyche *as such* is always an experience of ordered movement. Some psychologists have called neurosis one-sidedness – a disorder or disease of personality that occurs when the energies of opposing tensions no longer move freely within the psyche. When finally we seek out psychotherapy, it is likely to be because we feel stuck: there is no movement in our life, or we have lost any capacity to be moved. We have an e-motional disorder.[6] We seek 'medicine' ('dance was *medicine*,' writes analyst Tina Stromsted, describing her early experience, discussed later).

Movement in the psyche is slow. Forty years ago, near the end of my training, I woke from a dream of hearing a voice reciting the biblical story of Solomon's judgment, a story from the Hebrew Bible in which King Solomon of Israel ruled between women both claiming to be the mother of a child. Solomon revealed the true feelings of the women and their relationship to the child by suggesting that the baby be cut in two, with each woman to receive half. With this strategy of an archetypally impartial approach to justice, Solomon was able to discern the non-mother as the woman who approved of his proposal and the actual mother begged that the sword be sheathed, and the child committed to the care of her rival.

I still ached from my earlier separation from my children. At the time of this dream, the dream's voice bathed me in old collective wisdom, loosening, perhaps, the 'cramp' I had earlier described to Dr. E. as a 'cramp' in my middle that made me feel gutted, emptied, as if I couldn't stand tall or physically straighten up. As I emerged from hearing this dream voice, my tears flowed freely: I felt some recognition that my sacrifice, as terrible as it had been, had been made out of love. But it has taken me almost half a century to summon enough *personal* voice to write these words.

Seen through the attribute of movement, some dreams give us news of images that move through the psyche's depths over time. The outer form of such an image may change from dream to dream, but a kernel of meaning persists, as if such changes are simply iterations of an essential core. In turn, slow change in the core image portray a kind of deep, progressive process of transformation. For example, in one of my early dreams with Dr. P., an alarming black spider hovered above the white pages of an open book. Over time through many iterations, the symbolic meaning of the image of *spider* transformed into my dream visit from the Navajo goddess Spider Woman, where it appeared as a little brown spider with turquoise eyes and turquoise spinning ducts on her abdomen, sitting on a broom in a corner of my Zen meditation experience five decades later.

A kind of slow movement of personality integration can be tracked in a series of dreams as well. For example, early in training, I dreamed that a tall slender white-haired man and I were meeting in an open wildflower-spotted meadow. In the distance, mountains rimmed the meadow, but where *we* were, the sun shone, and the air was sweet. A small, full creek tumbled between the man and me, and each of us reached a hand out to the other across the stream. As we clasped our right hands together, I felt deeply confused: was I saying hello or goodbye?

This dream felt like a 'just-so' dream, and I almost let it go, but I noticed how changed the 'surround' or the environment presented in this dream was from earlier dreams: noticing this brought memories of earlier depictions of the earth on which I stood, and they varied, progressing from dream to dream: from being bare earth studded with shards of broken glass that made my bare feet bleed, for example, to being a barren hilltop in the dead of night on which I waited . . . and waited . . . to a depiction of a plowed, black earthen field across which I had to walk in order to reach a white horse (see Chapter 10), to this dream of a flower-strewn meadow divided by a sunlit tumbling stream. Might an enduring form behind this crystalline stream comment on a gradual transformation in an original crack in my earth, whatever that might mean: a fault in the foundation of personality? I've no way of knowing anything for certain, but changes in images like these are worth pondering. A slow movement of changing 'surround' continues even now.

Psyche moved on, and I moved on as well. Fifty-some years later, this same tall slender white-haired man appeared again: now he held me close as we danced.

The man's hand was so supportive of my spine that he could bend me backward until my hair brushed the floor, and then we rose upright again. Round and round we danced, bending and rising, bending and rising, all the while moving effortlessly. Then this dream scene shifted to bright green spider plants hanging from a ceiling, cascading down in front of an open, sunlit window, each pot spilling over with slender bending leaves, and plant after plant branching – as spider plants do – to the pot beneath them. I had spider plants like these in my smudged office window in the middle of Manhattan and more at home. But these dream plants differed from the dark green plants I had at home: every long, slender, delicate dark green leaf had a bone-white spine, a clearly embedded backbone from which each leaf branched effortlessly, as if from inside out.

In Chapter 11, I mentioned a dream of spirit as a white wind, clearing out every crevice, every place on the earth. And only a few months ago, I dreamed of looking at an opening in the dark earth where deep blue stone streaked with white showed through. I felt as if I might be seeing right through the earth, into deep blue sky streaked with white clouds on the other side. The alchemical *caelum* came to mind, as did Hillman's words: blue initiates 'the birth of the aesthetic sense'; 'the Caelum, then, is an aesthetic condition of mind, on which the entire opus depends' (2011, 10). But given my particular psychosomatic, personal history, I'm inclined to view this recent dream through a somatic lens: there, it simply stands as the latest in a long series of images that can be read to portray an ongoing redemption of 'my earth,' my environment, my physical surroundings – and my symbolic experience of physical embodiment. The opening slash in the dark earth, for example, resonates a bit with the dream of the scarred body of the Night Sky Woman, but through *this* opening, at *this* time in my life, I catch a glimpse of something quite transformed: a body of earth-sky together, something of beauty and value – if not exactly a 'diamond body' then a lapis body, a body of heavenly blue stone. The way I personally come to understand these 'environmental' dreams, dreamed over years, is far less important, however, than the way this series demonstrates over time the movement of a slow transformation *of* psyche, *in* psyche, and (I believe) *for* psyche's sake and how they suggest that from the psyche's perspective, I (me-ego – the dreamer) have been the necessary bystander.

Movement like this happens deep in a dreamer's unconscious, as Jung would say; or, in the 'somatic' personality, as others might say; or, as I experienced it then (for lack of better words), in a 'greater personality,' that was somehow also me. By way of such transforming images, a series of dreams can validate personality integration that transpires over years of experience. As deep inner movement like this takes place, consciousness must simply wait, for we (dreamers) are at a loss for words. We 'wait in the dark,' or (mostly) we sleep. Eventually, conscious experience of psyche's inner movements finds a home in metaphor, in images and dreams, in objects we create, and in conscious recognition of archetypal patterns. But in unconscious depths, psyche opens into soul and soul itself seems to move and deepen. In therapy, movement seems to slow as psyche and soul widen, everything becoming roomy, slightly dreamy, and spacious rather than speeding up.

I feel trust in inner movement like this, just as I feel trust in the language of dreams. Some 'moving presence' makes me cry, makes me relax, gives me solace and brings me peace. I can respond as if I were a child, spared from utter division by a present mother. Maybe, under the impact of a bungled spinal lumbar block, a difficult childbirth, and a personal betrayal all at once, my inner spine (the 'spine' of my personality?) had simply broken. I'd never considered myself a spineless person, but I now know what it feels like to 'be broken in two.' Was my psychic residue left over from earlier, broken twin-ness? I'll never know. Psyche can never be pinned down by 'clear understanding,' as if it were a butterfly the mind can pin to a board and label. Our dreams still stammer out images, one image resonating with the next, even nesting within one another, like Russian dolls, and shadowy images of these 'resonances' remind me of the shadowy structures enclosed in the stony depths of a shaman's quartz, transfixing liquid space. My alchemical spider plants grew me a dream vision of a vegetative soul.

Jung taught that manifestations of the animus like my white-haired stranger had to do with indwelling spirit. I remember my recent dream, of dancing in and out of the holograph of a great white snake. Such a dream snake is a timeless symbol of primitive life energy, of kundalini rising up the chakras and awakening consciousness. The object of the practice of kundalini yoga was to arouse the goddess by introverted concentration in order that prana would be released, and – by penetrating successive 'spinal' centers or chakras – eventually gain union with Shiva, The Lord of Light, or Consciousness itself (Baynes, 1969, 199). Perhaps we can say that the backbone of a woman's personality (like my own) resembles a physical backbone, a vegetative version of a symbolic vehicle of spirit that moves to the dance of life from the inside out.

Psychotherapy, authentic movement, and others

Whether one is in a psychotherapeutic situation or not, an ordering or a reordering of personality often begins with the discovery of a link between inner and outer worlds, a feeling of relevance to something unknown. This 'sense of personal relevance' heralds the appearance of the symbolic 'shaman' within the modern psyche, and it indicates an awakening shaman instinct. The essential experience of the psyche's reality and autonomy, however, is distilled within the *temenos* of an individual personality itself. Among themselves, therapists often talk of the work in which they engage as 'constellating' movement within a closed vessel, or they speak of the 'sacred space' of a specialized relationship, and conscious attention around the attribute of movement tends to emphasize inner, emotional movement in patients and in the psyche. We often describe therapy as deepening, broadening, integrating, differentiating, sorting, growth, development, and process, and all these refer primarily to manifestations of movement within the psyche rather than the body, even though psyche and body are never separate.[7] Only over time do we come to consciously experience our individual bodies as a symbolic personification of the microcosmic temple or 'temple of light' – the sacred space and container of the moving power of life. When I was experiencing the ongoing (about forty days and nights) uprush of ordering energies that were constellated in my work with Joseph and Dr. P., and later with Dr. E., I found myself walking mandalas in my tiny Manhattan apartment as I hummed my voice exercises ('keep your voice going, even without words,' Joseph warned): a walk-through like this was possible, from kitchen to bedroom to living room to kitchen, round and round and round – a small space, indeed, but more than adequate. Yes, my body itself was my container, but I found that my container 'formed' still other versions of containment (mandalas) over and over again. Both movement and sound comforted and reassured me as my circling body danced invisible 'dance houses' into space and moving time.

For Tina Stromsted, analyst and authentic movement therapist, the primary enclosure for human movement is the human body. Describing how she danced as a child, Tina opens her essay with these words:

> Dance was medicine, and nature my deepest container and first witness. . . . Little did I know at the time that I was treating my wounded soul with core elements of authentic movement, which would become a cornerstone in my life and work . . . in the natural way of childhood I had stumbled on the whirling dance practiced by the early Sufis. . . . Over the years I have come to see authentic movement as a 'safe enough' container.[8]

Alan Schore declares in his recent book, *Right Brain Psychotherapy* (2019), that from a neurobiological point of view, all psychotherapy happens under the auspices of our 'right brain,' so to speak, so it is not surprising that today several therapies specifically use and knowingly affect our entire psychosomatic selves. Authentic movement, which originated in the work of Mary Whitehouse[9] in Europe, is considered to be a form of active imagination in the body that deliberately uses the body. The work is done in dialogue with the therapist or in groups. With Marion Woodman's BodySoul approach, work is often done in couples of therapist and patient, and a third, witnessing presence also may be called into play. The witness watches for spontaneous, emergent gestures and movements in the mover, understanding these movements as expressions of the somatic unconscious, unlocking previously unknown or frozen feeling aspects of the mover's psyche/soma. The witness then informs the mover of what they saw.

In another form of movement therapy, Emilie Conrad's *Continuum*[10] groups gather in a spacious room for teaching purposes, but individuals work individually and alone. Continuum offers the slowest, most seamless bodywork I've ever encountered. As each person becomes their 'own therapist,' the work becomes embodied self-fulfilling (Conrad, xiv). My engagement in Continuum's breath work and bodywork brought my awareness so deeply into openly moving psychosomatic depths that I found myself listening for, more than seeing or feeling, a (my) body's slow meditation on becoming en-fleshed. That meditative awareness *of* embodiment body, amplified *in* and *by* my body, allowed sensations, organs, perceptions, and feelings of my 'whole self' to emerge from such depths that they seemed to 'move as *they – not I* – wished,' for hours at a time. Continuum 'body/psyche work' is silent, deep, inward, and slow, so that psyche and soma seem to meld, flowing seamlessly into one another. The octopus was Emilie's favorite animal, and she dedicated *Life on Land* to 'the Holy Spirit of water that undulates from the stars to us, anointing us with its pulsating mystery.' I could swear that the 99% of water of which I hear each of us is composed was – in my experience of Emilie's exercises – met and matched with an equally watery, personalized, individual experience of psyche's depths, molecule by molecule, and it is hard to imagine that the whole experience was just my imagination.

Slowing down

The more I practice what Allan Schore calls the art and science of psychotherapy, the more aware I am of how important it is to help my patients *slow down*; to do this, I have to slow down too. Even when we recognize that the body is a deep, ongoing source of authentic movement, several analysts remind us that we tend to 'live' elsewhere – that is, in our minds – in what D. W. Winnicott calls the false self. The false self *prefers* to be located in the mind, because our minds move much faster than our bodies, and rapid movements of the mind take us away from our feelings, which are often painful and disagreeable. Feelings also tend to drag the somatic unconscious along with them. As the Korean teacher and Zen practitioner Haemin Sunim reminds us throughout *The Things You Can See Only When You Slow Down: How To Be Calm in a Busy World* that if we spend the entirety of our lives resisting 'what is,' yet are constantly in motion trying to adjust to 'what is,' not only will we remain unhappy about 'what is,' but we can also never 'slow down' enough to notice what's really important (51).[11]

So while 'original movement' that emerges from psyche/soma remains practically synonymous with life itself, movement that is unconsciously identified with thought in our minds informs us of how psychological defenses protect us from deeper feelings than we want to know and from memories that we are unaware we carry. Movement that is unconsciously identified with thought leads to being 'ourselves' as we *think* ourselves to be, not to being *simply* ourselves, whoever we are.

An example of the 'slowing down' that Sunim alludes to came to me as I worked a supervisee, who was reporting on a session she had with a highly agitated, obsessive woman. This particular patient repeatedly spent her sessions talking a mile a minute, unable to calm or settle. Eventually my younger colleague asked her patient to close her eyes so that she could lead the woman through a simple body-scan – a method of progressive relaxation; she asked her to pay attention to her breath and breathe into various parts of her body, including her chest and shoulders. Suddenly, the patient's eyes popped open, and the startled woman said, 'I just saw myself as a little girl! I was so tiny – so vulnerable – so innocent!' Then came her tears, and the woman spent the rest of her session getting acquainted with a hitherto neglected 'part' of her inner world – an aspect of her 'inner child' that was able to reappear *only when both therapist and patient assumed a slower pace*, a body pace, a spaciousness that welcomes embodied self-reflection.

Notes

1 Buckley, Michael J. S. F.: *Motion and Motion's God: Thematic Variations in Aristotle, Cicero, Newton and Hegel*. Princeton, NJ: Princeton University Press. 1971. 221–229.
2 ibid. 229.
3 Van Lelyveld, T. B.: *La Danse dans le Theatre Javanais*. Paris. 1931, as quoted in Gerardus van der Leeuw: *Sacred and Profane Beauty: The Holy in Art*. Translated by David E. Green. New York: Holt, Rinehart and Winston. 1963. 26.
4 Kingsley, Peter: *In the Dark Places of Wisdom*. Point Reyes, CA: The Golden Sufi Center. 1999.
5 See the work of Mircea Eliade. See also Lewis, I. M.: *Ecstatic Religion: An Anthropological Study of Spirit Possession and Shamanism*. London, England: Penguin Books, Ltd. 1971. 51.
6 Guido Majno: *The Healing Hand: Man and Wound in the Ancient World*. Cambridge: Harvard University Press. 1975. 394.
7 Each therapy hour includes voluntary and involuntary physical movements made by two human beings in conversation. However, given the paradigm of psychotherapy used here – ego development by way of consciousness and companioning by another in creative dialogue – I found it helpful to organize small bodily movements that tend to shade into posture and gesture under gesture.
8 Stromsted, Tina: *Embracing the Body, Healing the Soul C. G. Jung Society of Atlanta Newsletter*. Atlanta, Georgia. 2018. 1–5.
9 Whitehouse, Mary: 'The Tao of the Body,' in *Authentic Movement: Essays by Mary Starks Whitehouse, Janet Adler, and Joan Chodorow*. Edited by P. Pallaro. London: Jessica Kingsley. 1958.
10 Conrad, Emilie: *Life on Land: The Story of Continuum: The World-Renowned Self-Discovery and Movement Method*. Forward by Valerie Hunt. Berkeley, CA: North Atlantic Books. 2007.
11 Sunim, Haemin: 'Mindfulness,' in The Things You Can See Only When You Slow Down: How To be Calm in a Busy World. Translated by Chi-Young Kim and Haemin Sunim. UK and US: Random House. Penguin Life. 2012.

Chapter 13

Sound

Dr. Tomatis visits the Abbey

Once upon a time, a noted ear, nose, and throat specialist was called to consult on a strange case at a Benedictine Abbey in France. The doctor found seventy of the Abbey's ninety monks 'slumped over in their cells, like wet dishrags' (Bloom, 1987, 58).[1] Mystified, because he could find no medical cause, Dr. Alfred Tomatis discovered that in attempting to modernize the centuries-old lifestyle of the monastery, a new abbot had eliminated most of the traditional six to eight hours of Gregorian chanting from the monks' daily schedule, feeling that it served no real purpose. Soon the monks began sleeping late and working less. Dr. Tomatis reasoned that the monks' ascetic lifestyle – particularly their vows of silence – made their chanting a crucial avenue of both auditory and oral expression. Tomatis also believed that although Gregorian chants resonate in a singer's head and are chock-full of harmonic overtones, the high frequencies actually supplied essential electrical charges to the brain.[2] So, he got the monks singing again, and within nine months, all but two were back on the job, vigorously engaged in prayer. 'We are creatures of sound,' Tomatis explained, 'we live and breathe in it . . . in giving these monks back their sounds – *their own stimuli* – we simply succeeded in reawakening them' (Bloom, 58, italics mine).

No single phenomenon seems to affect us by way of the unconscious more immediately or with greater potential intensity than sound. Hearing a sound is much more diffuse than seeing an image, because when we hear sound, we do not hear a 'thing,' with a clear spatial or temporal outline. Hearing sound is characterized by quality and intensity; otherwise, it is dimensionless, like smelling something. And because sound addresses our hearing sense, it touches us directly and remains tied to an instinctive, unconscious experience of reality all our lives long. We resonate with sound. Our ears are the most uninterruptedly receptive of all our sense organs: they are always open. Unlike our eyes, we cannot close our ears at will. In fact, we are sensitive to sound not just through our ears but also through our whole skin, even our bones. All our organs are affected by sound (Bloom, 59).

Sound in early history

Like the other attributes, sound has a spiritual as well as a secular history. According to the *Kalevala* – a Finnish folk epic that was chanted with closed eyes antiphonally around the Baltic Sea – the world was sung into existence. In India, the sound of Krishna's flute brought the world into Being. Pre-Hellenic maternal goddesses – depicted holding lyres – had a similar significance. Other traditional doctrines held that sound gave rise to all manifestations of Being, commencing with light, air, and fire. In early Hindu stories, God laughed the world into Being. In fact, the Indo-European root of the word 'God' is *gheu-*, which meant to 'invoke by calling.'

Some of the earliest beginnings of civilization were sung as songs: blind Homer singing the *Iliad* and the *Odyssey* gave voice to the Greek imagination. The *Bhagavad Gita* or *Song of God* was sung in response to the questions of a blind king. In ancient temples of India, China, and Tibet, healing through sound became highly developed – a 'science' based on the belief that vibrations emanating from a spiritual source actually create the physical universe. For thousands of years, Buddhist and Hindu traditions used prolonged chants, ecstatic rhythm, and ancient melodic patterns to awaken the chakras, centers of energy in the body. The Hindu system of chakras designated the throat chakra as the vital point of transition from the lower body chakras to higher head chakras: air (or spirit) traveling through our mouth, throat and lungs and returning into sound, connected lower with higher centers. It is apparent that Hindu yogis understood (as did Indigenous Peoples in what is now called the United States) that inner and outer realities of visible body and invisible spirit unite on elemental levels. For example, they understood that an activation of Shakti is accompanied by a deep *humming sound*, like that of a swarm of bees, just as they understood that ascending *prana* is a *bodily, kinetic* effect of the awakened goddess (Baynes, 1969, 199, italics mine).

From our earliest beginnings, then, sound has been recognized as causal and formative, able to bring about change in the nature and fabric of the world, in the social order, and in individuals. This has important psychological implications. We might say that because sound exists, we *know* our world is more than corporeal, tangible, and visible: our world contains invisible mysteries. Abraham Heschel puts it like this: 'our mind is like a fantastic seashell, and when applying our ear to its lips, we hear a perpetual murmur from the waves beyond the shore' (Heschel, 1990). Perhaps the sound of wind, rustling leaves, or thunder and rain first aroused our idea of nature itself, alive in all its parts. If an animating spirit could not be seen, it could be heard, whether through omen, a sign, sounds made by a human mediator, or a shell held to an ear. Early human beings believed that the magic power of spoken words gave evidence of a magic force that resided in someone, escaping only through that person's voice. Often this force was personified in a spirit who gave a shaman a healing song. Today, sound continues to be a potent pathway to an inner awareness of soul.

Sound and deep religion

In my experience, sound is the most important shamanic attribute for awakening individual religious experience today, and it has always been so. The theology-based religions that we know today – mostly religions of 'the book' – are only a few thousand years old, and characteristic of post-agricultural societies. In my book here, I have been suggesting that the archetype of the shaman, including shamanic attributes, takes us back further historically, and calls on psychological depths. When Jung wanted to put across the idea that the roots of the psyche are grounded in instinct, he spoke of the 'two million-year-old-[hu]man in us.' Progressing back through history to the time of the hunter-gatherers – perhaps 500,000 years ago – we come to *religions of experience*, where trance and travel in spirit worlds were the prerogative and special 'gift' of the archaic shaman. Thus, the archetype of the shaman as it is experienced and expressed through the attributes offers us a through-line back to the beginnings of individual religious experience and the instinctive roots of the psyche. When an archaic shaman beat drums, sang songs, shook rattles, and danced behind a mask, they – through sound and movement, rhythm and respiration – communicated directly with the spirit world within and a tribal community of mesmerized onlookers without. When a modern person is moved by beautiful music, dances to rock and roll, or sings in a church choir, they too, immersed in sound, participate in an awakening resonance with Jung's two-million-year-old-(hu)man alive in the psyche's primordial depths – the continuing source of individual religious experience today.

A beautiful example of how sound resonates in the psyche is seen in the following dream of a patient, reported by Marie-Louise von Franz (1973, 248–249):

> I heard the mighty, deep sound of a bronze bell, an extraordinary ringing, such as I have never heard or imagined, a sound from beyond, of extraordinary beauty, irresistible . . . the sound seemed sacred to me, I thought it could come from a church, and instantly I was in a church of the purest Gothic style, of white stone. . . . But everything changed. The church became a broad vault, like the nave of the cathedral made of a transparent living red-orange material, bathed in a reddish light and supported by a forest of pillars. . . . For a moment I saw myself as standing tiny and alone . . . dazzled with the sense that I had a whole world to explore there. It was my heart. I was standing in the interior of my own heart, and I realized at this moment that the wonderful bell sound, which I could still hear, was nothing other than the beat of my own heart, or that this external sound and my heartbeat were one and the same. They were beating with the same rhythm. Macrocosm and microcosm were synchronized: the rhythm of the world's heart and my own heart were identical.

In this remarkable dream, sound itself leads a woman – first into a collective chamber of religion, a beautiful Gothic Church – and then into the innermost chamber of her individual heart. Together, rhythm and sound carry her experience of *coniunctio* of inner and outer worlds. Such a unity is always numinous.

Shamans, emotions, and songs

The archaic shaman learned songs and chants inspired by direct access to the spirit world. First uttered by the shaman, these sounds affected both the shaman and those who listened. Magical words had to be sung under specific conditions, and with marked restrictions; for example, words had to be recited in exact order, or the person repeating them had to be in a special place. The supply of magical prayers was restricted by conditions of creative ownership: new phrases and sounds could not be simply invented. Only under certain circumstances could a shaman be inspired to create new magical songs.

'Sounding' played a large part in a shaman's self-induced states of trance, and humming was a means of sending oneself into trance to explore the spirit world. According to Rasmussen, a shaman practiced magic words simply by walking about at home and talking to themselves, although the best and most powerful words came inexplicably when the shaman as out alone in the mountains. One method of learning such words was as follows:

> When one sees a raven fly past, one must follow it and keep on pursuing until one has caught it. If one shoots it with bow and arrow, one must run up to it the moment it falls to the ground, and standing over the bird as it flutters about in pain and fear, say out loud all that one intends to do, and mention everything that occupies the mind. The dying raven gives power to words and thoughts.[3]

But archaic shamans had to feel pain and fear too – not just the ravens they killed. Joan Halifax writes,

> At the moment when the shaman song emerges, when the sacred breath rises up from the depths of the heart, the center is found, and the source of all that is divine has been tapped . . . pain of the body and loneliness of the soul can decay the husk protecting the song within the singer. At that moment when the shaman is most profoundly enmeshed in the experience of suffering or joy, at the moment of ecstasy when he or she is transported to a place that is beyond mortality, the poetry breaks forth to overwhelm. . . . This is an emotion-filled process . . . it occurs in the realm of the spirit. . . (in healing) the singer brings into play his or her past experience of affliction and transcendent realization in relation to the one who is now suffering . . . he or she 'sings into life' those who are plagued with disease and those who are facing death.
>
> (Halifax, 1979, 30–31)

Today we know that sounds can feel as if they are torn from us, like uncontrollable laughter, screams, cries, or uncontrollable tears. The archaic shaman experienced uncontrollable sounds. The shaman-poet Orpingalik described such moments as 'when the seed of song breaks open,' explaining to Rasmussen,

> Man is moved just like the ice floe sailing here and there out in the current. His thoughts are driven by a flowing force when he feels joy, when he feels sorrow. Thoughts can wash over him like a flood, making his blood come in gasps, and his heart throb. Something like an abatement in the weather will keep him thawed up, and then it will happen that we, who always think we are small, will feel still smaller. And we will fear to use words. But it will happen that the words that we need will come of themselves. When the words we want to use shoot up of themselves – we get a new song.[4]

Sound and the human voice

As an attribute or quality of human personality, sound refers us to the sound of the human voice. When we hum or sing, a peculiarly sensitive situation is created in which the sound of our own voice comes back to us as a feature of objective reality. The act of hearing (together with the physiological system that is brought into play)[5] belongs to us, but that which we experience – our own sound – is not *in* us because we encounter our own 'sound' outside of ourselves. This means that even when we listen to ourselves, *our attention is directed to the objective world* (Bloom, 59): we experience ourselves subjectively and objectively at the same moment.

Each of us comes into this world with a unique sound. Each individual makes a sound that is as objectively given as the color of their hair or the shape of their nose. Like instinct, our natural sound is subject to becoming psyche only as it is modified through our gradual ego development, including the development of psychological defenses. Sounds that issue from our individual throats can indicate matchings or mismatchings of a head ego and a body ego, or a false self and a true self. It is a collective given that our necks and throats (through which sound passes) connect our heads and bodies, and when psychological problems become acute, we feel hung up, as if we were somehow dangling by the back of the neck, our feet unable to touch the ground.

So, each person's sound voices the expressive qualities and capacities of one's entire personality, not just who we *think* we are. This means that how each of us sounds refers to the mystery of *who* each of us is (and isn't – i.e., some parts of us are audible to others but remain unconscious to ourselves): the result is our own idiosyncratic personal 'voice' – its tones, harmonies, and multiple forms of expression. Beyond one's personal voice, however, there also Jung's 'voice of the inner [hu]man,' by which Jung meant a voice that issued from a wider personality: 'The phenomenon of the voice having a strongly personal character, may also issue from a center – but a center which is not identical to the ego' (CW11:70, 67).

This is the kind of voice I heard in my dream (the previous chapter) wherein 'someone' told me the story of Solomon's judgment.

Objectively speaking, the uniqueness of one's personal voice is confirmed by the fact that the pattern of tones and modulations creates an unmistakable record of personal identity. A voiceprint is more accurate than a photograph, a footprint, or casts of the swirled skin formation on our fingers or thumbs. We remember and recognize familiar voices indefinitely. Long before we understand the content, we recognize the voice of someone important to us because it activates the unconscious immediately: that's what 're-cognition' means.

Sound animates and populates our inner worlds, creating a kind of original inner climate in and through which we experience the emotions of instinctively lived life. It is in the nature of sound to draw us into itself, and if what we hear is *our* sound, we are drawn into *ourselves*. Our own voice proceeds out of our throats from the depths of bodily being: therefore, our own sound has an orienting effect, pulling us back into ourselves. By remaining closely attentive to our own sounds, we can be taken away from feelings of pain, sorrow, agitation, or confusion. A similar effect happens when we listen to or follow the sound of a sacred word or mantra: through listening, the mind becomes centered and focused, no longer at sixes and sevens – darting from one thought or bodily sensation to another. In the context of Christianity, repeatedly singing psalms is understood to have a similar effect, giving the mind respite from its habitual meanderings and penetrating to the inner realm of the heart, where even our intentions and will may be purified. As a result of entering deeply into the center of sound, one's body may straighten and become comfortable right where it is, as it is. It is as if sound has a capacity to hold us in a calm, safe place, as if there were no difference between listener and song or singer and song as both partake of the same unity. Time seems to stop, unfolding into the fullness of the present. Eastern teachings tell us that certain sounds have the power to clear the mind of superficial layers of thought, making it receptive to inner promptings of spirit; perhaps that is why while practicing voice exercises I have sometimes found myself remembering forgotten dreams.

Sound and psychotherapy: listening

Psychotherapy is conducted through the medium of sound. Essentially, speech is 'an act' of voice – a human act – the instinctive purpose of which has always been to reach one another. However, our voices communicate both conscious and unconscious dimensions of our being – both conscious and unconscious emotion. When our voices betray unconscious emotion, the shaman is activated in the psychotherapeutic situation, for better or worse. If there is even a trace of condescension or judgment in a therapist's voice, it will be heard and will engage the analysand's unconscious with a therapist's unconscious attitude, opinion, or belief. Such unconscious attitudes, opinions, or beliefs can be picked up through the voice. Other forms of 'magical' communication occur when we say something as a way of not saying anything, not revealing even to ourselves what lies behind our communication or when we use spoken language defensively, eluding what we really want to say. When we talk in order to keep someone at a distance, we use words in place of actions: we can use words as weapons, as camouflage, as a cry for help, or a cry of rage – or perhaps we are simply attempting to communicate an intense emotional state of which we are but dimly aware. Whatever our conscious intent may be, with 'magical communication,' our feelings have little connection with what we recount. On the other hand, we can also use sound and verbal communication to magically maintain contact with – meaning be in relation to, or even part of – another person. Here, our words will be primarily inferential: we unconsciously use words as if they were the words of chants and melodies, as if we intend them as 'body' for unconscious 'psyche,' as deliberately formed containers for sound. In curing rituals of the Navaho, for example, shamans use chants, charms, and exorcisms to combat evil influences and expel diseases, just as in 2 Kings (in the Bible), Saul's servants used harp music to cure their king of despondency, or mothers hum lullabies to help their infants sleep. Aside from summoning spirits, shaman chants could also destroy enemies and endow objects with supernatural power.

In the psychotherapy situation, we must pay special attention to the repercussions of what we say, lest an unconscious identification with the shaman's profession of mediation excuse us from personal responsibility for the impact of our words, our sounds, or our voice. The shaman in the therapeutic situation may listen for patterns as they are revealed in the psyche of another, rather than to individual elements or contents, and the shaman instinct selectively seeks out whatever aspect of the 'sounding' personality seems most in need of integration and human companioning in the therapeutic endeavor. In a therapeutic dialogue, therapists try to listen with conscious receptivity to significations that pertain to the psychological reality of themselves as well as their patients – the music between the words. A capacity for symbolic listening means a capacity to hear the present consciously and with feeling, to synthesize the present with what is known of the past, with what is understood of archetypal depths, and with whatever can be glimpsed of the future – also consciously and with feeling. It also means to listen to sound. We listen for natural speech rhythm and diction and inflection; we listen for idiom and for the degree and quality of spontaneity, enthusiasm, and vigor in a patient's speech. Listening and synthesizing like this involves our personal, affective components as well as our conscious capacities, so to some degree, the shaman is always present in both therapist and patient: both of us inhabit the shaman complex as the symbolic process flows.

Marie-Louise von Franz comments on how important it is to become conscious of shamanic undertones:

> The terrible thing is that one should be humanized right down to the physical vibration, not only veiled in a polite form. One can say that one was quite polite and not aggressive – *but one's voice lowered or something – and the*

> *affect makes the atmosphere bad – for both persons are animal and the other gets the physical impact.* The humanization of such an archetypal dynamism (expression of unconscious emotion) is an aspect of individuation, for it means integration, becoming conscious . . . mythologically expressed, this is the great task of getting a bewitched person back into human life, the redemption motif which you find in all human mythologies. The characteristic of a religious redemption is that a human being can be brought back. That is the secret mystery of an inner evolution.
>
> (von Franz, 1972, 127, italics mine)

Sometimes a shamanic personality purposely uses what von Franz calls bewitchment; Jung, for example, once sang a lullaby to a young girl and tells us her insomnia completely disappeared. 'Enchantment like that is the oldest form of medicine,' he wrote (Jaffe, 2014, 122–123). But generally speaking, people fall under archetypal spells. They become what von Franz calls bewitched or what we call dissociated. So, as we listen to the sound of our patient's voices (and our own), we listen with multiple levels of attention: does the 'self' presented align itself with what we hear? Does the intellectual or conceptual content match the emotional tone and coloration? How deep are the unconscious feelings that signal from below, wanting to claim 'humanity'? Our ability to attend to multiple levels of what we hear constitutes therapeutic listening, and this ability becomes a gift of time, self, and service. At best, therapeutic listening leads to one's own ability to give complete and undivided attention to another person, while from the side of the other person, our undivided attention feels redemptive in its own right. Head and heart begin to communicate.

The possibility that the way we listen to our patients opens the heart is beautifully illustrated by a story from *The Secret of the Golden Flower*. Lu-tsu has this to say about listening to relevant sound:

> In the Book of the Elixir it is said: The hen can hatch her eggs because *her heart is always listening*. That is an important magic spell. The reason the hen can hatch the eggs is because of the power to heat. But the power of the heart can only warm the shells; it cannot penetrate into the interior. Therefore with her heart she conducts this power inward. *This she does with her hearing. In this way she concentrates her whole heart*. When the heat penetrates, the chick receives the power of the heat and begins to live. Therefore a hen, even when she has left her eggs, always has the attitude of listening with bent ear. Thus the concentration of the spirit is not interrupted. . . . [An] *awakening of the spirit is accomplished because the heart has first died*. When a man can let his heart die then the primordial spirit wakes to life. To kill the heart does not mean to let it dry and wither away, but it means that it is undivided and gathered into one.
>
> (*The Secret of the Golden Flower*, italics mine)[6]

This small story suggests that a (therapist's) capacity for inner attention or listening to oneself is crucial to the opening of the heart. Everyday levels of despair – experiences of birth and life, love and loss, and illness and death – can harden the hearts of the best of us, but this little image of a broody hen, listening with cocked ear, suggests that sound itself has a unique ability to penetrate a 'shell of despair,' so that hope can hatch like a chick from an egg – heart energy beginning all over again.

Under extreme circumstances, the human heart may shatter, and the spirit world (the archetypal world) steps in. When this happens in psychotherapy, not only does 'spirit' awaken, but also the shaman complex stirs. The time has arrived when *feeling anything at all has become more important to the patient than whether 'hurt' happens again or not.* Somewhere at the end of my training, I remarked to Dr. E. that 'the scar tissue over what happened feels almost worse than what happened'; in that moment, I signaled that a hardened inside shell was cracking, and the possibility of new life had begun to stir. This is what happens with hope.

In the homely image of a broody hen listening with a cocked head, letting the 'heart die' implies that the hen's heart 'died' to its usual restless wanderings and everyday divisions: 'flitting about' has been curtailed, stopped, caught, gathered, stilled, focused, and concentrated. Metaphors flock like hens to a coop to this image because a disciplined, concentrated attention to the heart brings the idea of the psyche to life. Insight through self-sounding can feel like the virgin birth of consciousness itself. Salvador Dali made this point by painting the Madonna and Child, each curled around the other and both curled together into the shell of an enormous (listening) ear: a psychological reading of the symbolic 'sound' that Dali's painting makes suggests that one part of the mind can have an extraordinary impact on the other. Certainly, the birth of my consciousness was cradled in an aural nest.

Singing: Joseph and me

We human beings are fed not only by food but also by experiences of feeling alive, and singing actualizes aliveness in sound. While we sing, body and mind balance naturally as a result of suspending all but the gentle effort that is required to maintain attention on sound, and music and sound become forms of subtle nourishment.

Like speaking in public, however, singing can make us feel vulnerable. There's an interesting correlation between the ability to make sound and one's instinctive 'soundness,' so to speak – perhaps it is the old alchemical 'as above, so below.' Without necessarily understanding how it happens, most of us are aware that the voice reveals a great deal. Fearing that we will expose more than we want others to know, we tend to hold back when we speak or sing, causing the sound to stop a few feet in front of our noses: our mouths go dry, our legs tremble, and we can suffer excruciating self-consciousness at reciting, speaking, or singing in public.

So great is our normal, unconscious identification with our native voice that we are especially sensitive to any criticism about it, particularly when we are young – for example, being told that we have no singing voice: we sing off-key; we can't hold a tune in a basket. Worse still is being told that we will ruin everything for a group of singers if our voice is heard. Painful impressions like these go deep, are far-reaching, and can damage the whole personality in a sense of self and self-esteem: early impressions like these twist us all out of shape and may permanently prevent us from attempting to find our own voice, let alone sing. As a teenager, I had sung in a church choir, but I hated the thought of public speaking and couldn't imagine singing solo. Such was my situation when I met Joseph.

Three years into my analytic training, on the casual recommendation of a friend, I began taking singing lessons from Joseph. Within months, I reached depths of experience of the unconscious that no training analysis (or drug experience) has ever approached. Perhaps the simultaneous combination of analytic work and voice training constellated the depth of these experiences, but work with Joseph literally dissolved me into a swirl of self-states. Eventually, I emerged as myself again, but in a different configuration.

One could say I fell into the preverbal dimensions of experience – useful in my analytic ponderings, because my particular psychological issues had their origins in preverbal dimensions to begin with. Indeed, I couldn't sing words for months and didn't talk much either. It was as if my right hemisphere finally had its way full speed ahead for forty to fifty days, during which I didn't sleep, tried to eat everything I could to 'bring me to earth' but still lost twenty pounds. Kundalini energies rose up and circulated, round and round and round (I had been doing yoga for many years). Two people, neither of which had any idea of what was happening to me internally, told me I had an aura of light.

It felt as if all my 'character armor' were dissolving, along with all bodily stiffness and muscular tightness, to a point where there were no resistances left, either psychological or physiological. Another way I thought about it was that I fell into the collective unconscious into spontaneous experiences of birth and rebirth, reliving over and over again all kinds of early memories, along with somatic memories that came and went as patches of early infant eczema, previously outgrown by the age of four.

Joseph was a voice coach. He called himself a teacher and an educator of the antique psyche, not a therapist or psychoanalyst. Gifted, intelligent, and serious, Joseph was as introverted as one could possibly be without disappearing altogether; at the same time, he was immensely, spontaneously, emotionally expressive – even charismatic – so he attracted people (and animals) in all walks of life. Once, attributing his grand public persona to the stars, Joseph told me that he was 'a triple Leo'; thus, he was a born performer. Joseph had a tremendously difficult personal history: he began life as an orphan and made his way in the world working as a singer and a writer for years. He had an extraordinary capacity for a kind of conscious identification with others that seemingly allowed him to imagine himself not only into another's shoes but into another's personality. I'm sure that this imaginative capacity, along with his intuitive vision, keen empathy, and an unusually acute ear were native to Joseph, but he honed these abilities over his lifetime and placed them to good use. He had no patience for pretension, so unless you were willing to have all your conscious and unconscious presumptions poked at until they rattled around like old bones in a closet or fell away of their own accord, hiding anything from Joseph was next to impossible. This could make Joseph highly uncomfortable to be around. At the same time, as outrageous as he could be, most of the time Joseph was uproariously funny, though it never seemed to be at someone else's expense. Out of our ten years of working together in two or three hour-long sessions per week, he and I spent at least seven of those years cavorting outlandishly around his big open studio and singing together at the top of our lungs. As we sang and played together, Joseph taught and I learned.

Entirely self-educated, Joseph had the most impressive personal library I've ever seen. In his spare time (and sometimes all night long, since he didn't sleep much), Joseph wrote extensively – novels, songs, journals, dreams – and he also destroyed everything he wrote, because the process of writing was important to him, not the product. He taught himself to write in several languages, 'in order to understand the spirit' of a culture – in order to 'feel' his way into Japanese or Arabic – and who knows what else.

Joseph had a rigorous regard for relational 'truth' between people and an intense dislike of crazy-making relational game playing. The most deeply moral person I've ever known (and the least moralistic), Joseph never lied to me, either by omission or commission. Because I never felt judged, criticized, tricked, maneuvered, exploited, or manipulated, I was able to trust him implicitly. I loved Joseph without fear, in a way that was purifying, clarifying, hurtful, and deeply healing, all at once. Because I felt loved, respected, supported, and understood (most of the time) in return – even sometimes admired – I allowed myself to enter an earlier dream image of my heart – a 'red tent' I'd been afraid to approach because it was too full of pain. All that had been locked up there over years came flooding into consciousness in Joseph's presence. Yes, it was odd to share so much of myself with another person – a man who was neither brother nor father nor lover – odd, but essential. I did endure, and I did survive, and I emerged as the same person I used to be, but different.

In addition to the instinctive and unconscious training that occurred during my years of psychotherapeutic training, studying voice with Joseph educated me in self-knowledge and self-acceptance. I learned how uniquely we hear ourselves and how subjective an experience of self is. I learned that no one else has that unique experience, even a teacher, who hears sound objectively. During lessons, as the energy, breath, sound, and vibration constantly cycled up through my body, out my throat and in through my ears, I felt how my subjective experience was an extraordinary blend of inner and outer reality.

Over time, my voice freed up, built strength and energy, and gathered integrity. Any voice – giving voice to its unique sound – embodies the unique individuality of the person through whom it sounds. I learned how a singer can learn, practice, grow, and develop over the whole range of personality if they persevere, reflecting on this gathering self-integrity of mind and body. I also learned that the respiratory work that is employed in a disciplined study of voice is as sustained as any meditation or yogic deep breathing practice; and, as in those pursuits, personal memories as well as depths of the collective psyche activate out of the muscular, neurological, even cellular depths of the body and the mind: the aboriginal self becomes present in all its aspects.

I returned feeling reborn, renewed, transformed, and transfigured. Able to share myself fully without fear, I learned much about myself, including my own desire to be desired. Joseph raised me up again, somehow – good fathering, I suppose. Later, I supervised difficult cases with him, because he had an extraordinary feel for dreams. After ten years, I went back to school for doctoral studies, and I stopped working with Joseph. We spoke by phone every now and again, but before his death, Joseph went into retirement for four years, meaning he wouldn't see anyone. So when Joseph died, I hadn't seen him for a long time.

In all that time, I rarely dreamed of Joseph, but in one rare dream, Joseph supported my back while I did a full backbend, like I used to do as a child; in a second dream, he blessed me with a kiss on my forehead. Joseph was my guide, mentor, and master teacher. Over the years, I sent all kinds of other people to study with him – friends, patients, actors, writers, and singers. Some people stayed with him for a long time, while others found him frightening and left. I wish my readers could have met him. He was a rare person, a rare human being.

Looking back, clearly my experience of the attribute of sound was of archetypal dimensions. Gradually, my experience of an aboriginal or implicit self that constellated simultaneously out of psychotherapy with Dr. E. and voice lessons with Joseph clarified into the archetypal pattern (constellation) of the shaman. Recall that early on, I had said to Joseph, 'it's as though the big shaman is healing the little shaman!' But at the time I made that comment, the *image* of a shaman per se, historical or otherwise, had yet to enter my ken.

Jung once described the dangers that accompany deep archetypal activation like this: 'Whenever an archetype appears things become critical, and it is impossible to foresee what turn they will take. As a rule this depends on the way *consciousness* reacts to the situation' (CW10:461, italics mine). In my situation, in order to develop, maintain, and strengthen the kind of consciousness that Jung implies, I needed all the help I could get. Joseph and my two analysts during those several years – Dr. P. and Dr. E. – were excellent, caring, rigorous psychotherapeutic companions who helped me uncover, train, and further develop my fragile sense of self and ego consciousness. It has been suggested that a slow 'approach to the numinous' may be the major curing factor of a neurosis (von Franz, 1993, 177), but my experience was anything but a 'slow approach': in the midst of repeated bouts of numinous overwhelm, I don't know how I would have survived during all that uproar and all that time without the caring, careful attention of Dr. P., Dr. E., and Joseph.

Jung also writes,

> Just as the great personality acts upon society to liberate, to redeem, to transform, and to heal, so the birth of personality in oneself has a therapeutic effect. It is as if a river that had run to waste in sluggish side streams and marshes suddenly found its way back to its proper bed, or as if a stone lying on a germinating seed were lifted away so that the shoot could begin its natural growth.
>
> (CW17:317)

Clearly, the attribute of sound played a large part in clearing a way for me back to an original course of life.

Notes

1 To further stimulate the monks' brains, Tomatis hooked them up to headphones and a cassette recorder programmed with baroque music, with the lower frequencies filtered out.

2 Bloom, 59. Studies done in India show that trees increase their yield under the influence of music: in response to what is played, plants grow toward or away from speakers, and with some music, plants withered and died. Nor does sound affect only organic matter: the Swiss scientist Hans Jenny vibrated inorganic matter like liquids, plastics, metal filings, and powders atop metal disks. As Jenny manipulated pitch, inorganic matter fashioned itself into organic shapes resembling spirals of a jellyfish, concentric rings of plant growth, or the pentagonal stars of sea urchins.

3 Rasmussen, Knud: *From the Intellectual Culture of the Igulik Eskimos*. Quoted in *The Coming and Going of the Shaman: Eskimo Shamanism and Art*. Winnipeg, Canada: The Winnepeg Art Gallery. 1979. 204.

4 Rasmussen, Knud: *The Netsilik Eskimos, Social Life and Spiritual Culture*. Translated by W. E. Calvert. *Report of the Fifth Thule Expedition*. 1921–24. Copenhagen: Glydendal. 1920. 321, quoted in Joan Halifax: *Shamanic Voices: A Survey of Visionary Narratives*. New York: E.P. Dutton. 1979. 30.

5 Ears, Nerves, and the Central Nervous System. Zukerkandl, Victor: *Sound and Symbol: Volume II: Man The Musician*. Translated by Norbert Guterman. Bollingen Series XLIV – 2. Princeton, NJ: Princeton University Press. 1973. 21ff.

6 *The Secret of the Golden Flower: A Chinese Book of Life*. Translated by Richard Wilhelm. New York: Harcourt, Brace and Company. 1952. 3, 46.

Chapter 14

Gesture

Definitions and history

In essence, a gesture is a bodily act, a physical motion that conveys or communicates ideas or emotions – an action, posture, or movement of an expressive, 'talking' body. Words may communicate facts and ideas, but where changing moods and emotional states are concerned, gestures are more important, because gestures 'put across' ideas and emotional states by miming them, whether a gesturing person is aware of what is being expressed or not. Each action is important: we say, 'one action speaks a thousand words'; and the actions of making – a book, a painting, a dance – are also gestures, manifesting our hunches, ideas, intuitions, and emotions in space.

Presumably, humankind's earliest form of communication took the form of gesturing. In 1941, anthropologist Adolphe Thomas wrote,

> Man thinks with his whole body, with his feet, his hands, his ears, as well as with his brain. . . . *Psychological activity is an activity of the total organism, not a local activity* . . . . A man dancing and gesticulating mimetically in the light of the sun or the hearth-fire must have seen how his body was projected on the rock walls surrounding him, and this drama may have given him the idea of fixing statically the most typical moments of the processes of nature. . . . [When] early man fixed objects and scenes in their characteristic moments, he described the mime of his body, and not his ideas. Thus the word '*mimogram*' should replace the false expression 'ideogram.' And these *mimograms* might be the most ancient graphic representations, with whose aid man tried in the darkness of those early centuries to make eternal the gesture of the moment.
>
> (italics mine)[1]

Because gesture is a historic precursor to language, we may understand gesture as an archaic mode of thought. Developmentally speaking, gestures imply acts of unconscious self-representation at the pre-symbolic or magical levels of the psyche, so for purposes of this chapter, we will assume that every gesture has a personal, developmental history, even if unknown. The title of Peter Levine's recent book, *In an Unspoken Voice: How the Body Releases Trauma and Restores Goodness* (2010), attempts to transform the older idea of gesture as an archaic mode of thought into a more modern, clinical, and conceptual shorthand idea of 'body language.' Rene Spitz, for example, suggests that the almost universal gestures of yes and no may be patterned by the reflex activities of a baby who is finding or failing to find the nipple to feed.[2]

Picture a crying four-year-old girl who needs a hug: beyond needing to feel loved and protected, this child also needs to feel a boundary around feelings of overwhelm. She needs to feel something that *informs* her: pain can't be the whole world because pain can be housed. When she is hugged, the child drops into her body. This is how a child's 'body of experience' comes to include a hugging world, or a world that can hug. Unconscious flesh and bones ground all of us in Being, because wholeness enters through the body's door. Writing about her toddler patient Deedee, whose native gestures are inhibited, relational therapist Tamsin Looker describes Deedee as moving stiffly and less steadily than her peers; she falls often, as if she cannot fully inhabit her little body while using her antennae to monitor her mother's moods. Noting that Deedee's capacity for empathy is overdeveloped, Looker suggests that the child isn't able to pay attention to her own insides, and sees Winnicott's (1949) 'premature ego development' in progress: 'Unable to rely on her mother's body and her mother's boundaries. . . [Deedee] takes care of herself with her mind' (Looker, 242).

Freud, Jung, and beyond

Freud, in his seminal work *The Ego and the Id*, struggled with the implications of phylogenetic roots of the mind, acknowledging the need to understand archaic mind in any therapeutic process. Jung also clearly recognized the need for the integration of our instinctual layering. Jung believed that in assimilating what he called the collective unconscious, each person moved toward wholeness, and he called this process of assimilation *individuation*. Understanding the collective unconscious as a concrete, physical/biological reality, Jung wrote,

> This whole psychic organism corresponds exactly to the body, which, though individually varied, is in all essential features the specifically human body (and mind) which all men have. In its development and structure, it still preserves elements that connect it with the invertebrates and ultimately with the protozoa. Theoretically, it should be possible to 'peel' the collective unconscious, layer by layer, until we came to the psychology of the worm, and even of the amoeba.
>
> (CW8:322)

I include this lengthy quote because it articulates the psyche's inclusiveness of *all* imagery, down to the lowly worm. Most of us know what someone means when they say, 'I felt like a worm,' but personal feelings alone may not indicate the psyche's collective allusions to the worm, particularly if an underlying process of individuation is relevant. And astute therapists are able to read images of gestures and posture in dreams as well as life, personal as well as collective. Therapists need wide imaginations.

Relational therapists write about how widespread psychosomatic disharmony is (practically ubiquitous), and how disconnection from the body means disconnection from one's truest feelings and core sense of self (e.g., Looker, 238). Attention to one's own and a patient's body-based experiences and to connections and disconnections between psyche and soma are critical to the analytic holding environment, so the more a psychotherapist is able to surrender to their own body-based experience and flow of bodily imagery before giving in to the inevitable pressure to abstract and verbalize, the less they will participate in a shared psychosomatic disharmony.

We know that when infant bodies go unheld ('unloved'), hatred can flow in, and we know that self-hate, stored in blood and bone, generates self-neglect. Many women with whom I've worked cannot inhabit their bodies with conscious care, nor do they live in bodies that gesture freely. One woman sat opposite me like a frozen doll, gesturing an unconscious history of trauma and defense that would take months or years to enter our mutual awareness, if ever it did. An hour later, a second woman – barely containing her enthusiasm for what she was telling me – gestured wildly, her body eloquent with psyche's secret text: for the second woman, gestures amplified her tumbling expressiveness, adding body to her words and weight to her ideas.

Like other attributes of our instinctively human bodies, gesture figures as an expressive mode. As adults, we express instinctive reactions as immediate physical responses, instinctively apprehending most gestures even when we don't understand them. If someone moves to strike us, we recoil without reflection: no conscious process need occur. It is as if the body's most basic knowledge happens in molds of kinesthesia and synesthesia where our muscles and senses pool their impressions, making us listen to music 'muscularly,' or 'watch' dance with our legs. A capacity for simple awareness best presents a gestural dimension of Being to therapists, because awareness opens us to an experience of self, of other people, and of the world. Awareness allows us to feel a gesture in another, and sense it for ourselves. Most of us are unaware of unconscious gestures that we engage in repeatedly: a jiggling foot, a raised shoulder, a head tilt now and then – and here is where training films of therapists at work have been so helpful: we catch ourselves engaging in them!

Gesture as a language

The vocabulary of gesture is both limited and profound, and most gestures communicate so imperatively that they are understandable beneath language differences. Funk and Wagnall describe the sign language of the Indigenous Peoples of the Great Plains as communicating beneath mutually unintelligible languages (tribal dialects) to the point of being able to recount myths and stories. Not only are such sign languages utilitarian, but they are full of rhythm and ritual, and they include in their graphic grammar signs for things, for actions and for emotions. So similar are some signs from culture to culture (particularly those for rain, the crescent moon, flowers, horns, fire, and erotic desire or copulation) that anthropologists suggest that the sign language of the Indigenous Peoples of the Great Plains might be related to the elaborate gesture codes of Asia, like the Hindu mudras or the derived gestures of the Hawaiian hula.[3]

In the language of the psyche, the precision, tempo, and quality of a gesture vary with the temperaments of the individuals who perform it: my handwriting will differ from yours, as will my mannerisms of speech. Yet if we keep in mind universally understood pantomime, we glimpse the basically communicative nature of gesture: always the outstretched hand either gives or receives, and gestures of hunger and thirst, gestures of homage or fear, are similar the world over. Collective gestures like these form a basic grammar of the psyche that each psyche recognizes, from the beginning of time to the present.

In our contemporary culture, many people who are deaf use a visual language of 'signing' with one's hands – American Sign Language (ASL) – and infants, who are anything but deaf, are taught baby signing, which is an authentic version of ASL that has been especially chosen to encourage early visual communication between infants and their parents. My niece was able to use ASL to fulfill part of her PhD language requirement, so gesture is far from dead in the world we know today.

Gesture as posture

Just as we can think of gesture as an act, we can think of a posture as the conscious or unconscious embodiment of the underlying attitude out of which an act or gesture happens. Formalized stage gestures and postures have their counterparts in meticulously observed postural attitudes of worship that have appeared all over the world: think of the movements of tai chi, the genuflections of Greek Orthodox believers, or Judeo-Christian *metanies* (from *metanoia*, meaning 'repentance') like the kiss or the kneeling posture for worship or prayer. In earlier times, solar and astronomically based religions taught – by means of sacred performance, musical rites, and symbolic gestures – information that we now come to know through scientific theory. Both Egyptian and early Indian priests walked around their temples in a circular path each day – for example, to suggest that the sun circles the heavens in the same way. Frequently, group gestures became rhythmic ceremonial dances. When certain mystery rites forbade the use of the spoken word, important lore would be mimed or danced. Greek history records that a famous Greek mime was said to have expressed the entire Pythagorean philosophy in a brief dance.[4] The Buddha is said to have once transmitted the essence of his teachings by *showing* a flower, and similar meaning was implied by the gesture of the High Priestess who *revealed* a single ear of corn in culmination of Eleusinian initiatory rites.

We might say that gestures that involve the entire body become symbolic postures. Odin hanging upside down from Yggdrasil and Jesus hanging from the cross are examples of symbolic postures that have carried religious significance for entire civilizations. Both of these images imply voluntary self-sacrifice, but they carry different psychological implications. Rather than sharing in the suffering of the world or saving humankind from death, as translators of the Christian crucifixion suggest, Odin's posture of self-sacrifice is an early example of a shamanically activated sacramental gesture. Odin's hanging does not refer to redemptive humanness but instead is oriented toward obtaining magical power for its own sake; intending to win the secret of magic by acquiring the hidden knowledge of a 'gnostic' quest, Odin hung from Yggdrasil headfirst and found the Runes, which were symbolic of the magical lore he sought. The tarot's image of the Hanged Man is similar.

Similarly, hatha yoga's asanas are sacramental – symbolic postures – and deliberately magical in intent. When practice of the asanas is accompanied by appropriate meditative and ascetic techniques, it is designed to open the magical levels of the psyche/soma and 'burn the rubbish of the mind,' healing the psyche of five errors of mind: error itself, knowledge, imagination, memory, and sleep.[5] The practice of hatha yoga can introduce us to a primary sense of bodily measure and proportion, as if we were learning to play our own bodies as our earliest instruments.

However, the pursuit of a deliberately magical discipline like hatha yoga may be problematic, as it was for me. My dream of Jung and the little white dog made this luminously clear. To briefly recap this dream, I am in a room with Jung, who is watching me meditate. Then Jung rises and leaves the room, saying, 'that's all well and good, but who will look after the little white dog in the kitchen?' (I tell this dream in more detail in Chapter 8.)

Jung's dream gesture – turning away and leaving the room – implied that an overly ascetic or yogic attitude that I was taking toward my life might ignore something important, might overlook something that needed attention. A little white dog in the kitchen needed looking after, and the situation portrayed by my mind-over-matter posture came too close to being an end run around issues that concerned looking after and caring for a small, loyal animal. Today's clinical shorthand refers to this kind of end run around something instinctively relevant as making a spiritual bypass – and spiritual bypasses hold no victories for either body or soul. In this dream, a little white dog (my instinctive nature?) needs caring for, and the psyche itself (whose reality I was discovering at the time of this dream) could be valorized only as my conscious sense of identity became stronger. Jung defined individuation as a *valorization by humanness* that becomes manifest as each person discovers their own grounding in embodied soul, so Jung's dream gesture and dream comment also suggest that an evolving capacity for undergoing ego enlargement can't be forced or brought about by isolation and denial (e.g., ascetic meditation). *A shamanic capacity for integrating aspects of the collective is won only under the direct fire of the instincts, in the 'kitchens' of everyday life.*

Gesture and the shaman

Gesture was centrally important to the archaic shaman and remains so in the shamanic arts, because not only do we gesture with bodies, but we also react to gestures by way of our unconscious bodies. Feeling the sensory isolation of the caves and painting that he envisioned on the walls, an archaic shaman called on a fathomless resource of psychic forces: the animals the shaman's gestures portrayed contained embodied 'gods' as they expressed themselves in terms of the tribe's mythic imagination. A shaman's individual (empathetic and aesthetic) imagination inspired them to put 'animals' on the walls in the first place, and the shaman's imagination allowed others (through identification) to similarly 'deepen' themselves, as if they too were 'becoming' gods, 'becoming' animals, enlarging first themselves and then other members of the tribe.

We can say that through the archaic shaman, spirit 'gestured' its own forms across a divide that early shamans knew of and we still feel, forming gestures that join human to animal, mind to body, doing to being, and other to self. Today, spirit dwells within the same egoless corridors. In being and in profession, a historical shaman embodied occupation of a mimetic space of archaic identity that still exists between a 'reality' that we know, and mystery: hence, a shaman's strange aura of alienation and feelings of exemption. Through postural depictions and gesturing enactments, shamans signified the borders of existence: all the unconscious postures of the archaic shaman – as artist, as visionary, as healer – reveal the shaman's unconscious identification with an archetypal configuration. In transitional space between sacred and profane, and individual and group, shamans enshrined their subjective inner realities as objective truths, just as artists do today. Gods, other worlds, and a shaman's songs and ordeals are what the shaman depicted to others as givens. The shaman's very presence among their people gave meaning and shape to a great unknown surround.

Recognizing this, Northrup Frye (1968) suggested that the animals that a shaman portrayed represented an extension of human awareness and power into the objects of greatest energy and strength that shamans found around them. In the gesture of 'making' animals on a rock, for example, a shamanic 'maker,' looking at animal forms with human eyes, identified with what they saw, virtually putting on its skin. That was how, from the outside in, they could assimilate the energy, beauty, and glory of what they found around themselves into their observing mind.

'Telling' in both being and behavior, shamans were our first narrators and storytellers, and from this perspective, a shaman's whole life constituted a gesture. Pre-egoic (at least as we understand a sense of ego identity today), a shaman's activity unconsciously expressed and articulated all that has been preserved for us by oral literature and traditions of prehistoric people. Communicating through the medium of the unconscious, they transmitted an abundance of meaning over which they had little command. Prelinguistic in communication, and reflecting neither exterior reality nor historical events, the life and profession of an archaic shaman enacted the dreams, interior dramas, tensions, and hopes of early human beings to themselves.

Gestures and psychotherapy

All bodies have the same vocabulary of physical movements from which to select, but the ways we use postures and gestures differs from one body to another. In some of us, the 'style' of bodily behavior is banal: in others, it is highly mannered; in some people, bodily behavior is vague, while others' behaviors are precise; occasionally a body is witty. As joy belongs to the spirit, pleasure belongs to the body, and pleasure responds to what only a body can provide – a kind of *sensate, felt insight* that can establish and recognize connection, resemblance, and relationship with the world in which we live. And because our bodies *are* the spirit's chemistry, only from our bodies can we learn the metaphors of spirit's rhetoric. This is to say that the immaterial psyche works through material means.

Consider the way we enter psychotherapy: usually we do so from the posture of what Donna Orange describes as a 'suffering stranger,' gesturing to another stranger across the room: we walk, sit, and speak gestures of coming for help with ourselves, our lives. What implicit assumptions do we display as we assume such a posture? That another person can help us (countering our characteristic self-sufficiency)? That we are lost (countering our usual confidence that we know where we are)? Both Freud and Jung turned to the body as a 'container' for symptoms of disturbed unconscious life. After Darwin, writes Peter Levine (286), 'Freud was one of the first thinkers in modern psychological times to insist that we are part of nature, that nature – in the form of instincts and drives – lies within us.' Carl Jung paid close attention to the body and the *dreaming body*, looking for meaning where others did not. Jung tells a lovely story about how his attention was caught by the mysterious hand gestures made over and over again by Babette in the back wards of the Burgholzli Hospital. The old woman, diagnosed with a catatonic form of dementia praecox, had made these gestures for over forty years, and no one had ever wondered what they meant. After Babette died, Jung went to her voluminous file and unearthed the fact that she had been in love with – and rejected by – a cobbler. Her repetitive gestures of sewing shoes were her unconscious way of keeping his memory alive. 'I regarded the main task of psychotherapy as understanding the things that were taking place within the sick mind.' Jung wrote, 'The shoemaker movements (gestures) indicated an identification with her sweetheart which had lasted until her death' (*Memories Dreams Reflections*, 1989, 124–125).

Gay and Kathlyn Hendricks list in their book *At the Speed of Life* what they call five flags, signs of disharmony between mind and body that they consider to be first-line methods of diagnosis and treatment. The five flags (which I think of as gestures of the psyche) are signals, say the Hendricks – signposts to essence, or 'winks' from the soul – that the stress of *separation from essence* has become too wearing. 'In our experience, recognizing [the five flags] is a skill . . . crucial to the therapist' (74). The flags indicate cracks in the persona, where the body shows through in a gesture, posture, or symptom. The first flag is the *breathing flag* – a change in breath that signals a shift to the fight-or-flight breathing mechanisms of the body, signaling the withholding of unexpressed emotion. A *movement flag* can be any movement the body makes – a sudden crossing or uncrossing of legs, a sudden shadow across the eyes. A *postural flag* is more static, usually signaling a chronic issue that has settled into the body itself: one shoulder lower than another, an habitual slump, or a sunken chest. *Verbal flags* appear in the tone of someone's voice, and the content of communication: a flat tone or a whine? Words clipped or mumbled? Words repeated, as if underscored? The fifth flag, the *attitude flag*, is made up of posture, voice, tone, and speech patterns.

Another approach that takes the body's gestures seriously is the sensorimotor approach of Pat Ogden and her collaborators (2006). Ogden focuses on the unconscious or implicit processes that are reflected in nonverbal behaviors such as gesture, posture, prosody, facial expressions, eye gaze, movement habits, and so on. She finds that careful and sensitive attention to these in the relationship to her patient often opens up somatic resources foreclosed by trauma, giving access to the 'implicit self' of her patient. Ogden's many sensitive case studies and films demonstrate how gestures, posture, and movements provide direct access to potential release from the defensive rigidities into which her clients have been forced by trauma.

Because it is always the body that gives access to any immediate experience of the 'valley of the shadow of death,' pain lives in the body too, and sometimes 'gathering wholeness' is painful. All the more reason for contemporary therapists to take pains to provide the sense of a shared safe space into which dissociated feelings can enter. In such spaces, even breathing slows down, as dissociated self-states gesture themselves back to life. Memory reclaims embodiment as feelings flow into arteries of time long past and symbolically embodied enactments free burdened hearts.

Internal postures and dream gestures

In this final section, I expand the notions of gesture and posture to include *internal attitudes*, linking them back to the shamanic sensibility and worldview with which I began this book. Most of the time, we think of ourselves as seeing through our eyes. But when we think about the shaman as a symbolic process, we see through our minds. That the term 'archetypal shamanic paradigm' might still be the best description of this internal posture was recently reconfirmed for me as I read Wade Davis's account of meeting a legendary naturalist in the Northwest Amazon of Columbia. Davis writes of his host,

> His most prized possession was a shaman's necklace, a single strand of palm fibre threaded through a 6-inch crystal of quartz. He described it as

> both the penis and crystallized semen of Father Sun, explaining that within were thirty colours, all distinct energies that had to be balanced in sacred ritual. The necklace was also the shaman's house, the place to which he went when he took *yage*, the hallucinogenic potion also known as *ayahuasca*. Once inside, the shaman looks out at the world, over the territory of his people and the sacred sites – the forests, waterfalls, mountainous escarpments, and black water rivers – watching and watching the ways of the animals.
>
> (Davis, 95, italics mine)[6]

Davis's description confirms that even today, a self-identified shaman 'enters his house' and from there directs his inner vision at the world, and watches 'the ways of the animals,' and this underscores my conviction that *in its healing aspect*, the shaman complex naturally and continually constellates out of the psyche's ongoing need to connect our human minds to our animal bodies and our human bodies to our animal minds in an archetypal fashion. At the same time, *under its creative aspect*, this same shaman complex constellates in every effort we make to connect the outer world with our human capacities for inner vision, and our all-too-human inner realities with our felt-wonder at the outer world. A shaman's *house* continues to be the shaman's *mind*, and from inward, psychological depths, the shaman complex comes into being that it may 'bridge two worlds,' whether we think of those two worlds as inner and outer, past and present, here and there, or now and then. Davis's posture as a storyteller informs us of creative gestures of writing and creating amazing photography out of his personal experience of journeying around the globe.

In a second book (*The Wayfinders*), Davis tells another tale, this story not of a shaman but of an individual person – a Polynesian wayfinder – named Nainoa, who was the navigator on the replica of an old seafaring canoe named the *Hokule'a*. In fact, Nainoa sailed the *Hokule'a* from Hawaii to Easter Island on a wildly ambitious journey that implied crossing the Doldrums and tacking into the wind for 2,300 kilometers, sailing a total distance of nearly 20,000 kilometers – all with no seafaring instruments other than his native feel and wisdom, so to speak. Davis tells us that at one point, close to their goal, Nainoa began to doze then snapped awake in a daze to realize that with the overcast skies and sea fog, he actually had no idea where they were. 'He had lost the continuity of mind and memory essential to survival at sea. [But] he masked his fear from the crew . . . and remembered Mau's [his teacher's] words: *Can you see the image of the island in your mind?*' (63, parentheses mine).

What really struck me was Davis's report of Nainoa's response to the memory of his teacher: Nainoa entered psyche's symbolic realm:

> He became calm, and realized that he had already found the island. It was the *Hokule'a* [the craft he was piloting], and he had everything he needed on board the sacred canoe. Suddenly, the sky brightened, and a beam of warm

> light appeared on his shoulder. The clouds cleared and he followed that beam directly to the island of Rapa Nui.
>
> (Davis, 2009, 63)

Like the earlier Amazonian shaman, Nainoa visited his inner house – the 'inside' of his mind – transported there not by *yage* (as earlier) but by the alarm and confusion that fueled his experience of existential crisis – feeling lost at sea. The centering, internal posture that Nainoa assumed in crisis bears some resemblance to what happens in many when they pray: Nainoa centered down, centered in, and tried to trust: this implies that as Nainoa found containment in his experience of *himself*, he found access to what he needed.

The ability to assume an internal posture of trust in oneself and one's surroundings is kin to an inner posture implied by an ancient alchemical dictum that Dr. E. once recommended I assume: 'Remember,' he said to me, 'you have all you need, and you need all you have.'

I have since used this little alchemical equation as a kind of diagnostic tool, because those who find it hard to believe that they already have all they need for a psychological journey differ greatly from those who cannot imagine that 'all that they have' – all the accumulated baggage, emotional or otherwise – is of any worth whatsoever, if only in the posture of beginning. Remembering my own experience, I made neither head nor tails of *either* side of this equation when I heard it, but the general idea of even assuming an inner, psychological posture gave me hope. The secret of this little alchemical dictum ultimately lies in embracing its 'both/and' nature, because choosing one side over the other is fruitless, whereas embracing both sides equally somehow calls forth an inner, uniting spaciousness. Perhaps spaciousness itself makes room for implicit wholeness. The experience of it feels something like being contained by the world around you, beyond pain, gain, or judgment of any kind. In fact, simply embracing this bit of 'alchemical gold' was – for me – like stumbling into Rumi's open field, 'beyond good and evil,' where parts of myself met and greeted each other, holding hands if they so wished, and rejoiced.

From time to time, we do tend to speak of a people's collective nature; we speak of one particular culture as being warlike, while another seems more peacefully inclined. Germanic peoples have been characterized as industrious, for example, and the French as culturally sophisticated. In a similar fashion, I wonder, can we speak of a whole people assuming a characteristic posture of Being? Though he did not name it as such, Wade Davis described such a posture of Being in Santa Fe last year when he told us about the Barasana of the Columbian Amazon. Characterizing the Barasana way of life as philosophically dazzling in its sophistication, profoundly hopeful in its implications, and radically different from our own, Davis writes (102),

> In Barasana there is no word for time, and the sacred sites are not memorials or symbols of distant mythic events. They are living places . . . that eternally

> inform the present. For (the Barasana people) the past is the present, and the sacred sites are to this day inhabited by mythic beings. . . . There is no beginning and end in Barasana thought, no sense of a linear progression of time, destiny, or fate. Theirs is a fractal world in which no event has a life of its own, and any number of ideas can coexist in parallel levels of perception and meaning. Scale succumbs to intention. Every object must be understood . . . at various levels of analysis. A rapid is an impediment to travel, but also a house of the ancestors, with both a front and a back door. A stool is not a symbol of a mountain, it is in every sense an actual mountain, upon the summit of which sits the shaman. A row of stools is the ancestral anaconda, and the patterns painted onto the wood of the stools depict both the journey of the ancestors and the striations that decorate the serpent's skin.[7]

Like the Barasana, the Indigenous Peoples of Australia also enter the world, seemingly prepared to *care* for what they find (meaning both each other *and* the world) by following 'song lines' in a reality they know as dreaming. And the Maori manage to clearly differentiate this all pervasive, ongoing state of dreaming within everyday life. Here again, the reality of two worlds is taken for granted and embraced, because it is understood that neither exists without the other. When I measure the deeply shared, communally enacted internal posture that the Barasana and Maori portray against the cultural milieu in which I grew up, my mind and heart ache since I am from a world like Davis's modern Canada, a world in which secular materialism seems to be the conceit of modernity itself (120). This secular materialism allows countries like mine to mindlessly assume an overall consumerist attitude that not only limits our care for each other but reduces our planet – indeed our entire environment – to the state of a *commodity*, as if it were nothing but raw resources to be consumed at whim (119). Perhaps it is only my imagination, but Davis's description of the collective wisdom inherent in a Barasana world offers us an outline of an imaginative, collective wisdom that we desperately need now in order to develop a sense of global consciousness that can counterbalance our old overweening postures of domination, ownership, dominion, and greed.

Whether our modern cultural postures are the result of the left-brain, evolutionary primacy over right-brain influence, as Ian McGilchrist suggests in *The Master and His Emissary*, or whether they are simply the price humans inevitably pay when we forget the gift of 'the intuitive mind,' as Albert Einstein suggests, is up to psychologists and philosophers to debate for as long as they wish. Einstein wrote, 'The intuitive mind is a sacred gift and the rational mind is a faithful servant. We have created a society that honours the servant and has forgotten the gift' (quoted in McGilchrist, 2009, 116).

Albert Einstein was a creative, shamanic personality. Most of us know how he thought in images, because pictures of elevators, clocks and trains moving past each other informed his (and still our) understanding of the theory of relativity. Less well-known, however, is how much Einstein 'thought' with his body. Peter Levine tells us that in Einstein's biography, Einstein reveals how some of his greatest discoveries seemed to come first from his body in the form of tingling, vibrating, and other enlivening sensations. 'In a process that appeared to have been mysterious, even to him,' writes Levine, Einstein's 'bodily sensations informed the images and insights that led him to his great discoveries' (Levine, 280). Realizing this returns me to the shamanic importance of reconnecting as fully as we can to our inner worlds and our embodied selves. More important even than understanding various *causes* of our shrinking, absolutistic, Western worldviews is – it seems to me – cultivating a widespread ability to summon human consciousness to counter it. I hope these seven meditations on psyche and suffering encourage others to find ways and means of transforming our cramping conscious minds by widening our awareness, widening our latent shamanic imagination – the poet's juniper fuse – so that it can light up inner and outer worlds together and deepen our conceptions of how we connect to each other.

All of us need creative lives, and like every artistic creation, a creative life is the outcome of many creative gestures. Just like the whole-life gesture of an archaic shaman, or the whole-life gesture of any piece of art, a creative life expresses the outcome of some individual *person's* response to the world – a particular person, whose expression has been determined by their world, including the earthly elements of work itself. Creatively lived lives are constructed out of the personally claimed, self-reflective consciousness that each person lives out over human-size time, and we 'fabricate' our creative works out of *things of this world* – paint, wood, paper, stone – even our written words.

Proto-shamanism may have been the first great spiritual impulse to gesture across a great divide that separates our human minds from our human bodies, a gulf that seemingly separates doing from being and 'other' from self. But I envision the evolving psyche as something that has recently emerged into that yawning abyss over time, as if to create a seam. Picture the shaman complex as an early star in a dark constellation, the outlines of which we are still struggling to comprehend. A shamanic personality that is unconsciously entangled in the shaman complex is simply an unconscious envoy of that dark emerging psyche – one among many others. On psyche's side of that dark seam, untangled unconscious energy matters because the depths and textures of the deep imagination matter, affecting the timbre and tenor of our collective wisdom. How well each individual person can work themselves free of unconscious entanglement in the shaman complex also matters (at least to us), because our small human work frees the dark energy of psyche for humanly creative living.

Meanwhile, psyche itself affects us all, in all that we know of time, streaming between the souls of each of us, pouring forth like starlight from the World Soul.

Notes

1 Thomas, Adolphe V.: 'L'Anthropologie du Gests, d'apres Marcel Jousse,' in *Revue Anthropol.* 51 (1941). Quoted in Gerardus van der Leeuw: *Sacred and Profane Beauty: The Holy in Art.* Translated by David E. Green. New York: Holt, Rinehart and Winston, Inc. 1963. 124.

2 Spitz, Rene: *No and Yes: On the Genesis of Human Communication*. New York: International Universities Press. 1957. 6.
3 Funk and Wagnall: *Standard Dictionary of Folklore, Mythology and Legend*. New York: Funk and Wagnall's, Inc. 1972. 1011.
4 Adzema, Robert, and Mablen Jones: *The Great Sundial Cutout Book*. New York: Hawthorne Books, Inc. 1978. 11.
5 Funk and Wagnall, ibid.
6 Davis, Wade: *The Wayfinders: Why Ancient Wisdom Matters in the Modern World*. Canada: House of Anasi Press. 2007. 95.
7 op. cit. 100–103.

Bibliography

Abram, David: *The Spell of the Sensuous*. New York: Vintage Books. 1997.

Adzema, Robert, and Mablen Jones: *The Great Sundial Cutout Book*. New York: Hawthorne Books, Inc. 1978. 11.

Alexander, Eliot: *Myths*. Maidenhead, England: McGraw-Hill Book Company, Ltd. 1976. 56.

Alhanati, Shelley: 'To Die and So to Grow,' in *The Psychoanalytic Review*. Volume 91. Number 6. December 2004. 760–778.

Alper, Gerald: *The Elephant in the Room: The Denial of the Unconscious Mind*. New York: iBooks. 2014.

Auden, W. H.: 'For the Time Being: A Christmas Oratorio,' 1944, in *Collected Poems*. New York: Random House, Modern Library Edition. 2007. 347ff.

Bachelard, Gaston: 'La Poetique de la Reverie,' in *On Poetic Imagination and Reverie: Selections from Gaston Bachelard*. Translated by Colette Gandin. Dallas, TX: Spring Publications. 1987. 97–98.

Bahn, Paul: *The Cambridge Illustrated History of Prehistoric Art*. Cambridge: Cambridge University Press. 1998.

Bahn, Paul, and Jean Vertut: *Journey Through the Ice Age*. London: Weidenfeld & Nicolson. 1997

Baker, Nicholson: *Human Smoke: The Beginnings of World War II, the End of Civilization*. New York: Simon & Schuster. 2008.

Balint, Michael: *The Basic Fault: Therapeutic Aspects of Regression*. New York: Brunner/Mazel. 1968.

Bataille, George: *Lascaux, or The Birth of Art*. Translated by Austryn Wainhouse. SKIRA: Great Centuries of Painting. Cleveland: The World Publishing Company. 17.

Baynes, H. G.: *Mythology of the Soul*. London: Rider and Company. 1969.

Benedict, Ruth: *Patterns of Culture*. New York: The New American Library. 1934.

Beston, Henry: *The Outermost House: A Year of Life on the Great Beach of Cape Cod*. New York: St. Martin's Griffin. 2003.

Bishop, Peter: *The Greening of Psychology: The Vegetable World in Myth, Dream, and Healing*. Dallas: Spring Publications. 1998.

Blakeslee, Sandra, and Matthew Blakeslee: *The Body has a Mind of Its Own: How Body Maps in Your Brain Help You do (Almost) Everything Better*. New York: Random House Trade Paperbacks. 2008.

Bloom, Pamela: 'Soul Music,' in *New Age Journal*. March–April 1987. 58.

Brandchaft, B., S. Doctors, and D. Sorter: *Toward an Emancipatory Psychoanalysis: Brandchaft's Intersubjective Vision*. New York: Routledge. 2010.

———: 'Systems of Pathological Accommodation and Change in Analysis,' in *Psychoanalytic Psychology*. Volume 24. 2007. 667–687.

Briffault, Robert: *The Mothers: A Study of the Origins of Sentiments and Institutions*. Volume 1. New York: The MacMillan Company. 1927. 4–11.

Buckley, Michael J. S. J.: *Motion and Motion's God: Thematic Variations in Aristotle, Cicero, Newton and Hegel*. Princeton, NJ: Princeton University Press. 1971.

Caldwell, Christine: *Bodyfulness: Somatic Practices for Presence, Empowerment, and Waking Up in This Life*. Boulder: Shambhala. 2018.

Campbell, Joseph: *Masks of God: Primitive Psychology*. New York: Viking Press. 1970. 384–385.

———: 'The Historical Development of Mythology,' in *Myth and Mythmaking*. Edited by Henry A. Murray. Boston: Beacon Press. 1969. 33.

Cassirer, Ernst: *Language and Myth*: (Meister Eckhart, as quoted in) Translated by Susanne K. Langer. New York: Dover Publications, Inc. Harper and Brothers. 1946. 74.

Chodron, Pema: *Comfortable with Uncertainty: 108 Teachings on Cultivating Fearlessness and Compassion*. Complied and Edited by Emily Hilburn Sell. Boston and London. Shambhala. 2008.

Coleman, Warren: *Act and Image: The Emergence of Symbolic Imagination*. New Orleans, Louisiana: Spring Journal, Inc. 2016.

Conrad, Emilie: *Life on Land: The Story of Continuum: The World-Renowned Self-Discovery and Movement Method*. Forward by Valerie Hunt. Berkeley, CA: North Atlantic Books. 2007.

Corbin, Henry: *Jung, Buddhism, and the Incarnation of Sophia: Unpublished Writings from the Philosopher of the Soul*. Edited by Michel Cazenave, with the assistance of Daniel Proulx. Translated by Jack Cain. Rochester, VT: Inner Traditions. 2014.

Coxhead, David, and Susan Hiller: *Dreams: Visions of the Night*. New York: Avon Publishers. 1976. Illustration 40.

Curtis, Gregory: *The Cave Painters: Probing the Mysteries of the World's First Artists*. New York: Anchor Books. 2007.

Damasio, Antonio: *Looking for Spinoza: Joy, Sorrow, and the Feeling Brain*. Orlando, FL: Harcourt. 2003.

———: *The Feeling of What Happens: Body and Emotion in the Making of Consciousness*. New York: Harcourt Brace. 1999.

———: *Decartes' Error: Emotion, Reason, and the Human Brain*. New York: G. P. Putnam's Sons. 1994.

Davis, Wade: *The Wayfinders: Why Ancient Wisdom Matters in the Modern World*. Canada: House of Anasi Press, Inc. 2009.

Edelman, Gerald: *Bright Air, Brilliant Fire: On the Matter of Mind*. New York: Basic Books. 1992.

Edelman, Gerald, and G. Tononi: *A Universe of Consciousness: How Matter Becomes Imagination*. New York: Basic Books. 2000.

Edelman, Sandra: *Turning the Gorgon: A Meditation on Shame*. Woodstock, CT: Spring Publications, Inc. 1998.

Edinger, Edward F.: 'The Vocation of Depth Psychology,' in *Science of the Soul: A Jungian Perspective*. Edited by Daryl Sharp and J. Gary Sparks. Toronto, Canada: Inner City Books. 2002. 81–98.

———: *Ego and Archetype: Individuation and the Religious Function of the Psyche*. New York: Pelican Series, Penguin Books. 1973.

Eliade, Mircea: *Ecstatic Religion: An Anthropological Study of Spirit Possession and Shamanism*. London, England: Penguin Books, Ltd. 1971.

———: *Shamanism: Archaic Techniques of Ecstasy*. Translated from the French by Willard R. Trask. Bollingen Series LXXVI. New York: Pantheon Books. 1964.

———: *Myths, Dreams, and Mysteries: The Encounter Between Contemporary Faiths and Archaic Realities*. Translated by Philip Mairet. New York: Harper & Row. 1957.

Ellenberger, Henri: *The Discovery of the Unconscious: The History and Evolution of Dynamic Psychiatry*. New York: Basic Books. 1970.

Erdrich, Louise: 'Asiniig,' in *Original Fire: Selected and New Poems*. New York: Harper Perennial. 2003. 153.

Eshelman, Clayton: *Juniper Fuse: Upper Paleolithic Imagination and the Construction of the Underworld*. Middletown, CT: Wesleyan University Press. 2003.

Ferguson, John: *An Illustrated Encyclopedia of Mysticism and the Mystery Religions*. London: Thames & Hudson Ltd. 1976.

Frankfort, Henri-Paul, and Hamayon, Roberte N., Editors, in collaboration with Paul G. Bahn: *The Concept of Shamanism: Uses and Abuses*. Vol. 10 of Bibliotheca Shamanistica, Edited by Mihaly Hoppal, published for the International Society for Shamanistic Research. Budapest: Akademiai Kiado. 2001.

Freesoul, John Redtail: 'The Native American Prayer Pipe: Ceremonial Object and Tool of Self-Realization,' in *Shamanism: An Expanded View of Reality*. Edited by Shirley Nicholson. Wheaton, IL: The Theosophical Publishing House. 1987. 204.

Frye, Northrop: *A Study of English Romanticism*. Chicago: University of Chicago Press. 1968.

———: *Fearful Symmetry*. Princeton, NJ: Princeton University Press. 1947.

Funk and Wagnall: *Standard Dictionary of Folklore, Mythology and Legend*. New York: Funk and Wagnall's, Inc. 1972. 1011.

Geertz, Clifford: 'Deep Play: Notes on the Balinese Cockfight,' in *Myth, Symbol and Culture*. Edited by Clifford Geertz. New York: W. W. Norton and Company. 1971. 29.

Giedion, Sigfried: *The Eternal Present: The Beginnings of Art*. Bollingen Series 35, Volume 6. 1 New York: Pantheon Books. 1962.

Govinda, Lama Anagarika: *Creative Meditation and Multi-Dimensional Consciousness*. Wheaton, IL: Quest Books. 1976.

Grof, Christina, and Grof Stanislav: *Holotropic Breath Work: A New Approach to Self-Exploration and Therapy*. New York: Excelsior Editions. 2010.

Grof, Stanislav: *The Adventure of Self-Discovery: Dimensions of Consciousness and New Perspectives in Psychotherapy and Inner Exploration*. New York: State University of New York Press. 1988.

Guthrie, Dale: *The Nature of Paleolithic Art*. Chicago: University of Chicago Press. 2005.

Haidt, John: *The Righteous Mind: Why Good People are Divided by Politics and Religion*. New York: Pantheon Books. 2012.

Halifax, Joan: *The Fruitful Darkness: A Journey Through Buddhist Practice and Tribal Wisdom*. New York: Grove Press. 1993.

———: *Shamanic Voices: A Survey of Visionary Narratives*. New York: E. P. Dutton. 1979. 16, 30–31, 321.

Harlow, Olivia (story) and Gabriela Campos (photos): 'Try . . . And Try Again: Ann Reinking Gives Lessons in Dance and Life,' in *The New Mexican. Pasatiempo*: March 1–7, 2019. 24–25.

Harpur, Patrick: *Daimonic Reality: A Field Guide to the Otherworld.* New York: Viking Arkana. 1994.
Hass, Robert: *A Little Book on Form: An Exploration into the Formal Imagination of Poetry*. New York: HarperCollins. 2017. 6.
Henderson, Joseph L.: *Cultural Attitudes in Psychological Perspective*. Toronto, Canada: Inner City Books. 1984. 42–43, 88–92.
Hendricks, Gay, and Hendricks, Kathlyn: *At the Speed of Life: A New Approach to Personal Change Through Body-Centered Therapy*. New York: Bantam. 1994.
Henriksen, Georg: *I Dreamed the Animals: Kaniuekutat: The Life of an Innu Hunter*. New York and Oxford: Berghahn Books. 2009.
Heschel, Abraham J.: *I Asked for Wonder: A Spiritual Anthology*. Edited by S. H. Dresner. New York: Crossroad Publishing Company. 1990.
Hillman, James: *Alchemical Psychology*, Kindle Edition. Uniform Edition of the Writings of James Hillman. Spring Publications, Inc. 2011. 10–10.
Hoagland, Tony: 'A Walk Around the Property,' in *Priest Turned Therapist Treats Fear of God: Poems*. Minneapolis, MN: Graywolf Press. 2018. 9–10.
Hooper, Walter: *C. S. Lewis: A Companion and Guide*. London: The Incorporated Catholic Truth Society. 1956. ix, 252.
Huizinga, Johan: *The Waning of the Middle Ages*. London: Routledge and Kegan Paul, Ltd. 1924. 116.
Ingham, Mary Beth: *Scotus for Dunces: An Introduction to the Subtle Doctor*. The Fran ciscan Institute. 2003. 53–66.
Ingher, Dina: 'Brain Breathing,' in *Science Digest*. June 1981. 75, 110–111.
Island Imagery: A Beginning. Exhibition publication organized by Memorial University Art Gallery. 1975.
Jaffe, Aniela: *From the Life and Work of C. G. Jung*. Daimon Verlag. Einseldeln, Switzerland 1989, 2014. 122–123.
James, William: *The Varieties of Religious Experience: A Study in Human Nature*. New York: The Modern Library. 1936.
Jest, Corneille: *Tales of the Turquoise: A Pilgrimage in Dolpo*. Translated by Margaret Stein. Boston and London: Snow Lion. 1998. 19.
Johnson, Don Hanlon, Editor: *Bone, Breath, & Gesture: Practices of Embodiment*. Berkeley, CA: North Atlantic Books. San Francisco: California Institute for Integral Studies. 1995.
Johnson, Mark: *The Meaning of the Body: Aesthetics of Human Understanding*. Chicago and London: University of Chicago Press. 2007.
Jung, C. G.: *Memories, Dreams, Reflections*, Revised Edition. Recorded and Edited by Aniela Jaffe. Translated from the German by Richard and Clara Winston. New York: Vintage Books. 1989.
———: *Nietzsche's Zarathustra: Notes of the Seminar Given in 1934–1939*. Edited by James L. Jarrett. Bollingen Series XCIX. Princeton, NJ: Princeton University Press. Volumes 1, 2. 1988.
———: *C. G. Jung Speaking: Interviews and Encounters*. Edited by William McGuire and R. F. C. Hull. Princeton, NJ: Princeton University Press. 1977.
———: *Collected Works*. Translated by R. F. C Hull. Bollingen Series XX. New York: Pantheon Books. 1964. (Quotations from Jung's *Collected Works* will be designated by *CW:* and followed by the volume number and the paragraph number, in parentheses, following the quotation throughout.)

———: *Modern Man in Search of a Soul*. New York: Harcourt Brace & Co. 1933. 197.

Jung, C. G., and K. Kerenyi: 'The Psychology of the Child,' in *Essays on a Science of Mythology*. New York: Pantheon. 1949. 105.

Kagge, Erling: *Silence in the Age of Noise*. Translated from the Norwegian by Becky L. Crook. New York: Pantheon Books. 2017.

Kahn, M. Masud R.: *The Privacy of the Self: Papers on Psychoanalytic Theory and Technique*. New York: International Universities Press, Inc. 1979.

Kalsched, Donald: *Trauma and the Soul: A Psycho-Spiritual Approach to Human Development and Its Interruption*. London and New York: Routledge. 2013.

Kingsley, Peter: *In the Dark Places of Wisdom*. Point Reyes, CA: The Golden Sufi Center. 1999.

Lakoff, George, and Mark Johnson: *Philosophy in the Flesh: The Embodied Mind and Its Challenge to Western Thought*. New York: Basic Books. 1999.

———: *Metaphors We Live By*. Chicago: University of Chicago Press. 1980.

Laugrand, Frederic, and Jarich Oosten: *Hunters, Predators and Prey: Inuit Perceptions of Animals*. New York and Oxford: Berghahn Books. 2015.

———: *Inuit Shamanism and Christianity: Transitions and Transformations in the Twentieth Century*. Montreal, Kingston, London and Ithaca: McGill-Queen's University Press. 2010.

———: *The Sea Woman: Sedna in Inuit Shamanism and Art in the Eastern Arctic*. Fairbanks: The University of Alaska Press. 2008.

Layard, John W.: 'Shamanism: An Analysis Based on Comparison with the Flying Trickster of the Malekula'; also, 'Malekula: Flying Tricksters, Ghosts, Gods, and Epileptics,' in *The Journal of the Royal Anthropological Institute of Great Britain and Ireland*. Vol ume 60. 530.

Leroi-Gourhan, Andre: *Treasures of Prehistoric Art*. New York: Harry N. Abrams. 1967.

Levine, Peter A.: *In an Unspoken Voice: How the Body Releases Trauma and Restores Goodness*. Berkeley, CA: North Atlantic Books. 2010.

Lewis-Williams, David: *The Mind in the Cave: Consciousness and the Origins of Art*. London: Thames & Hudson, Ltd. 2002.

Lewis-Williams, David, and David Pearce: *Inside the Neolithic Mind: Consciousness, Cosmos, and the Realm of the Gods*. London: Thames & Hudson, Ltd. 2005.

Lightman, Alan: 'Material,' in *Searching for Stars on an Island in Maine*. New York: Vintage Books. 2018. 18–31.

———: *A Sense of the Mysterious: Science and the Human Spirit*. New York: Vintage Books. 2005.

Lockhart, Russell A.: 'Eros in Language, Myth and Dream,' in *Quadrant*. Volume 2. Number 1. Summer. 1978. 41, 49, 54.

Lommel, Andreas: *The World of the Early Hunters*. Translated by Michael Bullock. London, England: Evelyn, Adams and Mackay, Ltd. 1967a. 10.

———: *Shamanism: The Beginnings of Art*. Translated by Michael Bullock. New York: McGraw-Hill Book Company. 1967b.

Looker, Tamsin: 'Mama, Why Don't Your Feet Touch the Ground? Staying with the Body and the Healing Moment in Psychoanalysis,' in *Relational Perspectives on the Body: Relational Perspectives Book Series*. Edited by Lewis Aron and Frances Sommer Anderson. Volume 12. Hillsdale, NJ and London: The Analytic Press. 1998.

Luce, Gay Gaer: *Biological Rhythms in Human and Animal Physiology*. New York: Dover Publications, Inc. 1971.

Mai-Mai, Sze: *The Way of Chinese Painting: Its Ideas and Techniques with Selections from the Seventeenth Century Mustard Seed Garden Manual of Painting*. New York: Random House. 1959. 191.

Majno, Guido: *The Healing Hand: Man and Wound in the Ancient World*. Cambridge: Harvard University Press. 1975. 39.

Marion, Jim: *Putting on the Mind of Christ: The Inner Work of Christian Spirituality*, 2nd Edition. Newburyport, Massachusetts: Hampton Roads Publishing Company. (2000) 2011.

Maritain, Jaques: *Creative Intuition in Art and Poetry*. Cluny Media Edition. (1953) 2018.

McGlashan, Alan: *Gravity and Levity*. Boston: Houghton Mifflin Company. 1976. 125.

McGilchrist, Iain: *The Master and His Emissary: The Divided Brain and the Making of the Western World*. New Haven and London: Yale University Press. 2009.

Mead, G. R. S., Editor: *Thrice-Greatest Hermes*. London: John M. Watkins.1964, Vol. II, pp. 6f.

Mellon, Nancy, and Ashley Ramsden: *Body Eloquence: The Power of Myth and Story to Awaken the Body's Energies*. Santa Rosa, CA: Energy Psychology Press. 2008.

Merchant, John: *Shamans and Analysts: New Insights on the Wounded Healer*. London: Routledge. 2012.

Merkur, Daniel: *Becoming Half Hidden: Shamanism and Initiation Among the Inuit*. New York and London: Routledge. 1992.

Merton, Thomas: 'Hagia Sophia,' in *A Thomas Merton Reader*. Edited by Thomas P. McDonnell. New York: Doubleday. 1989. 506.

———: 'To Each His Darkness,' in *Raids on the Unspeakable*. New York: New Directions. 1966. 11–12.

Montgomery, Sy: *Search for the Golden Moon Bear: Science and Adventure in Pursuit of a New Species*. White River Junction, VT: Chelsea Green Publishing. 2002.

Mukherjee, Siddhartha: *The Emperor of All Maladies: A Biography of Cancer*. New York: Scribner. 2010.

Mystical Rites and Rituals. London: Octopus Books, Ltd. 1975. 98.

Neumann, Erich: *Depth Psychology and a New Ethic,* Reprint Edition. Boulder, Colorado: Shambhala. 1990.

———: 'The Mystic Vision,' in *Mystical Man*. Bollingen Series XXX. Volume 2. Princeton, NJ: Princeton University Press. 1968. 375–415.

Oakes, Maud: *The Stone Speaks: The Memoir of a Personal Transformation*. Forward by William McGuire. Introduction by Joseph L. Henderson. Wilmette, IL: Chiron Publications. 1987.

Oates, Wayne: *Nurturing Silence in a Noisy Heart*. Garden City: Doubleday. 1979. 3.

Ogden, Pat, Kekuni Minton, and Clare Pain: *Trauma and the Body: A Sensorimotor Approach to Psychotherapy*. Forward by Daniel J. Siegel and Bessel A. van der Kolk. New York: W. W. Norton and Company. 2006.

Ogden, Thomas H.: *Subjects of Analysis*. London: Karnac Books, Ltd. 1994. 61–95.

Onians, Richard B.: *The Origins of European Thought*. New York: Arno Press. 1973. 168–172.

Orange, Donna M.: *The Suffering Stranger: Hermeneutics for Everyday Clinical Practice*. New York: Routledge. 2011.

Otto, Rudolf: *The Idea of the Holy: An Inquiry into the Non-Rational Factor in the Idea of the Divine and Its Relation to the Rational*. Translated by John W. Harvey. New York: Oxford University Press. 1970. 211–212.

Palmer, Parker J.: *On The Brink of Everything: Grace, Gravity and Growing Old*. Oakland, CA: Berrett-Koehler Publishers, Inc. 2018. 99.

———: *A Hidden Wholeness*. San Francisco: Jossey-Bass. 2004. 55.

'Myth and the Quest for Meaning: Earth and Spirit,' in *Parabola*. Volume VI. Number 1. Winter 1967. 7.

Picard, Max: *The World of Silence*. Translated by Stanley Godman. Chicago: Regnery. 1952. 219, 227, 229–230.

Prechtel, Martin: *The Smell of Rain on Dust: Grief and Praise*. Berkeley, CA: North Atlantic Books. 2015.

Pullman, Philip: *Daemon Voices: On Stories and Storytelling*. New York: Alfred A. Knopf. 2018.

Purce, Jill: *The Mystic Spiral: Journey of the Soul. (Art and Imagination)*. London: Thames & Hudson. Perfect Paperback. Illustration 1.

Quinan, Clarence: 'The American Medicine Man and the Asiatic Shaman: A Comparison,' in *The Annals of Medical History*. New Series. Volume 10. New York: Harper and Brothers. 1938. 509.

Rainer, Yvonne: *Feelings are Facts: A Life*. Writing Art Series. Cambridge, MA: MIT Press. 2006.

Rank, Otto: *The Trauma of Birth*. New York: Dover Public Inc. 1993.

Rasmussen, Knud: *Intellectual Culture of the Iglulik Eskimos*, quoted in *The Coming and Going of the Shaman: Eskimo Shamanism and Art*. Winnipeg: The Winnipeg Art Gallery. 1979. 182, 204.

———: *The Netsilik Eskimos, Social Life and Spiritual Culture*. Translated by W. E. Calvert. *Report of the Fifth Thule Expedition*. 1921–24. 7. Copenhagen: Glydendal. 1920. 321, as quoted in Joan Halifax: *Shamanic Voices: A Survey of Visionary Narratives*. New York: E.P. Dutton. 1979. 30.

Reed, William: 'Shamanist Principles of Initiation and Power,' in *The Shaman from Elko*. San Francisco: C. G. Jung Institute of San Francisco. 1978. 47.

Roethke, Theodore: 'In a Dark Time,' in *Collected Poems*. Port Townsend, Washington: Copper Canyon Press. 1965.

Roheim, Geza: *The Gates of the Dream*. New York: International Universities Press. 1952. 252.

———: *Magic and Schizophrenia*. Bloomington and London: Indiana University Press. 1970. 64.

Rohr, Richard: *The Divine Dance: The Trinity and Your Transformation*. New Kensington, PA: Whitaker House. 2016. 28–31.

Rovelli, Carlo: *Reality Is Not What It Seems: The Journey to Quantum Gravity*. New York: Riverhead Books. 2017.

Sacks, Oliver: *The River of Consciousness*. New York: Vintage Books. 2017.

———: *A Leg to Stand On*. New York: Touchstone. 1984.

Safina, Carl: *Beyond Words: What Animals Think and Feel*. New York: Henry Holt and Company. 2015.

Sardello, Robert: *Silence: The Mystery of Wholeness*. Benson, NC: Goldenstone Press. 2006.

Schore, Allan N.: *Right Brain Psychotherapy*. New York: W. W. Norton and Company. 2019.

———: *The Science of the Art of Psychotherapy*. New York and London: W. W. Norton & Company. 2012.

Scholem, Gershom: *On the Kabbalah and Its Symbolism*. New York: Schocken Books. 1965. 179.

Scott-Maxwell, Florida: *The Measure of My Days*. New York: Penguin Books. 1968. 42.
———: *Women and Sometimes Men*. New York: Popular Library. 1973.
The Secret of the Golden Flower: A Chinese Book of Life. Translated by Richard Wilhelm. New York: Harcourt, Brace and Company. 1932. 46.
Shampo, Marc A., and Robert A. Kyle: *Nei Ching – Oldest Known Medical Book*. Mayo Clinic Proceedings. Google.
Sheets-Johnstone, Maxine: *The Roots of Thinking*. Philadelphia: Temple University Press. 1990.
Sirotkin, Eric: *Witness: A Lawyer's Journey from Litigation to Liberation*. Ashland, OR: White Cloud Press. 2017.
Spitz, Rene: *No and Yes: On the Genesis of Human Communication*. New York: International Universities Press. 1957. 6.
Stern, Daniel: *The Interpersonal World of the Infant: A View from Psychoanalysis and Developmental Psychology*. New York: Basic Books. 1985.
Stone, Hal, and Sidra Winkelman: *Voice Dialogue: A Tool for Transformation*. Camarillo, California: Devorss and Company. 1985.
Stone, Michael, Editor: *Freeing the Body, Freeing the Mind: Writings on the Connections Between Yoga and Buddhism*. Forward by Robert Thurman. Boston and London: Shambhala. 2010.
Storr, Anthony: *Music and the Mind*. New York: Ballantine Books. 1992.
———: *Solitude: A Return to the Self*. New York: Random House, Inc. 1988.
Stromsted, Tina: *Embracing the Body, Healing the Soul. C. G. Jung Society of Atlanta Newsletter*. Atlanta, Georgia. 2018. 1–5.
Sunim, Haemin: 'Mindfulness,' in *The Things You Can See Only When You Slow Down: How To be Calm in a Busy World*. Translated by Chi-Young Kim and Haemin Sunim. UK and USA: Random House. Penguin Life. 2012.
Suzuki, D. T.: 'The Awakening of a New Consciousness in Zen,' in *Man and Transformation: Papers from the Eranos YearBooks*. Bollingen Series XXX. Volume 5. Edited by Joseph Campbell. New York: Pantheon Books. 1964. 201.
Symington, Neville: *Narcissism: A New Theory*. London: Karnac. 1993.
Taussig, Michael: *Shamanism, Colonialism and the Wild Man: A Study in Terror and Healing*. Chicago and London: The University of Chicago Press. 1987.
Taylor, Barbara Brown: *An Altar in the World: A Geography of Faith*. New York: HarperOne. 2010.
Taylor, Cory: *Dying: A Memoir*. Portland, OR and Brooklyn, New York: TinHouse Books. 2017.
Thomas, Adolphe V.: 'L'Anthropologie du Geste, d'apres Marcel Jousse,' in *Revue Anthropol*. 51 (1941), quoted in van der Leeuw, Gerardus: *Sacred and Profane Beauty: The Holy in Art*. Translated by David E. Green. New York: Holt, Rinehart and Winston, Inc. 1963. 124.
Tronick, Ed: *The Neurobehavioral and Social-Emotional Development of Infants and Children*. New York and London: W. W. Norton & Company. 2007.
Ulanov, Ann B.: *Receiving Woman: Studies in the Psychology and Theology of the Feminine*. Philadelphia: Westminster Press. 1981.
———: *The Feminine in Jungian Psychology and in Christian Theology*. Evanston, IL: Northwestern University Press. 1971.
Van der Kolk, Bessel A.: *The Body Keeps the Score: Brain, Mind, and Body in the Healing of Trauma*. New York: Viking. 2014.

Van der Leeuw, Gerardus: *Sacred and Profane Beauty: The Holy in Art*. Translated by David E. Green. New York: Holt, Rinehart and Winston. 1963.

Van Lelyveld. Th. B.: *La Danse dans le Theatre Javanais*. Paris, 1931, as quoted in van der Leeuw, Gerardus: *Sacred and Profane Beauty: The Holy in Art*. Translated by David E. Green. New York: Holt, Rinehart and Winston. 1963.

van Löben Sels, Robin: *A Dream in the World: Poetics of Soul in Two Women, Modern and Medieval*. London and New York: Brunner-Routledge. (2003) 2012.

———: *Dreamwork(ing): A Primer*. Truchas, NM: Trout & Mountain Press. 2010.

———: *Wanting A Country for This Weather and Other Poems*. Lampeter, Ceredigion, Wales: The Edwin Mellen Press, Ltd. (1993) 2003.

Vasilevich, G. M.: 'Early Concepts About the Universe Among the Evenks,' in *Studies in Siberian Shamanism*. Edited by Henry M. Michael. Toronto: University of Toronto Press. 1963. 46–83.

Von Franz, Marie-Louise: 'Some Aspects of the Transference,' (1973), in *Psychotherapy*. Boston and London. Shambhala. 1993. 248–249.

———: *Number and Time: Reflections Leading Towards a Unification of Psychology and Physics*. Evanston: Northwestern University Press. 1974. 65.

———: *The Feminine in Fairytales*. New York: Spring Publications. 1972. 127.

Watson, Lyall: *Elephantoms*. New York: W. W. Norton & Company, Inc. 2002.

Weigert, Edith: *The Courage to Love: Selected Papers of Edith Weigert*. Princeton, NJ: Yale University Press. 1970.

Wink, Walter: *The Powers: Volume 1: Naming the Powers: The Language of Power in the New Testament*. Philadelphia: Fortress Press. 1984. 124.

Winkelman, Michael: *Shamanism: A Biopsychosocial Paradigm of Consciousness and Healing*, 2nd Edition. Santa Barbara, CA: Praeger (An imprint of ABC-CLIO, LLC). 2010.

Winnicott, Donald W.: 'Transitional Objects and Transitional Phenomena,' in *Playing and Reality*. New York: Basic Books. 1971. 1–25.

———: *The Maturational Processes and the Facilitating Environment: Studies in the Theory of Emotional Development*. New York: International Universities Press, Inc. (1948) 1965. 184–185.

———: 'Mind and Its Relation to the Psyche-Soma,' in *Through Pediatrics to Psychoanalysis*. New York: Basic Books. (1949) 1958. 243–254.

Wittgenstein, Ludwig: *The Tratatus Logico-Philosophicus*. New York: Dover. 1922. 4.1212.

Wood, James: *How Fiction Works*. New York: Farrar, Straus and Giroux. 2008.

Woodman, Marion: *Conscious Femininity: Interviews with Marion Woodman*. Toronto: Inner City Books. 1993.

The Works of Thomas Traherne (complete set). Edited by Jan Ross. D. S. Brewer. 2020 (not yet published).

Yeats, William Butler: 'Crazy Jane Talks with the Bishop,' and 'The Circus Animals' Desertion,' in *The Collected Poems of W. B. Yeats*. Wordsworth Poetry Library. Hertfordshire: Wordsworth Editions Limited. 1994. 221, 296.

Zaleski, Carol: *Otherworld Journeys: Accounts of Near-Death Experience in Medieval and Modern Times*. New York: Oxford University Press. 1987.

Zuckerkandl, Victor: *Sound and Symbol: Man The Musician*. Volume II. Translated by Norbert Guterman. Bollingen Series XLIV – 2. Princeton, NJ: Princeton University Press. 1973. 21ff.

———: *Sound and Symbol: Music and the External World*. Princeton, NJ: Princeton University Press. 1969.

Zweig, Paul: *Three Journeys: An Automythography*. New York, New York: Basic Books. 1976.

Index

Note: Page numbers in *italic* indicate a figure on the corresponding page.

For Product Safety Concerns and Information please contact our EU representative GPSR@taylorandfrancis.com Taylor & Francis Verlag GmbH, Kaufingerstraße 24, 80331 München, Germany

Batch number: 10726493

Printed by Printforce, the Netherlands